Biomedical Engineering for Global Health

Explore the fundamentals of biomedical engineering technologies with this thought-provoking introduction, framed around modern-day global cancer inequities. Connecting engineering principles to real-world global health scenarios, this textbook introduces major technological advances in cancer care through the lens of global health inequity, discusses how promising new technologies can address this inequity, and demonstrates how novel medical technologies are adopted for real-world clinical use. It includes modular chapters designed to enable a flexible pathway through the material for students from a wide range of backgrounds; boxed discussion of contemporary issues in engineering for global health, encouraging students to explore ethical questions related to science and society; supplementary lab modules for hands-on experience in translating engineering principles into healthcare solutions; and over 200 end-of-chapter problems targeting multiple learning outcomes to solidify student understanding. Designed to equip students with all the critical, technical, and ethical knowledge they need to excel, this is the ideal introduction for students in biomedical engineering and global health.

Nirmala Ramanujam is the Robert W. Carr Professor of Engineering and Professor of Cancer Pharmacology and Global Health at Duke University, and Founder of the Duke Center for Global Women's Health Technologies. She is a Fellow of the National Academy of Inventors, Optica, SPIE, and AIMBE.

Brian Crouch is Assistant Research Professor of Biomedical Engineering at Duke University and Assistant Director of Research at the Duke Center for Global Women's Health Technologies.

CAMBRIDGE TEXTS IN BIOMEDICAL ENGINEERING

Series Editors
W. Mark Saltzman, Yale University
Shu Chien, University of California, San Diego

Series Advisors
Jerry Collins, Alabama A & M University
Robert Malkin, Duke University
Kathy Ferrara, University of California, Davis
Nicholas Peppas, University of Texas, Austin
Roger Kamm, Massachusetts Institute of Technology
Masaaki Sato, Tohoku University, Japan
Christine Schmidt, University of Florida
George Truskey, Duke University
Douglas Lauffenburger, Massachusetts Institute of Technology

Cambridge Texts in Biomedical Engineering provide a forum for high-quality textbooks targeted at undergraduate and graduate courses in biomedical engineering. They cover a broad range of biomedical engineering topics from introductory texts to advanced topics, including biomechanics, physiology, biomedical instrumentation, imaging, signals and systems, cell engineering, and bioinformatics, as well as other relevant subjects, with a blending of theory and practice. While aiming primarily at biomedical engineering students, this series is also suitable for courses in broader disciplines in engineering, the life sciences and medicine.

Biomedical Engineering for Global Health

Cancer, Inequity, and Technology

Nirmala Ramanujam
Duke University, North Carolina

Brian Crouch
Duke University, North Carolina

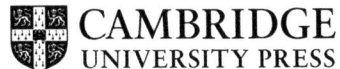

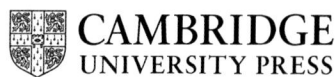

Shaftesbury Road, Cambridge CB2 8EA, United Kingdom

One Liberty Plaza, 20th Floor, New York, NY 10006, USA

477 Williamstown Road, Port Melbourne, VIC 3207, Australia

314–321, 3rd Floor, Plot 3, Splendor Forum, Jasola District Centre,
New Delhi – 110025, India

103 Penang Road, #05–06/07, Visioncrest Commercial, Singapore 238467

Cambridge University Press is part of Cambridge University Press & Assessment, a department of the University of Cambridge.

We share the University's mission to contribute to society through the pursuit of education, learning and research at the highest international levels of excellence.

www.cambridge.org
Information on this title: www.cambridge.org/highereducation/isbn/9781108833448

DOI: 10.1017/9781108980746

© Nirmala Ramanujam and Brian Crouch 2025

This publication is in copyright. Subject to statutory exception and to the provisions of relevant collective licensing agreements, no reproduction of any part may take place without the written permission of Cambridge University Press & Assessment.

When citing this work, please include a reference to the DOI 10.1017/9781108980746

First published 2025

Printed in the United Kingdom by TJ Books Limited, Padstow Cornwall

A catalogue record for this publication is available from the British Library

Library of Congress Cataloging-in-Publication Data
Names: Ramanujam, Nirmala, 1968– author. | Crouch, Brian, 1990– author.
Title: Biomedical engineering for global health : cancer, inequity,
and technology / Nirmala Ramanujam, Brian Crouch.
Other titles: Cambridge texts in biomedical engineering
Description: Cambridge, United Kingdom ; New York :
Cambridge University Press, [2025] | Series: Cambridge texts in
biomedical engineering | Includes bibliographical references and index.
Identifiers: LCCN 2024000018 | ISBN 9781108833448 (hardback) |
ISBN 9781108980746 (ebook)
Subjects: MESH: Biomedical Technology – methods | Biomedical Engineering |
Point-of-Care Systems | Neoplasms – therapy | Health Inequities | Global Health – trends
Classification: LCC R856.15 | NLM W 82 | DDC 610.28–dc23/eng/20240404
LC record available at https://lccn.loc.gov/2024000018

ISBN 978-1-108-83344-8 Hardback

Additional resources for this publication at www.cambridge.org/ramanujam

Cambridge University Press & Assessment has no responsibility for the persistence or accuracy of URLs for external or third-party internet websites referred to in this publication and does not guarantee that any content on such websites is, or will remain, accurate or appropriate.

Contents

Preface	*page* ix
1 How Technology Has Shaped Evolution of Healthcare	1
Changes in Healthcare Practice Over Time	2
Advances in Energy Generation Spurred Medical Innovation	8
Evolution of Medical Technologies Changed Care Delivery and Payment	13
Looking Ahead	25
Summary	26
Problems	27
2 Technology and Cancer in the Twenty-First Century	31
Cancer Control in the US	32
Imaging Technologies for Screening, Diagnosis, and Treatment of Cancer	39
Molecular Testing, Omics, and Imaging	48
Classes of Systemic Therapies	58
Looking Ahead	68
Summary	69
Problems	70
3 Cervical Cancer: The Face of Inequity	74
The Cervix and Cervical Cancer	76
The Evolution of Modern Gynecology	81
The Virus That Causes Cervical Cancer Has Revolutionized Primary and Secondary Prevention	90
Cervical Cancer Is a Disease of Health Disparities	99
Looking Ahead	110
Summary	111
Problems	112
4 Point-of-Care Assays for Examining Body Fluids and Cells	118
The Origins of Point-of-Care Testing	120
Point-of-Care Molecular Testing	128

Point-of-Care Testing and Cancer	137
Looking Ahead	144
Summary	145
Problems	146

5 Point-of-Care Technologies for Imaging Applications — 150

POCT for Microscopy of Cells and Tissues	152
POCTs for Imaging Internal Body Cavities	161
Ultrasound Imaging and POCTs	170
Looking Ahead	179
Summary	180
Problems	182

6 New Approaches to Vaccination and Cancer Treatment — 185

Cancer Prevention and Treatment	186
Thermal Ablation	196
Chemical Ablation	205
Looking Ahead	213
Summary	214
Problems	215

7 From Technology to Translation — 219

Basic Concepts for Statistical Analysis	220
Determining Statistical Significance	227
Calculation of Key Metrics for a Clinical Study	246
Looking Ahead	257
Summary	258
Problems	259

8 Making Decisions Using Data Analytics — 265

Data Analytics for Classification	267
Supervised and Unsupervised Learning	273
Dimension Reduction and Generalizability	289
Looking Ahead	301
Summary	302
Problems	304

9 Deep Learning — 309

Artificial Neural Networks	311
Convolutional Neural Networks	321

Algorithm Bias	330
Looking Ahead	337
Summary	338
Problems	339

10 The Evolution of Healthcare in the Twenty-First Century   344

The Growing Shortage of Healthcare Experts in Rural and Low-Resource Settings	345
Addressing the Shortage of a Skilled Healthcare Workforce Through eHealth	351
Addressing Healthcare Disparities in Low- and Middle-Income Countries	357
Looking Ahead	364
Summary	364
Problems	365

Index   369

Preface

Today we have unprecedented capabilities to create technologies that transform the way we live. Modern technologies allow consumers greater access to resources that were once out of reach. One notable example is the computer. Over 50 years ago, computer workstations were complex, expensive, and inaccessible to the public. Now, almost everyone has access to computing technologies of some kind. The great demand for such devices has spurred competition and lowered the cost to a point where they are affordable to most of the world's population. As with computing devices, there has been an explosion in biomedical innovation over the last century that has been instrumental to establishing the modern healthcare system. Despite this, half the world will slither down the precipice toward increasing morbidity and mortality.

Having previously developed technologies targeted at improving access to cancer screening and treatment both locally and globally, we have seen firsthand these challenges and, at the same time, compelling opportunities for a new generation of educators, innovators, and entrepreneurs. We have had the opportunity to teach students what we have learned through research and design projects, as well as through traditional and project-based courses. The creation of a rich tapestry of materials from these courses has been essential to developing this book.

This book examines the intersection between the global burden of cancer, health inequities, and technology innovation. It addresses three overarching questions: *How have advances in medical innovation led to healthcare inequities? How can new biomedical engineering solutions extend the reach of healthcare to a broader, more diverse population? What is required to translate these innovations for far reaching impacts?* These themes position biomedical engineering innovations in a historical, medical, and societal context.

Why does this book begin with the US as a case study? The US healthcare system serves as an important example of how unaffordability of healthcare has been shaped by advances in medical technologies. Today, healthcare expenditures in the US far exceed those of other high-income countries, without a concomitant increase in life expectancy. By studying the role technology has played and continues to play in shaping the way healthcare is delivered in the US, we can use these important lessons to inform future models of healthcare delivery in different socioeconomic settings globally.

Why does this book focus on cancer? Cancer is one of the twenty-first century's significant health and development challenges regarding human suffering and the damage it causes to a country's socioeconomic fabric. Cancer, like other noncommunicable diseases (NCDs), has created enormous health disparities. Today, it disproportionately affects populations in low- and middle-income countries (LMICs); these countries account for the vast majority of cancer deaths. Though high-income countries like the US have advanced diagnostic and treatment options, these are out of reach to the poorest populations of the world. It is important to note that even though cancer is a recurring theme in this book, the core content applies to other healthcare challenges – for example, other NCDs.

Why does this book discuss policy? Many have decried health insurance as one of the major forces leading to unequal access to care in the US. Health insurance policy was created in the early twentieth century to subsidize the increasing cost of healthcare, primarily spurred by specialized medical technologies and specialists. As healthcare costs grew, health insurance became less affordable, *or* it did not sufficiently cover certain medical expenses. Today, technology in the form of telehealth has made healthcare more accessible. Recent legislative changes and revised telehealth reimbursement policies have also made telehealth more affordable. Technology and healthcare policy are inextricably linked.

TEXTBOOK DESCRIPTION

This book illustrates the interconnectedness between biomedical engineering, humanities, medicine, and policy, how this has led to the current state of healthcare, how to reverse course, and the challenges of translating technologies for societal benefit. It begins with a thought-provoking introduction framed around modern-day cancer inequities in the US healthcare system. Through a systems-thinking approach, it equips students with critical, technical, and ethical knowledge to connect engineering principles to real-world healthcare scenarios. An ideal book for students in biomedical engineering and global health, it discusses how technological advances can address health challenges across high-, middle-, and low-income countries. The book includes modular chapters designed to enable a flexible pathway through the material for students from a wide range of backgrounds. Boxed discussions, examples, and end of chapter problems explore ethical questions. Key engineering concepts are connected to real-world scenarios reinforcing understanding of multiple learning objectives. Supplementary labs, homework assignments, discussion questions, and software promote hands-on experience and open-ended problem-solving.

The textbook is divided into three modules. Module 1, consisting of Chapters 1–3, describes the role of medical technologies in the evolution of healthcare over the last 100 years (the twentieth century) and how it has shaped modern-day cancer care. Module 1 conveys a vital message: *Sophisticated technologies have increased healthcare expenditures and inequities.* Module 2, consisting of Chapters 4–7, covers a range of point-of-care innovations based on molecular medicine, imaging, and minimally invasive treatment. In addition, it covers the design of clinical trials, which are essential to demonstrating the clinical value of a test or treatment. The main message here is: *Point-of-care solutions can transition a significant portion of healthcare services from hospitals to primary care facilities and even homes.* An apt example is the COVID-19 rapid antigen home test. Module 3, consisting of Chapters 8–10, focuses on data analytics and telemedicine, with the ultimate goal of turning observations into action. Advances in machine learning coupled with telemedicine can augment, complement, or, in some cases, substitute physician-based care. The final message is: *The power of computing combined with internet and communication technologies enables precise and personal interventions across a broad and diverse population.* The topics covered in each module are enumerated below.

MODULE 1: THE EVOLUTION AND ROLE OF TECHNOLOGY IN CANCER CONTROL IN THE TWENTIETH CENTURY

- The Industrial Revolution spurred the evolution of healthcare in the US over the twentieth century.
- Advances in modern technologies and drugs have helped to establish modern cancer screening, diagnosis, and treatment.
- Point-of-care technologies can detect the earliest signs of and prevent cancer progression.

MODULE 2: NEW POINT-OF-CARE TECHNOLOGIES FOR CANCER SCREENING, DIAGNOSIS, AND TREATMENT

- Molecular tests provide precise diagnosis of diseases such as cancer.
- Point-of-care modalities enable imaging of cells, tissues, and organs.
- Different types of low-cost therapies can be leveraged for use in point-of-care treatments.
- Statistical testing and clinical design are essential to demonstrating the efficacy and safety of tests and treatments.

MODULE 3: DIAGNOSTICS, INTERPRETATION, AND COMMUNICATION

- Different analytic data techniques can be used to identify patterns that differentiate diseased tissues from nondiseased tissues.
- Machine learning and deep learning methodologies can be used to create automated algorithms for disease diagnoses.
- Telemedicine can efficiently and effectively extend care to hard-to-reach populations.

HOW DO STUDENTS BENEFIT FROM THIS BOOK?

Biomedical engineering impacts healthcare through contributions to fundamental knowledge in medicine and biology and the translation of engineering innovations to healthcare delivery. This textbook focuses on the latter. The material covered in the text enriches student knowledge on topics that exemplify cross-cutting themes of technology, healthcare systems, and society. Not only do science and engineering affect society, but society's decisions influence the role of technology and, thereby, the role of scientists and engineers. These relationships inform what healthcare solutions are needed. We need to understand the principles behind new technological advances to know how to develop them to solve pressing healthcare challenges. Technologies offer little value when used in isolation. A well-organized ensemble of engineering solutions is needed to ensure access to the full continuum of care. Moreover, we need to examine engineering solutions in the context of clinical, regulatory, and policy frameworks in order to translate idea to impact.

The book explores the fundamentals of global health with an introduction framed around modern-day cancer inequities in the US healthcare system. Using a systems-thinking approach, it equips students with the critical, technical, and ethical knowledge they need to connect engineering principles to real-world scenarios. It is an ideal introduction to biomedical engineering and global health for students.

This textbook is structured to emphasize systems thinking, an important skill for understanding the complex interdependencies between medical technologies and healthcare. With engineering serving as the backbone, students learn various concepts related to systems thinking. The examples below exemplify this approach.

- Students learn that medical technologies improve healthcare, which they indeed do. However, students also recognize that they can do the opposite – increase healthcare costs and worsen health disparities.
- Students learn how to develop point-of-care diagnostic tests and the capability of these technologies to reach the patient's community or even their homes. However, early disease detection, though necessary, is only one rung of the health systems ladder. Innovations in point-of-care treatments are necessary to ensure access to the continuum of care.
- Students learn that artificial intelligence algorithms are powerful and can transform healthcare by leveraging vast amounts of health data to make future predictions. However, they recognize that algorithms will not serve the intended purpose without adequate data to represent diverse populations.
- By examining the past, students can begin to shape the future where modern technology can revive a once common feature of medicine – the house call – to deliver much of the care that many patients need, and to many more patients.

HOW CAN INSTRUCTORS USE THIS BOOK?

The modular nature of the book reflects its flexibility for use in various courses, such as introduction to biomedical engineering, courses on biomedical engineering and global health, and engineering design. The modules can be taught in order or independently. For example, a course on medical technologies may benefit from Module 2. Module 3 can be used across various engineering courses as this material is foundational to interpreting, analyzing, and transmitting data. Module 1 will be valuable in a course that covers topics at the intersection of technology, healthcare systems, and society.

There are three or four chapters in each module. The chapters are structured similarly to provide a clear and consistent structure. Learning objectives and a summary add clarity. Example boxes reinforce the learning objectives. Deeper Look boxes connect engineering principles to real-world scenarios by emphasizing science and society, providing the historical context for different scientific innovations, and discussing emerging technologies that are simpler, faster, and better. Detailed Explanations boxes delve further into mathematical concepts and derivations. Bolded words in the chapters expand readers' scientific vocabulary.

Each chapter presents four types of problems: (1) compare and contrast – helps students draw connections between or distinguish two different concepts; (2) interpret new data – helps students understand how new data fits within the context of the material in the chapter; (3) calculations/graph interpretation – helps reinforce concepts through a calculation or interpretation of a graphic; and (4) synthesis of information – helps students combine multiple concepts and apply them to a new problem.

Supplemental resources extend the material covered in the book. Homework questions provide a growing repository for assignments. Open-ended discussion questions serve as additional topics for in-class activities. Lab modules paired with the engineering chapters give students hands-on experience constructing simple prototypes. Additionally, computer programs allow students to simulate different scenarios related to topics covered in the book.

1 How Technology Has Shaped Evolution of Healthcare

Improved energy generation during the Industrial Revolution led to major breakthroughs in medicine. Advances in medical technologies and, in particular, medical innovations, have shaped healthcare delivery over the last 100 years, specifically in the approximately 40 **high-income countries** (HICs), which were the first to develop during the Industrial Revolution. Today, modern healthcare practice is further enhanced by the digital revolution. Medical innovations have improved the way diseases such as cancer are screened, diagnosed, and treated.

As medical technology advanced, so too did hospitals from sub-par care facilities riddled with infection and outbreaks to their modern, sterile counterparts. Improvements in technology came at a cost, however, necessitating changes in how healthcare was paid for, which led to subsidized payments in the form of health insurance. What started as a homegrown effort eventually became widely adopted. The increased costs of how care is delivered and how it is paid for has created barriers to healthcare access, particularly in **low- and middle-income countries** (LMICs). **Middle-income countries** (MICs) have limited industrialization, while **low-income countries** (LICs) are those with poor rural economies, and comprise 50 percent of the global population.

This chapter sets the stage by discussing how the Industrial Revolution and subsequent medical innovations transformed the way healthcare is accessed in the US, yet increased the disparity in the healthcare received by different populations. The next chapter will describe medical innovations in the context of breast cancer. Chapter 3 will explicitly highlight access disparities, using cervical cancer as an example, and the promise of a new generation of technologies to change this trajectory. Chapters 4–7 will focus on the next generation of medical tests and treatments and their translation to clinical care. Chapters 8 and 9 will focus on data analytics, which, when coupled with medical technologies, can rapidly expand the reach of healthcare. Finally, Chapter 10 will highlight the ways in which telemedicine can be used across different healthcare systems and ultimately bring personalized care to end users in clinical deserts. The power of technology, data analytics, and telemedicine is poised to not only democratize healthcare but actually make current medical care even more effective and efficient.

2 How Technology Has Shaped Evolution of Healthcare

This chapter sets the stage for the rest of the book. Before discussing healthcare in the context of health disparities, it is important to understand how we have come to where we are, with the US serving as an example. Why is the US a good example? It has healthcare expenditures that far exceed those of other HICs, without a concomitant increase in life expectancy. Specifically, we will look broadly at the role technology has played and continues to play in shaping the way healthcare is delivered in the US. By contextualizing the history of healthcare, we can begin to imagine the future.

LEARNING OBJECTIVES

Changes in Healthcare Practice Over Time
- Intuitive, evidence-based, and precision medicine and the differences between them;
- key discoveries that led to the transition from intuitive to evidence-based to precision medicine;
- health disparities that can result from the practice of precision medicine.

Advances in Energy Generation Spurred Medical Innovation
- The energy sources that became accessible during the different industrial revolutions and how improvements in energy production spurred advances in medical technology;
- the efficiency of different energy sources and the diversification of energy sources between high, middle-, and low-income countries;
- the renewable energy sources that are being used for electrification in LMICs, where the electricity grid is limited or unavailable.

Evolution of Medical Technologies Changed Care Delivery and Payment
- The impact of technology innovations on the US healthcare system;
- the relationship between health insurance, life expectancy, and health expenditures, and the evolution of health insurance;
- the increasing cost of cancer care and impact on affordability.

Changes in Healthcare Practice Over Time

What prompted changes in healthcare practice over time? In large part, increased knowledge and understanding of disease improved diagnosis, treatment, and outcomes for patients. There are three main periods in medical practice, dictated by **intuitive medicine** or decision-making based on intuition, **empirical medicine** or **evidence-based medicine** based on population data, and **precision medicine**, which is tailored to the individual patient.

Changes in Healthcare Practice Over Time

In this section we will explore the differences between these medical eras and how technology has influenced movement from one method to the next.

For most of human history, the practice of medicine was primarily intuitive medicine. Figure 1.1 shows the Canon of Medicine (1025 CE) and the Kahun Gynaecological Papyrus (~1800 BCE), examples of early medical texts. The Canon of Medicine, written by Avicenna in Persia around 1025 CE, is a collection of five books that comprehensively describe medical practice, available drugs, and types of diseases and treatments (Smith, 1980). The Kahun Gynaecological Papyrus, a much older text written in Egypt around 1800 BCE, contains 34 paragraphs, each devoted to a particular medical condition (Smith, 2011). Both of these texts provide maps of illnesses and treatments commonly seen by medical experts of the time. Though the boundaries between eras of medical treatment are hazy and at many points the approaches overlapped, intuitive medicine was still the primary source of diagnostic and treatment strategies at the turn of the twentieth century.

In intuitive medicine there were many unknowns with respect to how to solve a medical problem. Skilled experts combined their own knowledge with that of others nearby to patch together solutions. For example, if a patient presented with a cough, in the absence of modern-day tests the cough might have been attributed to a cold or a flu and not treated for the underlying cause, which, in fact, could be lung cancer. It is important to note that disease outcomes were often unpredictable with intuitive medicine.

Under intuitive medical practice, the relationships between diagnosis, treatment, and outcomes were limited by communication between physicians,

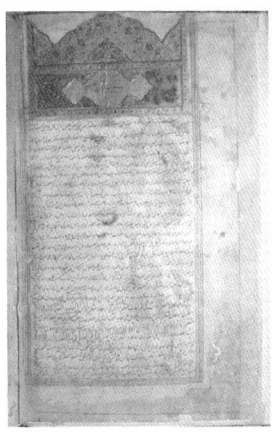 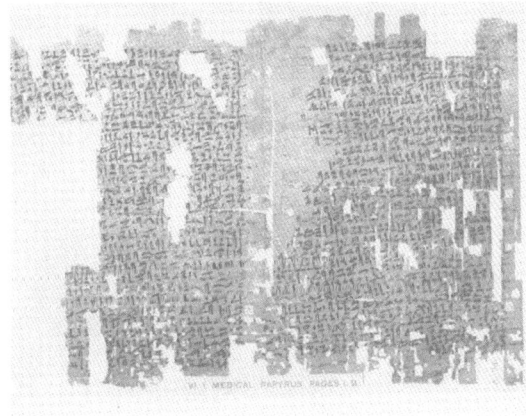

Figure 1.1 The Canon of Medicine and the Kahun Gynaecological Papyrus are examples of early medical texts. The Canon of Medicine, written by Avicenna in Persia around 1025 CE, is a collection of five books that comprehensively describe medical practice, available drugs, and types of diseases and treatments (Smith, 1980). The Kahun Gynaecological Papyrus, a much older text written in Egypt around 1800 BCE, contained 34 paragraphs, each devoted to a particular medical condition (Smith, 2011).

small numbers of patients, and limited numbers of medical innovations available, if any. As a result, the underlying causes of disease were widely unknown, leading to use of ineffective treatments. Staying with the lung cancer example, treatment of a cough using cough suppressants may only provide symptomatic relief even as the cancer progresses.

As mentioned above, intuitive medicine remained the primary form of medical practice until the turn of the twentieth century. Empirical medicine, using population-level data to treat disease, arose as industrial revolutions in many regions early in the twentieth century prompted a development cascade of diagnostic and treatment technologies coupled with population growth. Increased use of medical technologies on a larger population allowed previously unexplored disease patterns to emerge over time. Ultimately, disease patterns showed a correlation between the treatments used and the desired outcomes. This population-level data was amassed to create a collection of outcomes-based treatment and diagnostic strategies that could be more broadly disseminated.

Though empirical medicine demonstrated that specific ways of diagnosing or treating patients were on average better than others, the root cause of symptoms was still poorly understood. Evidence-based medicine, an evolution of empirical medicine, leveraged improvements in medical technologies to gather more sophisticated data that refined diagnosis and treatment of particular diseases. Using the patient with lung cancer as an example, evidence-based medicine established the presence of lung cancer not by symptoms alone, but rather by imaging and pathology of a biopsy sample.

While evidence-based medicine provided new opportunities to understand the underlying causes of disease, development of more specific therapies to target root causes lagged. Staying with lung cancer, the standard treatment was chemotherapy and radiation therapy. **Chemotherapy** is a class of medicines used to treat cancer in a nonspecific manner. **Radiation therapy** uses high-energy waves to produce DNA damage. Historically, both of these treatments used a one-size-fits-all approach based on evidence generated at a population level, rather than tailored to the individual. In other words, while population-level evidence-based medicine made great strides with treatment strategies and outcomes, patients did not benefit equally. Further research would be required to elucidate the underlying causes of disease.

How can therapies be improved so that patients will more predictably benefit from them? An example is helpful to illustrate how this may occur. For lung cancer, scientists discovered that the epidermal growth factor receptor gene (*EGFR*) is frequently overexpressed in nonsmall-cell lung cancer (NSCLC) (Prabhakar, 2015) and can be targeted for treatment. This means that a patient's tumor could be tested for this **cellular receptor** (the cellular protein that binds to a molecule for signaling) and, if positive, treated with a targeted therapy that inhibits the EGFR receptor. Understanding the link between causality and disease manifestation in a specific individual or subset of individuals, as with the *EGFR* example, can make medicine more precise. Precision medicine tailors the interventions through molecular therapies to the individual's characteristics – for example, the EGFR receptor – rather than providing treatment based on population characteristics. Today there are at least half a dozen drugs that target *EGFR* gene mutations in NSCLC.

Example: Intuitive, Evidence-Based, or Precision Medicine?

Question: A patient goes to a primary care physician for an annual checkup. She complains of stomach pain and the physician does a physical. When the physician presses against the area above the pelvic region the pain worsens, raising suspicion of a growth in that part of the body. Next, the physician orders an imaging test and confirms there is indeed a mass in the area around the left ovary. To determine if additional procedures are needed (such as biopsy), a blood test is used to look for a cancer-specific marker, CA 125, which is related to increased risk of ovarian cancer. Which of the tests is intuitive and why? Which test is evidence-based and why? Which test is the most precise and why?

Answer: Pressing against the pelvic region is an intuitive test, as the physician is using their knowledge of human anatomy to identify what is causing the symptom. The imaging test is evidence-based, where the physician is using information based on the interpretation of images to establish whether there is an abnormality and what type it could be. The blood test is the most precise, as it is looking at a specific marker for cancer. The imaging test is not precise as a mass in the image could be benign or cancer.

Figure 1.2 summarizes the medical advances that led to the evolution from intuitive to precision medicine, using lung cancer as an example. The advent of imaging as well as molecular diagnostics and therapeutics was key to the evolution from intuitive to empirical, and ultimately precision, medicine. Intuitive medicine relied solely on a provider's individual knowledge and experience working with disease. Increased population growth and wider communication networks permitted the evolution of empirical medicine, using population-level data to provide better diagnoses and therapies. Innovations in technology eventually promoted precision medicine, which uses individual patient data to characterize disease more precisely. But why was it not until the turn of the twentieth century that we first saw changes in medical practice? The next section will explain how improvements in energy consumption during the industrial revolutions spurred advancements in medical technology that would ultimately improve medical practice.

6 How Technology Has Shaped Evolution of Healthcare

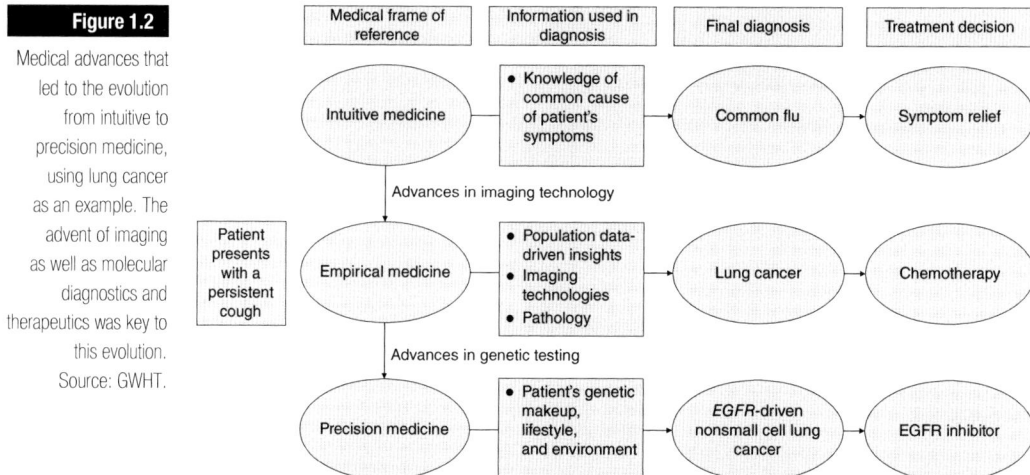

Figure 1.2
Medical advances that led to the evolution from intuitive to precision medicine, using lung cancer as an example. The advent of imaging as well as molecular diagnostics and therapeutics was key to this evolution. Source: GWHT.

Deeper Look: The Similarities Between Precision Medicine and the *Titanic*

The sinking of the Titanic *exposed income inequality. The highest loss of life was among passengers with tickets in second and third class. Passengers with money were in the upper decks closest to lifeboats, while those with the least amount were located in the lower decks, making it difficult to escape to the top, where the lifeboats were stored.* In 1912 the *Titanic*, which set sail from Southampton, England for New York, was considered the ultimate passenger liner with the best available technology and highest level of luxury according to Joseph Vadus, who led the team that discovered the *Titanic*. The *Titanic* had a sophisticated electric control panel, four elevators, a master clock that would update all clocks in new time zones, and an advanced wireless communications setup for Morse code.

Just as the *Titanic* was pushing the boundaries of oceanic travel, precision medicine is transforming the way we can treat diseases such as cancer, like never before. It is the modern *Titanic*. Breast, melanoma, lung, leukemia, and colorectal cancer patients now often have molecular testing as a standard of care practice, which provides treatment options tailored to their specific tumor, allowing for improved survival outcomes and fewer and less severe adverse events (Brown et al., 2012)

In spite of its promises, precision medicine also entails the risk of exacerbating health disparities, just as the *Titanic* did with survival. For example, precision medicine is leading the charge against different cancers (Geneviève et al., 2020), owing to technological advances made in genomics, allowing the identification of a huge number of variants (Blumenthal et al., 2016). Molecular-based and individualized approaches for treatment of primary tumors as well as metastatic and recurrent tumors are now possible

Changes in Healthcare Practice Over Time

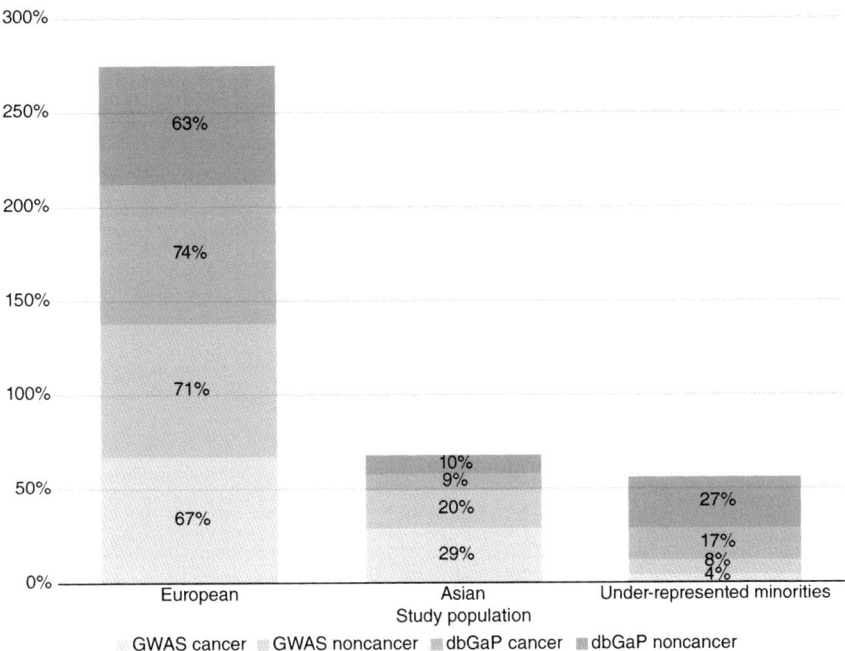

Figure 1.3 The number of GWAS as well as genotype and phenotype (dbGaP) studies broken down by disease and ancestry background in 2017 (Landry et al., 2018). A lack of genetic data for nonmajority populations has far-reaching implications; for example, establishing the risk of developing certain cancers will be next to impossible if benign and pathological variants cannot be distinguished from one another due to a dearth of data. Under-represented minorities here are African and Latin American.
Source: Authors' analysis of data from the GWAS Catalog and the database of Genotypes and Phenotypes (dbGaP).

(Geneviève et al., 2020). However, molecular and genomic testing have not been practiced uniformly. For example, in a genome-wide association study (GWAS) conducted in 2009, 96 percent of the samples were taken from participants with European ancestry. Seven years later, 81 percent of the samples collected were still of European ancestry (Patel et al., 2020). This is a striking reflection of disparities in research that has significant implications for the treatment of under-represented minorities. Figure 1.3 shows the number of GWAS as well as genotype and phenotype (dbGaP) studies broken down by disease and ancestry background in 2017 (Landry et al., 2018). A lack of genetic data for nonmajority populations has far-reaching implications; for example, establishing the risk of developing certain cancers will be next to impossible if benign and pathological variants cannot be distinguished from one another due to a dearth of data. The far-reaching implication is inequitable benefit in high-quality disease prevention even in the case where minority groups have access to prevention measures (Geneviève et al., 2020).

Advances in Energy Generation Spurred Medical Innovation

Efficient ways to generate energy were necessary for technological development. Each of the three major industrial revolutions (beginning in the mid eighteenth century through today) contributed in different ways to energy production and subsequently consequential innovations. The industrial revolutions also marked a time when prolific inventors laid the important groundwork for modern medical innovations and practices. Two specific examples (though there are numerous others that are equally important) are communication and transportation (Figure 1.4). The telegraph machine was critical for long-distance communication, and trains and automobiles for long-distance transportation. How did this all start?

The first Industrial Revolution in 1765 marked the discovery and use of natural resources, in particular coal, for energy generation. Notable inventions from this period were only made possible through the use of steam (e.g., the steam engine), a by-product of coal combustion, as a source of energy. The defining feature of an **internal combustion engine** is that expansion of hot gases moves pistons to cause the engine to perform useful work.

Nearly a century later, the second Industrial Revolution began in the mid nineteenth century, leading to new sources of energy – electricity, gas, and oil. The internal combustion engine, which was originally powered by coal and air, was impractical for widespread public use. With the availability of liquid fuels, the internal combustion engine became more practical, and was

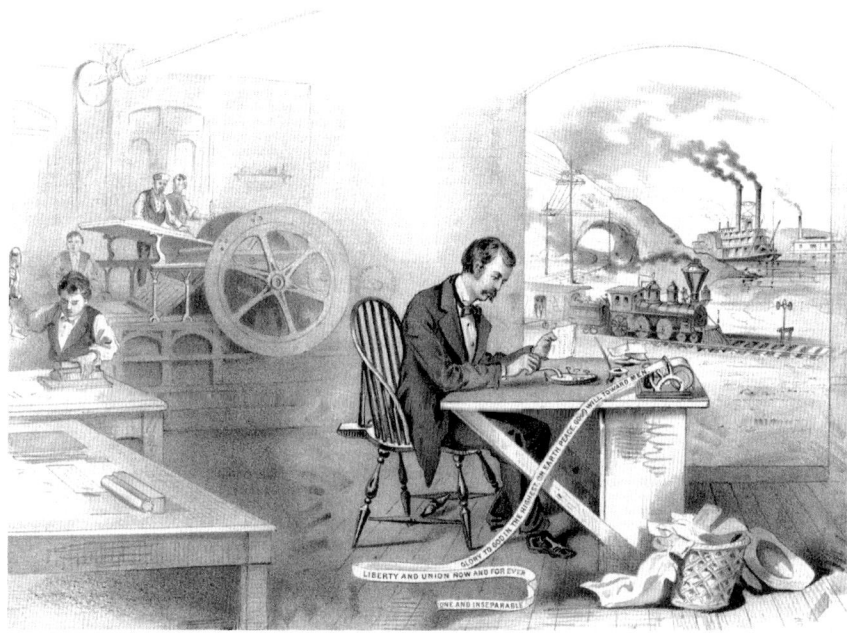

Figure 1.4
Two key inventions that paved the way for information transfer were communication and transportation. The telegraph machine was critical for long-distance communication, and trains and automobiles for long-distance transportation.
Source: © Keith Lance / DigitalVision Vectors / Getty Images.

9 Advances in Energy Generation

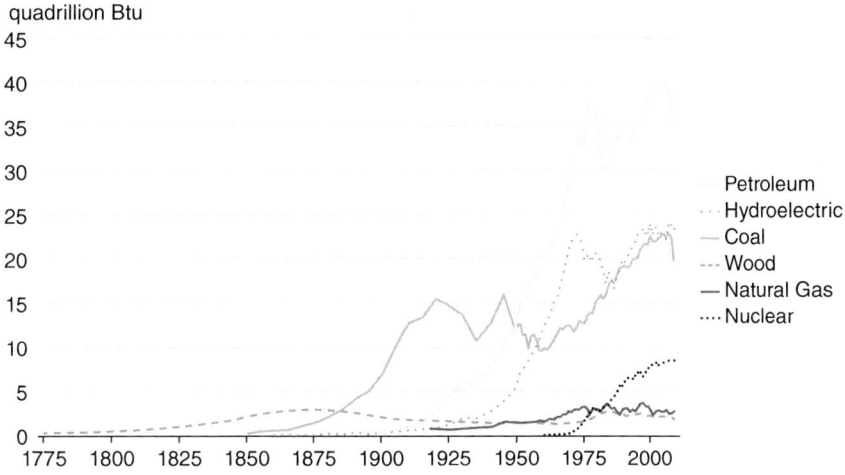

Figure 1.5 Changes over time in how energy generation was fueled. The main sources of energy today are coal, natural gas, petroleum, nuclear energy, and, most recently, renewables. The unit of British thermal units (Btu) corresponds to how much energy is used to produce useful work. Coal, the first natural resource to be used in the industrial revolution, has fallen out of favor in the twenty-first century.
Source: U.S. Energy Information Administration (Feb 2009).

later used to power automobiles and planes. The **telegraph machine** transmitted electrical signals over a wire laid between stations to revolutionize long-distance communication. The internal combustion engine also played an important role in electric power generation.

The second half of the twentieth century, referred to as the third Industrial Revolution, saw the emergence of yet another source of untapped energy – nuclear energy. The first major use of nuclear energy outside of warfare was power generation for submarines; however, commercial nuclear power development quickly followed (None, 1995). The transition from coal to nuclear power dramatically increased the efficiency of energy generation.

Figure 1.5 shows the change over time in how energy generation was fueled. The main sources of energy today are coal, natural gas, petroleum, nuclear energy, and, most recently, renewables. The unit of British thermal units (Btu) corresponds to how much energy is used to produce useful work. Coal, the first natural resource to be used in the Industrial Revolution, has fallen out of favor in the twenty-first century. How did the use of these sources for energy generation change between the 1950s and 2019? In 1950, the major sources of energy consumed were petroleum (38 percent) and coal (36 percent), with no nuclear energy and very limited renewable energy (9 percent). By 2019, coal decreased to just 11 percent of consumed energy, nuclear increased to 8 percent, and renewable energy marginally increased to around 12 percent, while natural gas (32 percent) and petroleum (37 percent) served as the major consumed energy sources.

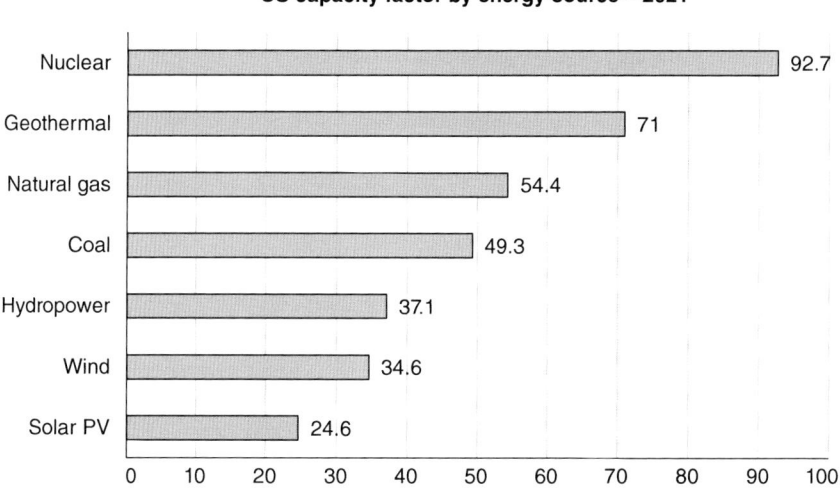

Figure 1.6 The capacity factor for different energy sources. The capacity factor is the amount of power generated at maximum capacity for a given energy source. The capacity factor is typically measured in megawatts (MW) or kilowatts (kW). Utilities can use the capacity factor to project the electricity load that a generator can handle. For reference, 1 kW of power is equivalent to 3,412 Btu.
Source: U.S. Energy Information Administration, www.energy.gov/ne/articles/what-generation-capacity.

The efficiency of a particular energy source is important to consider. Figure 1.6 shows the capacity factor for different energy sources. The **capacity factor** is the amount of power generated at maximum capacity for a given energy source. The capacity factor is typically measured in megawatts (MW) or kilowatts (kW). Utilities can use the capacity factor to project the electricity load that a generator can handle. For reference, 1 kW of power is equivalent to 3,412 Btu. The thermal efficiency is the ratio of the actual power generated divided by the capacity factor. For example, if a coal power plant has a heat rate of 10,000 Btu/kWh, but produces approximately 3,412 Btu/h, the thermal efficiency of the power plant is 3,412 Btu divided by the capacity factor, or 3,412/10,000, or 0.3412 (34.12 percent).

Deeper Look: Disparities in Energy Sources Across the Globe

Access to adequate sources of energy is necessary for development, as total primary energy demand increases with industrialization (Arto et al., 2016). High-income countries, which were the first to be industrialized two centuries ago, have a highly diversified energy portfolio consisting of coal, petroleum products, natural gas, nuclear, renewable, and other energy sources. Conversely, MICs, which have limited industrialization, have less diverse energy portfolios.

Low-income countries – which are mostly poor, rural economies – typically depend heavily on one type of energy (e.g., countries in Sub-Saharan Africa depend heavily on biomass fuel sources) (Karekezi et al. 2003).

According to the 2018 IEA *World Energy Outlook*, there are currently one billion people in the world – 13 percent of the total population – with no access to electricity, mostly in regions of Africa and South Asia that lack electricity grids. These regions have an opportunity to reduce the electricity gap by offering off-grid renewables, just as cell phones reduced the communication gap. According to H.E. Ambassador Omar Hilale at the Panel on Climate Action and Energy Transition, "Integrating and designing an energy mix largely reliant on renewable energy would simultaneously support strong growth, low emissions, and ecologically sustainable development."

Figure 1.7 shows the cost of solar and wind energy and the contribution of these sources to renewable energy growth in Africa. Solar energy has seen a precipitous decline in cost, followed by wind energy, over the period 2010–2018; Africa has increased its solar and wind energy power generation, which dominate its energy growth.

Example: What Is the Thermal Efficiency of an MRI Machine?

Question: Suppose the aggregated energy consumption of performing MRIs on 40,276 patients amounts to 614,825 kW/h. Solar photovoltaic energy is becoming more widely used and more cost-effective to generate. Calculate the per-patient cost for an MRI powered solely by solar photovoltaic power in 2010 vs. 2018.

Answer: The cost per kW/h for solar photovoltaic power in 2010 and 2018 was ~$0.37 and ~$0.08, respectively. To get the total cost, we simply multiply the cost per kW/h and the total number of kW/h:

$$\text{Total cost} = \frac{\$}{\text{kW/h}} \times \text{kW/h}.$$

Therefore, in 2010 and 2018:

$$\text{Total cost 2010} = \frac{\$0.37}{\text{kW/h}} \times 614{,}825 \frac{\text{kW}}{\text{h}} = \$227{,}485,$$

$$\text{Total cost 2018} = \frac{\$0.08}{\text{kW/h}} \times 614{,}825 \frac{\text{kW}}{\text{h}} = \$49{,}186.$$

The cost per patient can be calculated by dividing the total cost by the number of patients:

$$\text{Cost per patient 2010} = \frac{\$227{,}485}{40{,}276 \text{ patients}} = \$5.65 \text{ per patient},$$

$$\text{Cost per patient 2018} = \frac{\$49{,}186}{40{,}276 \text{ patients}} = \$1.22 \text{ per patient}.$$

Figure 1.7 Cost of solar and wind energy and the contribution of these sources to renewable energy growth in Africa. (a) Solar energy showed a precipitous decline in cost, followed by wind energy (2010–2018). (b) Africa is showing an increase in generation of power owing to solar and wind energy dominating growth. Source: (a) Data: Lazard Levelized Cost of Energy Analysis, Version 13.0 Image: OurWorldinData.org; licensed under CC-BY by the author Max Roser; (b) Pwc Image: Statista.

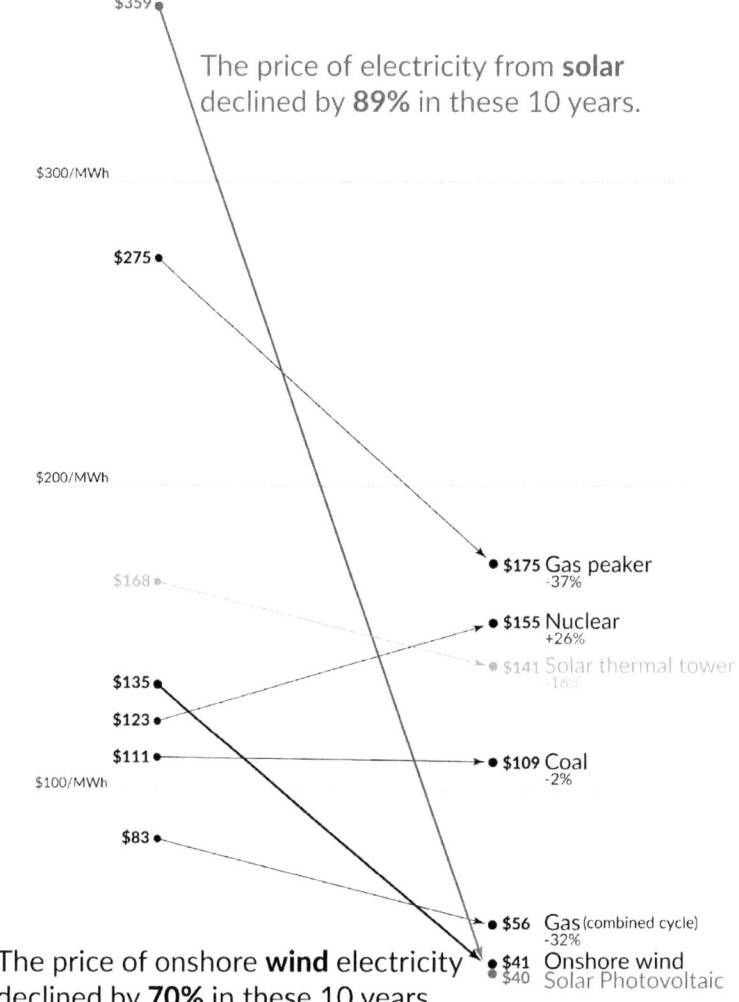

Figure 1.7 (cont.)

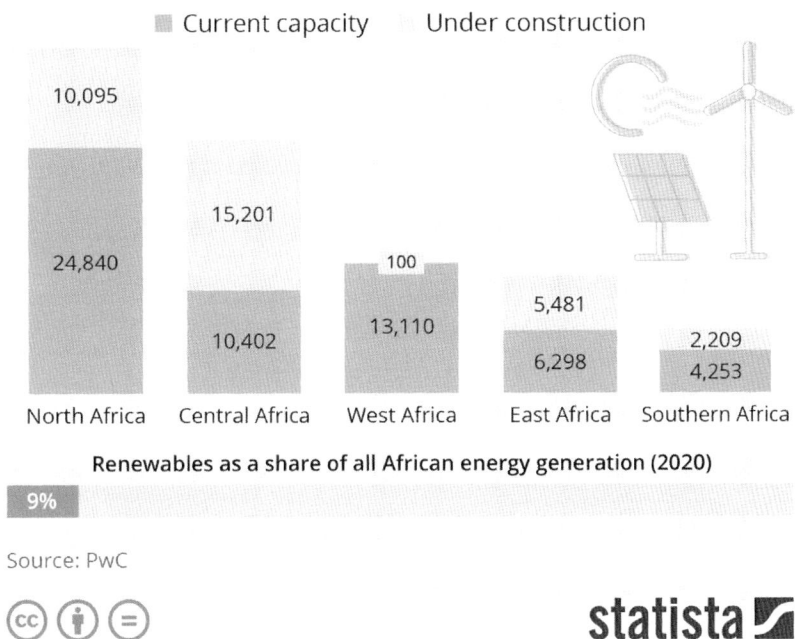

Evolution of Medical Technologies Changed Care Delivery and Payment

Shortly after the second Industrial Revolution, major strides in medical innovations began to take shape. With increased energy production, as well as empowered scientific discovery, the world was primed for a medical technology revolution. It is important to note that microscopes were invented prior to the industrial revolutions; however, improvements in energy generation spurred not only the refinement of the original microscope, but also the development of new imaging technologies.

The evolution of energy sources fueled many of the early innovations. Just before the turn of the twentieth century, German physicist Wilhelm Roentgen discovered X-rays, which you will learn more about in Chapter 2. **X-rays** allowed physicians, for the first time, to see anatomical structures deep inside the body without the need for exploratory surgery, reducing risk of infection and complication rates for patients. Figure 1.8 shows an X-ray view of the hand and wrist of a four-year-old child $c.1895$. After discovering the use

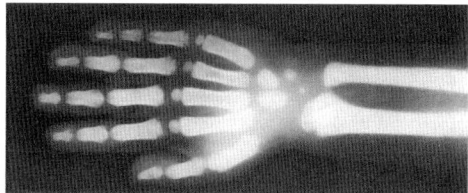

Figure 1.8 An X-ray view of the hand and wrist of a four-year-old child c.1895. After discovering the use of X-rays for imaging in 1895, additional uses for the technology rapidly evolved, including the first reported treatment of cancer with radiation in 1896 (Connell and Hellman, 2009).
Source: © George Eastman House / Contributor / Premium Archive / Getty Images.

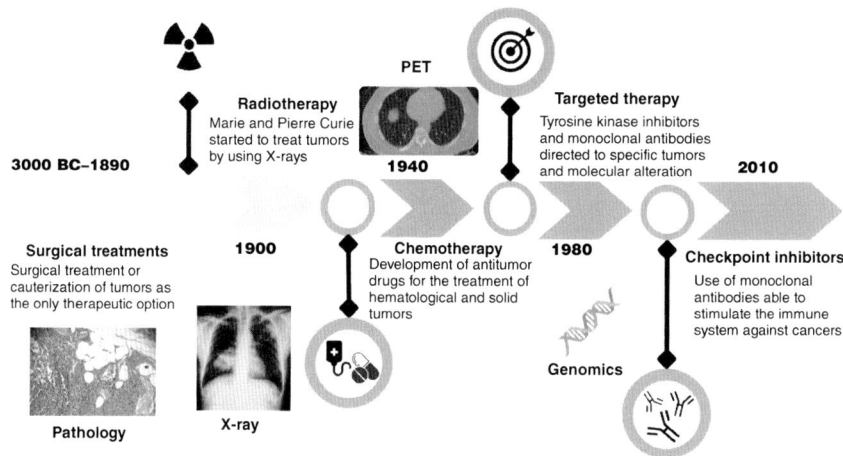

Figure 1.9 Major medical advances for development of cancer therapies. Since the first uses of X-rays to treat tumors near the turn of the twentieth century, the development of chemotherapeutic drugs in the 1940s, targeted therapies in the 1980s, and modern therapies such as checkpoint inhibitors in the last 10 years have improved treatment outcomes for patients.

of X-rays for imaging in 1895, additional uses for the technology rapidly evolved, including the first reported treatment of cancer with radiation in 1896 (Connell and Hellman, 2009). X-ray-based imaging remained the main modality until the 1970s. Other imaging techniques have since been developed and are now routinely used in hospitals. These technologies include **computed tomography** (CT), **ultrasound**, **positron emission tomography** (PET), and **magnetic resonance imaging** (MRI), all of which provide information on different features of the body – specifically, internal structures and biological processes.

Figure 1.9 shows major medical advances in the development of cancer therapies. Since the first uses of X-rays to treat tumors near the turn of the twentieth century, the development of chemotherapeutic drugs in the 1940s, targeted therapies in the 1980s, and modern therapies such as checkpoint inhibitors in the last 10 years have improved treatment outcomes for patients. Even today, surgery, albeit performed much more precisely than it was thousands of years ago, remains a mainstay for cancer treatment. It was the discovery of X-rays that opened up radiation therapy. Similar to surgery, radiation therapy is still widely used today to treat a variety of cancers, though radiation delivery is now more precise. Radiation therapy marked a transition from intuitive medical practice for cancer treatment to evidence-based medical practice.

Surgery and radiation are nonsystemic treatments. Evidence-based medical practice in cancer treatment continued with the development of systemic therapy, in particular chemotherapeutic drugs, capable of treating a number of cancers, though not all patients benefited equally. It wasn't until the development of targeted therapies in the 1980s that cancer treatment moved into the era of precision medicine, largely as a result of advances in imaging and other technologies allowing physicians and researchers to better understand cancer biology. Checkpoint inhibitors, which activate a patient's own immune system to attack the tumor directly, came onto the cancer therapy stage in the last decade, and represent the latest and most impactful form of precision medicine in cancer therapy. We will take an in-depth look at these technologies in Chapter 2.

It is important to note that, although these innovations radically increased the ability of the physician to make more precise diagnoses and prognoses and were available shortly after their discovery, it took time before many were widely adopted. For example, physicians questioned whether X-ray imaging of the chest would be as reliable as a physical examination, a hesitation potentially fueled by the impending threats of lost wages and decreased respect for their expertise through the mechanization of their profession. Even once physicians trust a new technology, other significant barriers to wider distribution include cost and infrastructure. Continuing the X-ray example, initial X-ray imaging units in production were expensive to purchase and had one enormous stipulation attached: access to electricity. Electricity was first commercially available in the US in 1882, only a few years before the discovery of X-rays, further impeding X-ray implementation (Woolf, 1987). Even today, researchers are always innovating new and better ways to diagnose and treat diseases like cancer; however, there is a significant lag between the introduction of a new discovery or technology and its broad adoption into clinical practice, owing to limited initial trust by physicians, as well as infrastructural restrictions.

Though sophisticated technologies were ultimately adopted, there was a concomitant increase in the associated costs. As a result, hospitals became central hubs for new medical equipment, transforming the healthcare landscape. With medical technology costs rapidly increasing, many patients simply did not have the means to afford new and better forms of healthcare, creating disparities in access. Health insurance was born out of these

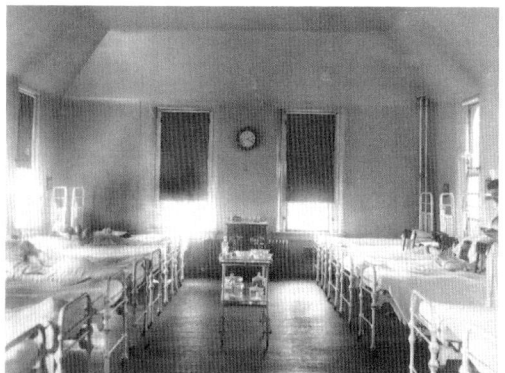 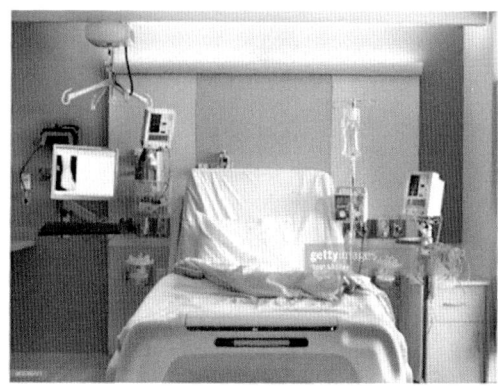

Figure 1.10 Differences between hospital wards in the early twentieth century and their modern-day counterparts. Hospitals in the early 1900s resulted in widespread infection owing to crowding of patients and lack of disinfection procedures. In the modern hospital, patients are typically housed in private rooms, and experts and modern technology have completely transformed care.
Source: © Bettmann / Contributor / Bettmann / Getty Images.

inequities in access, first as a grassroots effort, and eventually becoming the ubiquitous enterprise it is today.

In striking contrast to modern hospitals, at the turn of the twentieth century, hospitals were shelters for the needy and chronically ill patients. These hospitals were primarily funded by donations from wealthy individuals, and physicians volunteered to treat poor people as a way to gain practice and prestige. Affluent people received care from private physicians in their own homes. Examinations included general checkups – the use of a stethoscope to check the chest, lungs, and digestive tract, and/or the analysis of blood or urine. As anesthesia was still under development for most of the nineteenth and early twentieth centuries, most surgeries were limited to the surface of the body owing to patients' limited tolerance of pain. Figure 1.10 shows the similarities and differences between hospital wards in the early twentieth century and their modern-day counterparts. Hospitals in the early 1900s resulted in widespread infection owing to crowding of patients and lack of disinfection procedures. In the modern hospital, patients are typically housed in private rooms, and experts and modern technologies have completely transformed care.

Nearly three decades after Roentgen's discovery of X-rays, the American hospital began a rapid transformation into a modern, sophisticated institution through the development and adoption of more advanced medical technologies. In fact, innovations in diagnostic imaging, better therapies, and improved surgical practices from the 1930s spurred medical efficacy to previously unachievable heights. Advances in medical technology fueled by the rapidly growing American energy sector, the growing acceptance of medicine as a science, and improved standards of care made hospitals credible centers for care (Moseley III, 2008).

17 Medical Technologies Changed Care

In the early twentieth century, Americans experienced not only a rapid change in the technologies and treatments available, but also a shift in the way medical care was financed. It started out as an inclusive system that accommodated poor people, but became inaccessible to this population due to increasing demands and costs. Over time, insurance (a service that provides payments for defined expenses in exchange for a paid premium) changed the way care costs were covered; however, not everyone could afford health insurance because this service was largely provided through employers.

To counter the rising cost of healthcare, as well as the rapidly evolving landscape of care, health insurance was created as the primary way to subsidize expenses. Blue Cross and Blue Shield, the first major private health insurance options for Americans, were developed in the 1920s and 1930s to cover hospital and physician expenses, respectively. As the century progressed, so did the evolution of insurance. By 1960, employer-sponsored health insurance was the most common option, and in 1965 both Medicare and Medicaid were created to provide insurance to the elderly and to those who were unable to secure insurance otherwise. This incentivized providers to deliver care to elderly (Medicare) and socioeconomically disadvantaged (Medicaid) populations through a fee-for-service model, which will be discussed later in the chapter.

Health insurance is one of the largest employment benefits and one many prospective employees look closely at when choosing an employer. How do people who are unemployed receive health insurance? Medicaid and Medicare remain the two major government-sponsored health insurance programs in the US. Medicaid is implemented differently by each state, with each state having different eligibility standards. Currently, Medicaid provides health insurance to more than 70 million individuals in the US, predominantly from lower-income populations. Medicare, established in 1965, primarily supplies health insurance to individuals of age 65 or older. Today, Medicare provides health insurance to nearly 60 million individuals. Combined, Medicaid and Medicare pay for some health expenses for over 130 million people in the US, which is approximately 40 percent of the US population.

Figure 1.11 shows the uninsured rate for 1963–2016. The uninsured rate dropped dramatically following the creation of Medicare and Medicaid in the 1960s. Uninsured rates increased slightly from the mid 1970s until around 2010. In spite of this broad-reaching program, many people remained ineligible for either Medicaid or Medicare and had no alternative form of insurance. After the Patient Protection and Affordable Care Act (ACA) was passed in 2010 and open enrollment began, uninsured rates dropped to their lowest levels since health insurance was first implemented. The ACA, signed into law by President Barak Obama in 2010, significantly expanded government spending for Medicaid and Medicare to improve access for particularly vulnerable

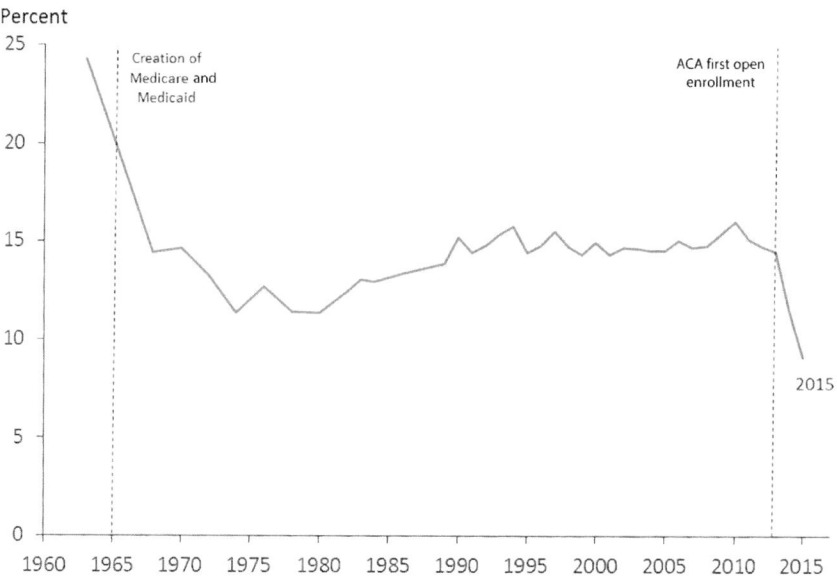

Figure 1.11 Uninsured rate 1963–2016. The uninsured rate dropped dramatically following the creation of Medicare and Medicaid in the 1960s. Uninsured rates increased slightly from the mid 1970s until around 2010. After the ACA was passed in 2010 and open enrollment began, uninsured rates dropped to their lowest levels since health insurance was first implemented.
Note: For years 1989 and later, data are annual. For prior years, data are generally but not always biannual.
Source: CEA analysis of National Health Interview Survey and supplement sources.

populations. One of the major features of the ACA was the prohibition of denying health insurance coverage for people with pre-existing health conditions or in certain high-risk occupations. Additionally, the ACA implemented a marketplace for purchasing health insurance coverage to increase competition, drive down insurance rates, and improve access to insurance coverage. The ACA has been praised by many for increasing access to affordable healthcare; however, opponents frequently cite the ACA as being responsible for overall rising medical costs.

We often think of health insurance from the perspective of an individual consumer – that is to say, we think about the benefits an individual receives by purchasing health insurance. It is important, however, to also think about health insurance from the perspective of a care provider. Healthcare providers (i.e., doctors and hospitals) are reimbursed by insurance companies for the services they provide to patients. There are two main models for determining how much a healthcare provider is reimbursed after care is completed: (1) fee-for-service; and (2) value-based care. Under the fee-for-service model, providers are reimbursed for the services they provide at a fixed rate negotiated between the provider and the health insurance company, regardless of what the outcome of the service was. For example, if a patient undergoes

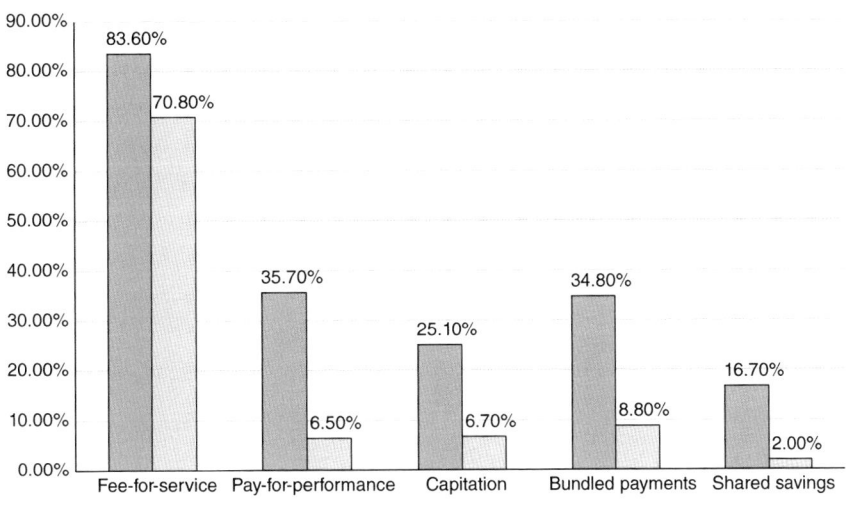

Figure 1.12 Physician revenue generated from five different reimbursement models (2016). The revenue is represented as the percentage of physicians receiving any payment from the particular reimbursement model shown and their share of practice or total revenue from that method. The **fee-for-service** model generates the highest revenue for physicians.
Source: www.ama-assn.org/sites/ama-assn.org/files/corp/media-browser/public/health-policy/prp-medical-home-aco-payment.pdf; Data: AMA 2016 Physician Practice Benchmark Survey.

surgery to remove a breast tumor, the hospital will be reimbursed by the insurance company at a fixed rate, regardless of whether the surgery was successful or unsuccessful. In this model, providers are rewarded for performing services, even if the service does not end up ultimately benefiting the patient. In simple terms, a sick patient provides more revenue to a care provider than a healthy patient. Value-based care models, conversely, reimburse providers based on patient outcome metrics or some hybrid model rather than the service provided. In other words, a healthcare provider will be reimbursed based on the quality of care provided rather than the number of services performed.

Figure 1.12 shows physician revenues generated from five different reimbursement models. The reimbursement models are fee for service, pay for performance, capitation, bundled payment, and shared saving. The overall revenue is represented as the percentage of physicians receiving any payment from the particular reimbursement model shown and their share of practice or total revenue from that method. The fee-for-service model generates the highest revenue. **Fee-for-service**, which provides a fee for each service, does not limit the number of procedures performed for a particular illness. **Capitation** (fixed, prearranged monthly payments per patient enrolled in a health plan, or per capita) appropriates payment by patient rather than by procedure.

Bundled payments (providers financially accountable for the total cost of a patient's treatment and recovery) is determined by both procedure and the patient. **Pay for performance** (reimburses based on how they perform their job) and **shared savings** (share percentage of net savings with providers to recognize their effectiveness in managing patients) incentivizes providers to prioritize quality of care

Deeper Look: Providers and Hospital Profit from Unnecessary Expenses for Patients

Resources that are widely available and profitable are more likely to be used by a physician or a hospital. A Dartmouth Atlas Project study found that patients were more likely to be admitted to hospital in regions where more hospital beds were available. The same held true for intensive care units. Most often, this equates to greater revenue for the physicians and hospitals, at increased cost to a patient. Patients who can afford to pay may get more procedures than may be required. On the other hand, patients who can't pay or pay less may not get the services they need as the revenue from these patients may be low or minimal.

This is compounded by the fact that specialists earn significantly more than primary care physicians (Steinwald et al., 2018). As a result, we have a shortage of primary care physicians, which limits access for patients (this will be covered in greater detail in Chapter 10). When access to primary care providers is limited, patients may not be diagnosed with an illness until it is more advanced, requiring more expensive care. This further amplifies undertreatment. If patients are not able to afford expensive treatment for advanced disease, they will definitely be undertreated.

Figure 1.13 shows the barriers to healthcare among nonelderly patients by insurance status in 2019. The major barrier to healthcare is lack of insurance, as uninsured individuals are significantly less likely to see a doctor or healthcare professional.

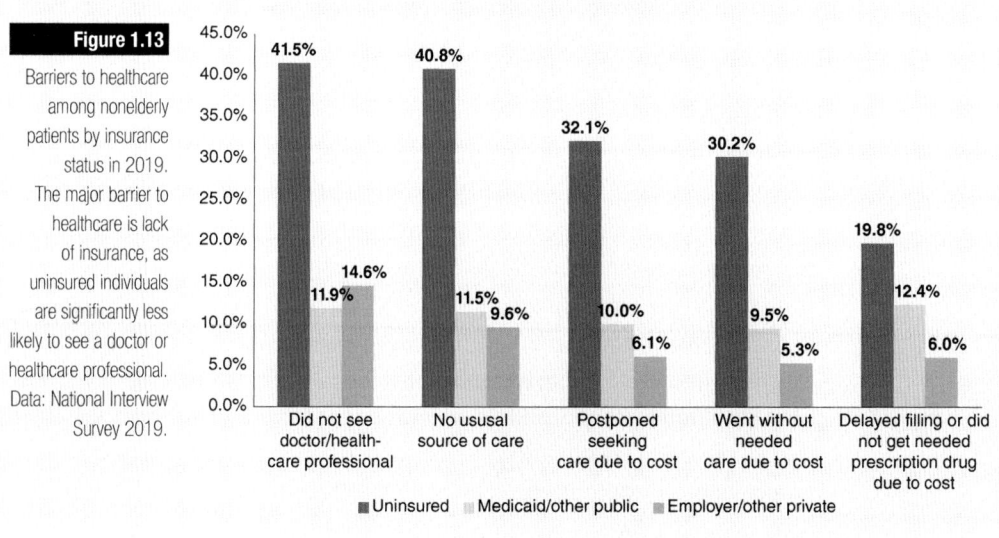

Figure 1.13 Barriers to healthcare among nonelderly patients by insurance status in 2019. The major barrier to healthcare is lack of insurance, as uninsured individuals are significantly less likely to see a doctor or healthcare professional. Data: National Interview Survey 2019.

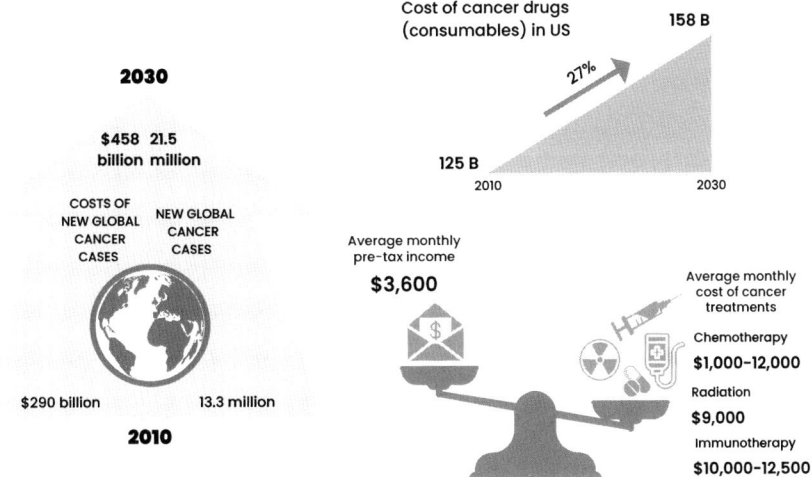

Figure 1.14 The increasing cost of cancer care. The number of new cancer cases is projected to almost double to 21.5 million globally, with associated costs booming to over $450 billion in 2030. The cost of cancer drugs is projected to increase by 27 percent from 2010 to 2030 in the US alone. The average pre-tax monthly income of $3,600 is far below the cost of the cancer therapies, which can cost over $10,000 per month.

We are at the precipice of enormous breakthroughs in both cancer diagnostics and treatment. New drugs such as imatinib for leukemia have shown unprecedented and promising results by converting a once deadly diagnosis into a "manageable condition" (Iqbal and Iqbal, 2014). A variety of imaging and therapeutic modalities are involved in patient care and opportunities for innovation abound. However, a less appealing side of this innovation is also present: increasing cost. Figure 1.14 shows the increasing cost of cancer care. The number of new cancer cases is projected to almost double to 21.5 million globally, with associated costs booming to over $450 billion in 2030. The cost of cancer drugs is projected to increase by 27 percent from 2010 to 2030 in the US alone. The average pre-tax monthly income of $3,600 is far below the cost of cancer therapies, which can be over $10,000 per month. Many of these drugs, however, do not provide significant clinical benefit, with patient survival following treatment measured in months rather than years (Vokinger et al., 2020). In short, while administrative costs account for 5 percent of healthcare expenditures, a significant driver of healthcare expenditures in the US is the increasing cost of medical drugs and devices.

Example: Cost of Breast Cancer Care

- The average household monthly income is $3,600.
- The average cost of radiation therapy is $9,000 per month.
- The average cost of chemotherapy is $3,000 per month.
- The average cost of breast cancer surgery is $8,000.

> Question: How much would the total cost of care be for a patient undergoing breast cancer treatment, assuming they have one surgery followed by 6 weeks of radiation therapy (1.5 months) and 12 months of chemotherapy? How many months of income would be required to cover the 6 weeks of radiation?
>
> Answer: To get the total cost of care, we add the costs of each individual portion of care:
>
> $$\text{Total cost} = \text{surgery} + 1.5 \text{ months of radiation} + 12 \text{ months of chemo},$$
>
> $$\text{Total cost} = \$8,000 + 1.5 \times \$9,000 + 12 \times \$3,000,$$
>
> $$\text{Total cost} = \$57,500.$$
>
> To get the number of months of income to cover 6 weeks of radiation therapy, we divide the cost of radiation by monthly income:
>
> $$\text{Number of months} = \frac{\text{Cost}}{\text{Income per month}},$$
>
> $$\text{Number of months} = \frac{1.5 \times \$9,000}{\$3,600 \text{ per month}} = 3.75 \text{ months}.$$

Getting care in a hospital also adds to the cost. Hospitals not only charge for the services; they also charge for the steep overhead compared to that of a smaller facility. The prices negotiated between insurers and healthcare providers are based on what is known as a hospital's **chargemaster** price. Hospital chargemaster rates are the equivalent of manufacturer's suggested retail price (MSRP) in car-buying markets. They are little more than the price a seller would ideally like to charge a consumer. Chargemaster rates are unlikely to be accurate reflections of actual hospital expenses. This price can vary from hospital to hospital (laterally) as well as from more centralized facilities to decentralized facilities (vertically). For example, the cost of an MRI is significantly higher when performed at a hospital compared to that at a freestanding health center. Further, the costs associated with services performed at a hospital may be significantly higher than services performed at the primary care level due to more advanced infrastructure and personnel training.

At first glance it might seem logical to house more advanced medical technologies in centralized facilities – after all, the majority of the population will never use them. Since costs can be covered by sufficient usage, these facilities are located in urban areas where there is a high density of potential patients. What if patients have to travel for long periods of time and what

Medical Technologies Changed Care

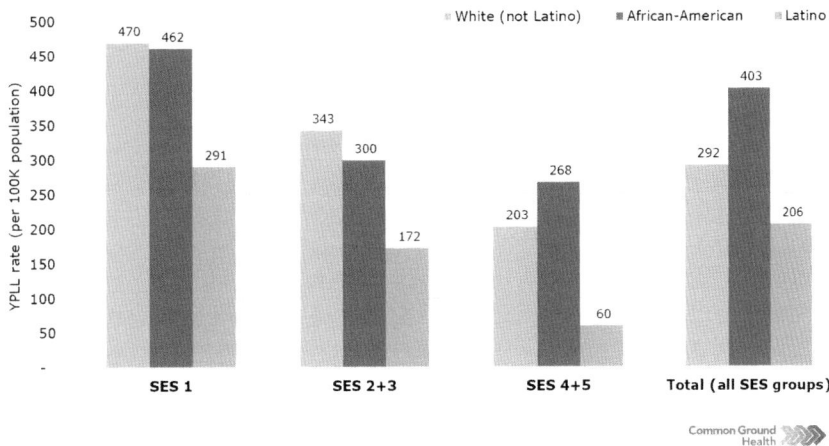

Figure 1.15 Years of potential life lost from lung cancer stratified by socioeconomic status and race. People of lower SES are more likely to lose a greater number of life years than people of higher SES. People of lower SES and minorities are more likely to die from diseases such as lung cancer than are people of higher SES.
Source: NYSDOH Vital Statistics for Finger Lakes nine county region; Age-Sex Adjusted Analysis by Common Ground Health.

if repeat visits are required, as is the case with cancer treatment? Travel to a centralized facility is needed, which further adds to the exorbitant cost of cancer care.

How does a combination of the dominant payment model, fee-for-service, the rising costs of cancer treatment, hospital fees, and distance to care impact uninsured individuals and those with low-cost insurance with high deductibles? It directly increases mortality and morbidity. Uninsured and underinsured populations are disproportionately overrepresented among minorities and people of lower socioeconomic status (SES). Figure 1.15 shows the years of potential life lost (YPLL) from lung cancer, stratified by SES and race. People of lower SES are more likely to lose a greater number of life years than people of higher SES. People of lower SES and minorities are more likely to die from diseases such as lung cancer than are people of higher SES. In fact, in 2012, 12 percent of the US population had no insurance, either because they did not have employer-based coverage and/or were not eligible for Medicare or Medicaid owing to the fact they did not meet the age criterion for Medicare and the income level for Medicaid. Health insurance programs originated to help prevent people from facing an enormous financial burden all at once by spreading the cost of care over time. Ironically, it has done the opposite, increasing racial and ethnic disparities in healthcare.

Figure 1.16 shows the changes in deaths per 100,000 people over time for different chronic diseases. Despite high investment in cancer therapies, the relative change in mortality is much lower than for stroke and heart disease.

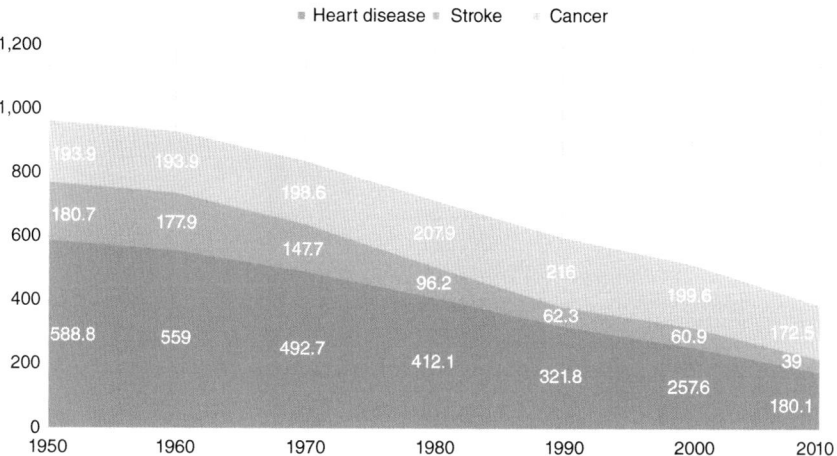

Figure 1.16 Changes in deaths per 100,000 people over time. Despite high investment in cancer therapies, the relative change in mortality is much lower than for stroke and heart disease.

In 1950, nearly 600 people per 100,000 died from heart disease compared to under 200 people per 100,000 in 2010, representing a 70 percent reduction. Similarly, stroke declined from almost 200 people per 100,000 in 1950 to just 39 per 100,000 in 2010, an almost 80 percent reduction. Cancer, on the other hand, went from just under 200 deaths per 100,000 in 1950 to just over 170 deaths per 100,000 in 2010, only an 11 percent reduction. In part, this disparity in improvement can be explained by the intricacies of cancer and the need for more research into the biological mechanisms underpinning cancer formation and growth.

Increased percentages of those with health insurance do not keep pace with rising healthcare expenditures, and rising healthcare expenditures do not improve life expectancy. Over the last 100 years, healthcare expenditures have increased from 2 to 20 percent of **gross domestic product** (GDP), the total value of goods and services produced or provided by a country during one year (Getzen, 2017). In the early 1900s, the US spent roughly the same share of GDP on health as other high Human Development Index (HDI) countries. By 1960, US health expenditures rose to 30 percent above the average and remained stable for the next 20 years. During the 1980s the gap widened, exceeding 160 percent of the average. Figure 1.17 shows the relationship between health insurance, life expectancy, and health expenditures. The data shows that the percentage of Americans with health insurance does not keep pace with healthcare expenditures, and that healthcare spending per capita is more than three times higher than in many other HICs, yet the populations of countries with much lower healthcare spending than the US enjoy considerably longer lives.

Americans with health insurance and health expenditures 1960–2010

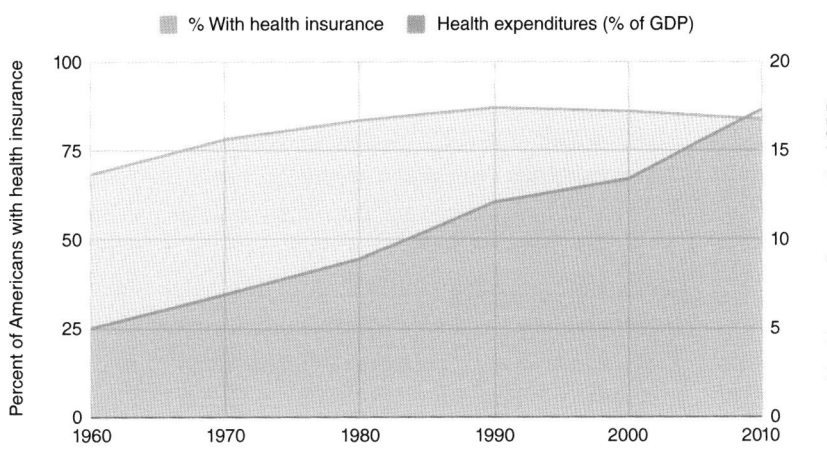

Health expenditures and life expectancy, 1960–2010

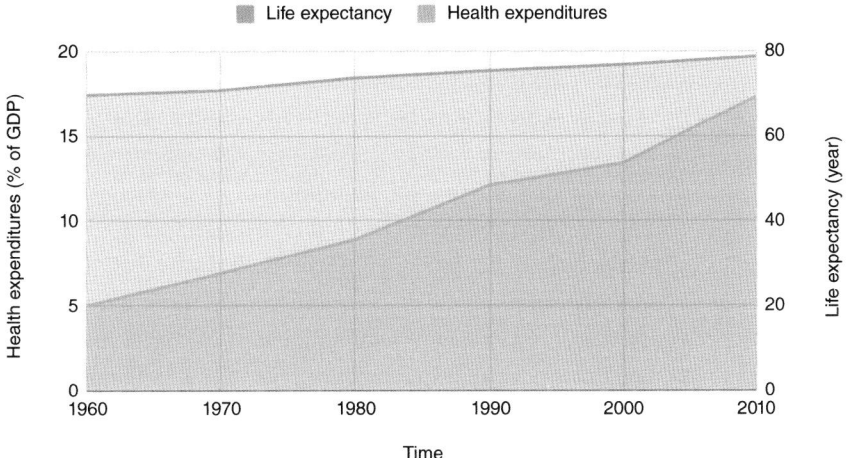

Figure 1.17 The relationship between health insurance, life expectancy, and health expenditure. The data shows that (a) the percentage of Americans with health insurance does not keep pace with healthcare expenditures, and (b) healthcare spending per capita is more than three times higher than in many other HICs, yet the populations of countries with much lower healthcare spending than the US enjoy considerably longer lives.
Source: Data from Kochanek et al. (2019) and Centers for Medicare & Medicaid Services (2015)

Looking Ahead

With the American healthcare system already bursting at the seams from elevated costs and increased stress, the COVID-19 pandemic really pressure-tested our healthcare system in unprecedented ways. In spite of the development of internet-based telemedicine in the late 1990s, adoption has been slow in many US healthcare settings. The COVID-19 pandemic caused a surge in its popularity and use, as many patients avoided public spaces such as clinics and hospitals due to fear of infection. Further, the COVID-19 pandemic has shown the ability of the US healthcare system to rapidly adapt in the face of adversity (Betancourt et al., 2020).

A trickle-down approach has been taken to advancing healthcare in regions and countries with under-resourced health systems. For example, developments in technology and treatment strategies in the global north eventually migrate to the global south. Unfortunately, this trickle-down approach does not take into account differences in healthcare and insurance systems between these regions. As a result, the solutions used in higher HIC settings (the focus of Chapter 2) are often not suitable for adoption in LMIC settings. This necessitates new innovations to improve access to healthcare that fit within the context-specific scenarios seen in LMIC settings. Telemedicine is essential but not sufficient.

Point-of-care technologies (POCTs) (Chapters 4–6) have the potential to signal a reversal in the healthcare paradigm, wherein inequitable care, owing to astronomical healthcare costs, could be lowered by bringing services traditionally offered in hospitals to the community or even home setting, as was done in the early twentieth century, akin to what we are seeing with telemedicine. Unlike the past, where technology innovation has resulted in sophisticated technologies that are confined to hospitals, there is now an opportunity to develop disruptive technologies that would not only replace their hospital counterparts, but also provide high-quality, affordable solutions in settings where access to healthcare is woefully lacking. The 2020 COVID-19 pandemic, both in HICs and LMICs, has made the need for these types of technologies and healthcare delivery systems more urgent than ever before.

SUMMARY

Medical practice has changed greatly throughout time, with the majority of changes occurring in the past 200 years. Early clinical practice for diagnosing and treating disease was primarily based on intuitive medical practice, or intuitive medicine. As the industrial revolutions improved energy generation, newer and better medical technologies were developed. When coupled with increased population growth and more widespread use, population-level data emerged, connecting diagnosis and treatment with outcomes. Eventually, empirical medicine or evidence-based medicine evolved out of use of population-level data. In the last century, with increased computational power and novel technologies becoming more widely available following the industrial revolutions, medical practice evolved to precision medicine, which uses characteristics of an individual rather than population-level data.

The dramatic changes in medical practice and improvements in technology over the last 100 years led to the creation of more centralized care facilities, such as hospitals. For example, improved imaging technologies such as MRI and CT require expensive equipment and highly trained technicians and physicians, which drives up the cost of care. At the same time, the high cost of these technologies leads to housing in centralized facilities, which are often further from suburban and rural areas. Ultimately, as cost of care has increased, changes in the way healthcare is paid for have developed, leading to modern-day health insurance programs.

PROBLEMS

Changes in Healthcare Practice Over Time

1. Explain how an imaging test can be empirical rather than precise.
2. How can precision medicine exacerbate health disparities?
   Use the following information for questions 3–5:

   A patient presents with intense stomach pain and is nauseated. They complain that the issue has been going on for several months and has recently gotten worse, as they are now also experiencing debilitating headaches.

3. Suppose a physician was diagnosing the patient 100 years ago without any ability to perform imaging or a blood test. How would the physician likely have diagnosed the patient if they had recently seen other patients who had stomach flu?
4. Now suppose a physician in 2022 has access to advanced imaging and blood tests and finds that the patient has masses in their stomach. Would this change the diagnosis?
5. How could precision medicine help, and in doing so inform treatment?

Advances in Energy Generation Spurred Medical Innovation

6. What are the different types of energy available during the first and second Industrial Revolutions?
7. What type of energy source is least used in 2022?
8. What would have been the main way to provide electricity to power an X-ray machine in the early 1900s?

9. What additional sources of energy would likely be used to power the X-ray machine in 1950?
10. In 2019, hydropower and natural gas were both used in equal amounts to provide 500,000 kW/h to power an X-ray machine. What is the difference in cost for each power source?
11. One way to reduce health disparities in LMICs is improved access to energy. Many African countries rely on biomass, whereas HICs have diverse energy portfolios. One way to address this issue is to not rely on old infrastructure but to pave new pathways to generate power. The two most popular options are solar and wind. What is the energy generated per unit cost of solar voltaic and offshore wind? Which is more economical?

Evolution of Medical Technologies Changed Care Delivery and Payment

12. What were two driving factors that led to the introduction of health insurance in the US?
13. What healthcare policies have led to a decrease in the uninsured rate in the last 70 years?
14. Which policy or policies most benefit a patient, but not a provider or hospital? Why?
15. Which policy or policies most benefit a hospital and provider, but not the patient? Why?
16. Which policy or policies most benefit an insurance company? Why?
17. A patient comes in for a breast cancer surgery. The tumor is removed and the patient is sent home. The pathologist determines that the tumor was not completely removed, and the patient needs to return for a second visit. The first surgery cost $5,000. The second surgery (i.e., re-excision) costs $2,500. What type of compensation model does this represent?
18. What payment methods of the five described in this chapter are incentive based?

Use the following information to answer questions 19 and 20.

- The average household monthly income is $3,600.
- The average cost of radiation therapy is $9,000 per month.
- The average cost of chemotherapy is $3,000 per month.
- The average cost of a breast cancer surgery is $8,000.

19. Assuming insurance covered 80 percent of the costs associated with care, what would the total cost be to a patient with breast cancer if they had 3 months of chemotherapy, surgery, 6 weeks of radiation therapy, and another 12 months of chemotherapy?
20. How many months of income would be required to cover the total cost of treatment? Assuming the average household spends 90 percent of their monthly income and puts 10 percent into savings, how many months of savings would be required to pay for the entire cost of treatment?

REFERENCES

Arto, I., Capellán-Pérez, I., Lago, R., Bueno, G., & Bermejo, R. 2016. The energy requirements of a developed world. *Energy for Sustainable Development*, 33, 1–13.

Betancourt, J. A., Rosenberg, M. A., Zevallos, A., Brown, J. R., & Mileski, M. 2020. The impact of COVID-19 on telemedicine utilization across multiple service lines in the United States. *Healthcare (Basel)*, 8, 380.

Blumenthal, G. M., Mansfield, E., & Pazdur, R. 2016. Next-generation sequencing in oncology in the era of precision medicine. *Jama Oncology*, 2, 13–14.

Brown, G. D., Patrick, T. B., & Pasupathy, K. S. 2012. *Health Informatics: A Systems Perspective*, Health Administration Press, Chicago, IL.

Centers for Medicare & Medicaid Services 2015. NHE summary including share of GDP, CY 1960–2013.

Connell, P. P., & Hellman, S. 2009. Advances in radiotherapy and implications for the next century: a historical perspective. *Cancer Research*, 69, 383–392.

Geneviève, L. D., Martani, A., Shaw, D., Elger, B. S., & Wangmo, T. 2020. Structural racism in precision medicine: leaving no one behind. *BMC Medical Ethics*, 21, 1–13.

Getzen, T. E. 2017. The growth of health spending in the USA: 1776 to 2026. Available at https://papers.ssrn.com/sol3/papers.cfm?abstract_id=3034031.

Iqbal, N., & Iqbal, N. 2014. Imatinib: a breakthrough of targeted therapy in cancer. *Chemotherapy Research and Practice*. doi: 10.1155/2014/357027

Karekezi, S., Kithyoma, W., & Energy Initiative. 2003. Renewable energy development. In Workshop on African Energy Experts on Operationalizing the NEPAD Energy Initiative, June.

Kochanek, K. D., Murphy, S. L., Xu, J., & Arias, E. 2019. Deaths: final data for 2017. *National Vital Statistics Report*, 68, 1–77.

Landry, L. G., Ali, N., Williams, D. R., Rehm, H. L., & Bonham, V. L. 2018. Lack of diversity in genomic databases is a barrier to translating precision medicine research into practice. *Health Affairs*, 37, 780–785.

Moseley III, G. B. 2008. The US health care non-system, 1908–2008. *AMA Journal of Ethics*, 10, 324–331.

None, N. 1995. *The History of Nuclear Energy*. USDOE Office of Nuclear Energy (NE), Washington, DC.

Patel, K., Patel, M., & Mukhi, H. 2020. Despite advances in precision medicine, disparities persist. *Targeted Therapies in Oncology*, 9, 16.

Prabhakar, C. N. 2015. Epidermal growth factor receptor in non-small cell lung cancer. *Translational Lung Cancer Research*, 4, 110–118.

Smith, L. 2011. The Kahun Gynaecological Papyrus: ancient Egyptian medicine. *BMJ Sexual & Reproductive Health*, 37, 54–55.

Smith, R. D. 1980. Avicenna and the Canon of Medicine: a millennial tribute. *Western Journal of Medicine*, 133, 367.

Steinwald, B., Ginsburg, P., Brandt, C., Lee, S., & Patel, K. 2018. *Medicare Graduate Medical Education Funding Is Not Addressing the Primary Care*

Shortage: We Need a Radically Different Approach. The Brookings Institution, Washington, DC.

Vokinger, K. N., Hwang, T. J., Grischott, T., et al. 2020. Prices and clinical benefit of cancer drugs in the USA and Europe: a cost–benefit analysis. *The Lancet Oncology*, 21, 664–670.

Woolf, A. G. 1987. The residential adoption of electricity in early twentieth-century America. *The Energy Journal*, 8, 19–30.

2 Technology and Cancer in the Twenty-First Century

According to the Centers for Disease Control (CDC), the top three causes of death in the early 1900s in the US were infectious diseases: pneumonia, tuberculosis, and gastrointestinal illnesses. Scientific discoveries, such as antibiotics, led to dramatic declines in deaths from infectious diseases during this period, particularly in **high-income countries** (HICs) such as the US. As the incidence of these diseases was reduced and/or eliminated, mortality rates from other ailments, especially chronic diseases such as heart disease, cancer, and diabetes, increased (Habib and Saha, 2010).

Today, cancer is the second leading cause of death globally, closely following cardiovascular disease; however, globally cancer is steadily increasing as a cause of death (Dagenais et al., 2020). High-income countries have made major strides in cancer control over the last 100 years. However, each year approximately 10 million people die from cancer, and 70 percent of these deaths are in **low- and middle-income countries** (LMICs). Undoubtedly, HICs are better able to prevent and control cancer, compared to less affluent countries, largely due to the availability of trained specialists, technologies, and drugs that are part of routine cancer care.

This chapter will cover the different technologies used in cancer control in the US, as well as how these technologies are used. Breast cancer is used as a specific example. The end of the chapter will briefly examine the ways in which technological advancements in countries like the US have left LMICs behind in terms of accessibility and affordability of care. This provides a frame of reference for the discussion of a new generation of technologies in later chapters, which promise to provide innovative solutions to cancer screening, diagnosis, and treatment in LMICs.

LEARNING OBJECTIVES

Cancer Control in the US
- The anatomy of the breast and breast cancer, and progression through the different stages of the disease;

- the steps involved in identifying and treating cancer or its precursors;
- a comparison of the sensitivity, specificity, negative predictive value, and positive predictive value of screening and diagnostic tests and the rationale for their differences.

Imaging Technologies for Screening, Diagnosis, and Treatment of Cancer
- The different types of electromagnetic waves that are used in medical imaging;
- the differences in the energy contained within the electromagnetic waves and how that impacts interactions with tissue;
- the different types of information about the tumor that can be obtained from medical imaging.

Molecular Testing, Omics, and Molecular Imaging
- The types of samples that can be used for molecular testing and the different types of molecular testing methods;
- the connections between molecular testing, "omics," and molecular imaging;
- understanding how the molecular underpinnings of cancer has revolutionized cancer treatment.

Classes of Systemic Therapies
- Different treatment options for cancer, differences between them and the specificity of therapies for the different subtypes of breast cancer;
- metrics and measurements of the benefit/impact of cancer treatment;
- the role of the immune system in cancer and the transformation of cancer treatment with immunotherapy.

Cancer Control in the US

What does a typical care prevention or treatment paradigm look like in the US? Figure 2.1 shows the three main steps for cancer control, using breast cancer as an example. A **screening** test is used to survey a region of the body, typically an organ, for cancer. **Diagnosis** is used to confirm the presence of cancer. **Treatment** is designed to kill or remove the cancer, and often involves more than one method. Screening tests are generally performed on presumed healthy individuals. Diagnostic tests are generally performed on individuals who have already had a screening test. Diagnosis is performed with pathologic assessment of a biopsy to confirm the presence or absence of cancerous or precancerous cells. Pre-invasive disease treatment requires excision or surgery, whereas treatment of cancer includes surgery, drugs, and radiation. In the case of breast cancer, imaging is used during both screening and diagnosis.

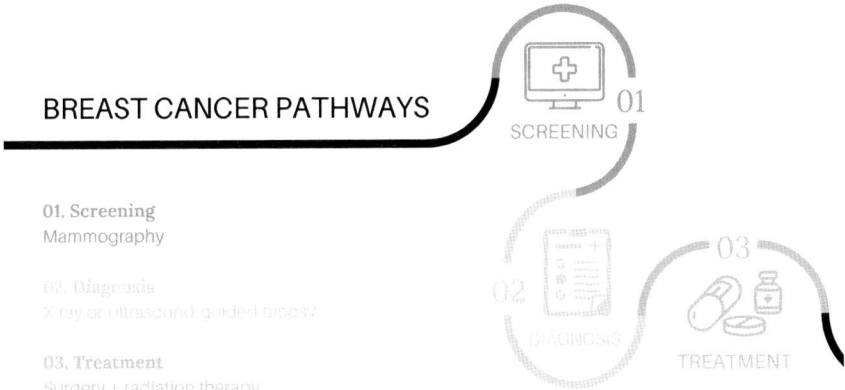

Figure 2.1 The three main steps for cancer control, using breast cancer as an example. A screening test is used to survey a region of the body, typically an organ, for cancer. Diagnosis is used to confirm the presence of cancer. **Treatment** is designed to kill or remove the cancer, and often involves more than one method.

Figure 2.2 shows the basic anatomy of the breast and the different stages of breast cancer. The breast duct produces milk following childbirth. Most Breast cancers originate in the ducts (though some develop in lobules). **Ductal carcinoma in situ** (DCIS) is confined to the duct and becomes **invasive ductal carcinoma** (IDC) if it makes it past the duct lining into the breast. **Stage** defines how advanced the cancer is, and **prognosis** is the predicted clinical outcome. The stage of disease is determined by multiple factors, including the size of the tumor, where the tumor is located, and whether cancer cells have spread outside of the breast. Prognosis is based on a variety of factors related to the patient demographics (e.g., age, body mass index), tumor characteristics (e.g., tumor size), and other factors (e.g., genetics). In breast cancer, stage 0 cancer is DCIS. As breast cancer stage increases, the five-year survival rate decreases from nearly 100 percent at stage I to only 20 percent at stage IV.

The earlier the breast cancer diagnosis, the better the prognosis and the chances for successful treatment. Figure 2.3 shows key procedures to find and treat the earliest signs of breast cancer. Imaging is used for screening (mammography) and diagnostic biopsy (ultrasound or multiangle mammography), and surgery is the most common treatment. Screening is performed on a general population and annual exams are recommended for women over 50 years of age. Anywhere from four to six samples are collected during diagnostic biopsy to ensure that the suspicious mass is adequately sampled. The images are read by a radiologist and the diagnosis of the tissue samples is performed by a pathologist. The specific tests and treatments will be discussed in greater detail later in this chapter.

The performance of both mammography and image-guided biopsy are characterized by the terms **sensitivity** (Equation 2.1) and **specificity** (Equation 2.2). **Sensitivity** indicates the true positive rate, and specificity

Figure 2.2

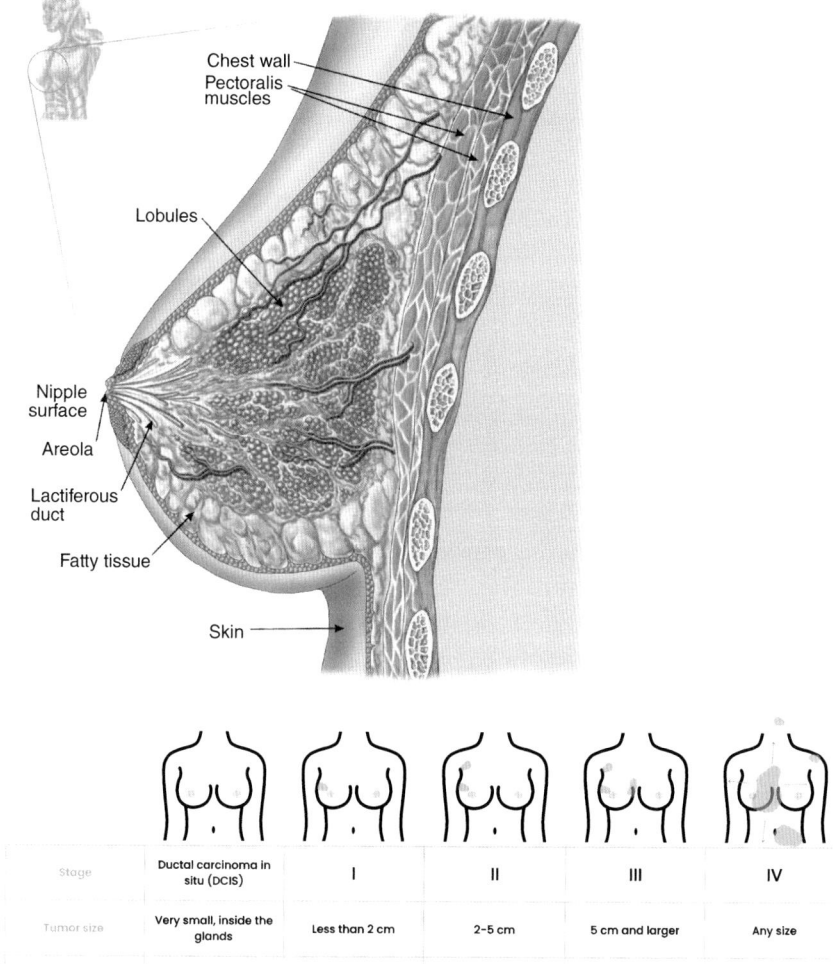

(a) The basic anatomy of the breast; and (b) the different stages of breast cancer. The breast duct produces milk following childbirth. Most Breast cancers originate in the ducts (though some develop in lobules). Ductal carcinoma in situ is confined to the duct and becomes invasive ductal carcinoma if it makes it past the duct lining into the breast. Stage defines how advanced the cancer is, and prognosis is the predicted clinical outcome. Source: (a) © Stocktrek Images / Stocktrek Images / Getty Images.

indicates the true negative rate. The sensitivity and specificity of mammography ranges from 70 to 90 percent and 90 to 95 percent, respectively, with sensitivity being on the low end for women less than 40 years of age who generally have dense breast tissue (mammograms provide the breast contrast of the tumor in a fatty tissue background). On the other hand, sampling multiple biopsies from the suspicious mass reflects high sensitivity, but the oversampling leads to low specificity as most of the biopsies are normal. The complementary attributes of the two techniques ensures that the majority of the general population does not undergo unnecessary procedures, and at the same time no cancers are missed in the diagnostic stage. The sensitivity, albeit

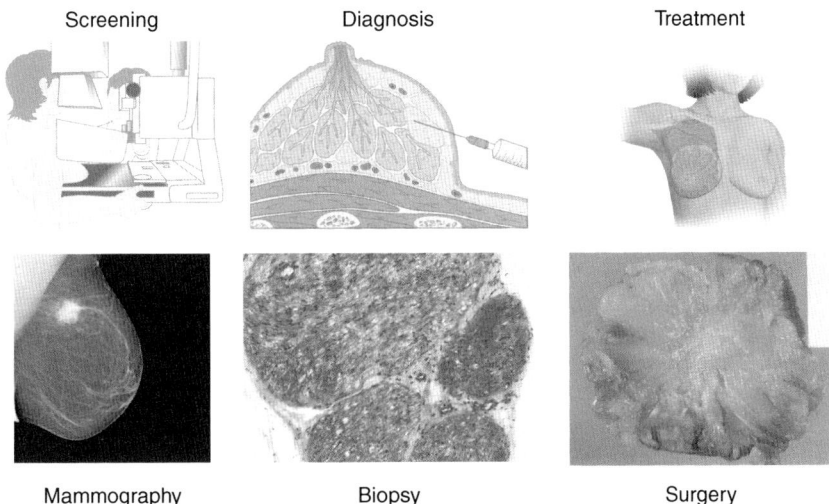

Figure 2.3 Key procedures to find and treat the earliest signs of breast cancer. The process entails cancer screening, diagnosis, and treatment. Imaging is used for screening and diagnostic biopsy, and surgery is the most common treatment.
Source: (a) Cancer Research UK / Wikimedia Common; (b) © Dorling Kindersley / Dorling Kindersley RF / Getty Images; (c) © Lauren Shavell / Design Pics / Getty Images; (e) © Sebastian Condrea / Moment / Getty Images; (f) Image: John Hayman.

low, can be countered by annual screening. While an ideal test would have a high sensitivity and specificity, it may be acceptable to have lower cutoffs, depending on the prevalence of the disease in the screening population.

Equations 2.1 and 2.2 are for test sensitivity and specificity, respectively:

$$\text{Sensitivity} = \frac{\text{\# of true positives}}{\left(\text{\# of true positives} + \text{\# of false negatives}\right)} \times 100, \quad (2.1)$$

$$\text{Specificity} = \frac{\text{\# of true negatives}}{\left(\text{\# of true negatives} + \text{\# of false positives}\right)} \times 100. \quad (2.2)$$

In addition to sensitivity and specificity, it is important to introduce two further terms – positive and negative predictive values (Equations 2.3 and 2.4, respectively). The **positive predictive value** (PPV) is the probability that subjects identified as having the disease by the test truly have the disease. The **negative predictive value** (NPV) is the probability that subjects who are identified as not having the disease by the test truly do not have the disease:

$$\text{Positive predictive value} = \frac{\text{true positive}}{\left(\text{true positive} + \text{false positive}\right)} \times 100, \quad (2.3)$$

$$\text{Negative predictive value} = \frac{\text{true negative}}{\left(\text{true negative} + \text{false negative}\right)} \times 100. \quad (2.4)$$

Example: Trade-Off between Sensitivity and Specificity

Question: A biomedical engineer is designing a new method for analyzing mammogram images to try to improve the sensitivity for detecting breast cancer compared to an expert physician's interpretation of the mammogram image. They test their algorithm on 100 mammogram images, 50 of which are positive for breast cancer and 50 of which are negative. The physician provides interpretation for the same 100 images. The results are tabulated below. Calculate the sensitivity, specificity, PPV, and NPV for the algorithm and the expert physician.

	Actually positive	Actually negative
Predicted positive	Algorithm: 45 Physician: 40	Algorithm: 15 Physician: 5
Predicted negative	Algorithm: 5 Physician: 10	Algorithm: 35 Physician: 45

Answer: To calculate the sensitivity, specificity, PPV, and NPV, we first must determine the number of true positives, true negatives, false positives, and false negatives. The number of true positives is the number that the algorithm or physician predicted positive that were actually positive (top left corner of the table); therefore, the number of true positives for the algorithm and physician are 45 and 40, respectively. The number of true negatives is the number that the algorithm or physician predicted negative that were actually negative (bottom right corner of the table); therefore, the number of true negatives for the algorithm and physician are 35 and 45, respectively. The number of false positives is the number that the algorithm or physician predicted positive that were actually negative (top right corner of the table); therefore, the number of false positives for the algorithm and physician are 15 and 5, respectively. The number of false negatives is the number that the algorithm or physician predicted negative that were actually positive (bottom left corner of the table); therefore, the number of false negatives for the algorithm and physician are 5 and 10, respectively. We can calculate the statistics using Equations 2.1–2.4 for each:

$$\text{Sensitivity}_{\text{algorithm}} = \frac{45}{45+5} \times 100 = 90\%,$$

$$\text{Sensitivity}_{\text{physician}} = \frac{40}{40+10} \times 100 = 80\%,$$

$$\text{Specificity}_{\text{algorithm}} = \frac{35}{35+15} \times 100 = 70\%,$$

$$\text{Specificity}_{\text{physician}} = \frac{45}{45+5} \times 100 = 90\%,$$

$$PPV_{algorithm} = \frac{45}{45+15} \times 100 = 75\%,$$

$$PPV_{physician} = \frac{40}{40+5} \times 100 = 89\%,$$

$$NPV_{algorithm} = \frac{35}{35+5} \times 100 = 88\%,$$

$$NPV_{physician} = \frac{45}{45+10} \times 100 = 82\%.$$

Breast cancer diagnosis is followed by a variety of treatment options, including surgery, radiation therapy, and/or chemotherapy, depending on the stage and severity of the disease. If the biopsy shows DCIS, surgery is typically the only procedure required. If the patient has invasive cancer, the surgeon will remove appropriate portions of the tumor and surrounding breast tissue to ensure the complete removal of cancerous cells. If the cancer has spread into the lymph node near the breast, the surgeon will also likely excise the axilla (area under the armpit) to remove the diseased lymph nodes. Depending on the type of tumor and how large it is, systemic therapy may be administered prior to surgery in an attempt to shrink the tumor to a more manageable size before excision. Surgery is typically followed by radiation and/or systemic therapy, again dictated by the cancer stage. In combination, these treatment strategies are modern-day medicine's most commonly successful techniques for reducing and eliminating cancers.

Deeper Look: Saving the Breast Also Saves Lives

The treatment of breast cancer with surgery extends back to the work of the late nineteenth-century William S. Halsted. Halstead popularized the **radical mastectomy**, which involved removing not only the cancerous breast but also the underarm lymph nodes and the chest wall muscles on the side of the cancer. He believed removing all tissues that allowed cancer cells to spread would save the lives of women with breast cancer. The radical mastectomy was devastating women, leaving them extremely disfigured and in a lot of pain.

In the late twentieth century, another surgeon, Bernard Fisher, would transform the way in which breast cancer surgery would be performed. He observed that cancer cells entered the blood early in their course, probably before they were discovered, and therefore radical mastectomies did little to save lives. Through prospective randomized trials (which you will learn more about in Chapter 7), Dr. Fisher demonstrated that a simple mastectomy (removal of the breast) or lumpectomy (removing a small portion of the breast localized to the cancer) followed by radiation was just as effective as more disfiguring forms of surgery. He published these findings in the *New England Journal of Medicine* (Fisher et al., 2002). Figure 2.4 shows the difference between a mastectomy and lumpectomy. **Mastectomy** removes the entire breast regardless of the amount of normal tissue surrounding the tumor. **Lumpectomy** removes just the tumor and a small ring of surrounding normal tissue, conserving as much healthy breast tissue as possible. Today the standard procedure for treating early breast cancers is lumpectomy followed by radiation therapy.

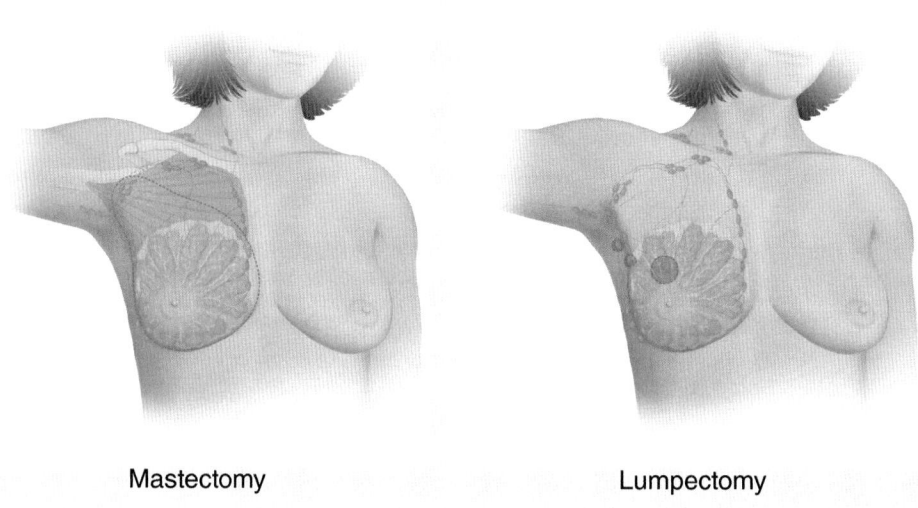

Mastectomy | Lumpectomy

Figure 2.4 The difference between a mastectomy and lumpectomy. Mastectomy removes the entire breast regardless of the amount of normal tissue surrounding the tumor. Lumpectomy removes just the tumor and a small ring of surrounding normal tissue, conserving as much healthy breast tissue as possible.
Source: © Lauren Shavell / Design Pics / Getty Images.

Changes in surgical practice, particularly the lumpectomy, have been driven in large part by improvements in imaging technologies. Transitioning from performing primarily mastectomies to lumpectomies was made possible in part because of mammographic screening of breast cancer. Improved screening using mammograms allowed breast cancers to be caught at earlier stages, therefore allowing for a less invasive procedure – lumpectomy – to be performed. The synergy between two distinct technologies used in the cancer control paradigm – imaging methods and treatment methods – is the foundation of cancer care. The next section will provide a more detailed discussion of imaging technologies for the screening, diagnosis, and treatment of cancer, using breast cancer as an example.

Imaging Technologies for Screening, Diagnosis, and Treatment of Cancer

In the example of breast cancer, we see that many different types of imaging and therapeutic technologies are used throughout the cancer control paradigm. These technologies are the basis of most cancer diagnostics today. They are medicine's most well-vetted and well-received approaches to diagnosis, prognosis, and treatment. Here, we are going to assess the different types of imaging technologies for screening, cancer diagnosis, and treatment, and take a closer look at how the complexity of these technologies frequently increases their cost and dictates how they are accessed.

What serves as the basis for modern medical imaging? With the exception of ultrasound, which uses sound waves, medical imaging technologies rely on the use of **electromagnetic (EM) radiation** (Bushberg and Boone, 2011). Electromagnetic radiation is an electric and magnetic disturbance traveling through space at the speed of light (3×10^8 m/s). Stated another way, EM radiation is the emission of energy from waves that have both electric and magnetic fields. As shown in Figure 2.5, EM radiation ranges from very low frequencies and energies (radio waves and microwaves) to very high frequencies and energies (gamma rays and X-rays). Different regions of the EM spectrum can be leveraged for either medical imaging or therapy. **Gamma rays** are used in positron emission tomography (PET). **X-rays** are used in a range of technologies, including computed tomography (CT) (Buzug, 2011) and mammography. Mid-level energy waves, such

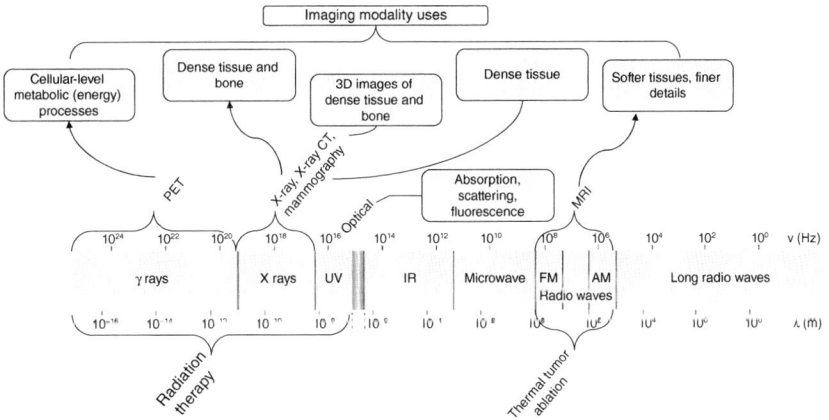

Figure 2.5 Electromagnetic (EM) radiation ranges from very low frequencies and energies (radio waves and microwaves) to very high frequencies and energies (gamma rays and X-rays). Different regions of the EM spectrum can be leveraged for either medical imaging or therapy. Gamma rays are used in PET. X-rays are used in a range of technologies, including CT (Buzug, 2011) and mammography. Mid-level energy waves, such as visible light, are used for light microscopes. Low-energy radio waves are employed in MRI (Hesselink et al., 1990).
Source: Adapted from https://commons.wikimedia.org/wiki/File:EM_spectrumrevised.png.

as **visible light**, are used for light microscopes. MRI uses low-energy radio waves (Hesselink et al., 1990).

What features in the body can these medical imaging techniques see? PET imaging using injected contrast agents that emit high-frequency gamma rays to visualize glucose uptake by tumors. X-rays can create contrast between bone or highly dense tissue and surrounding soft tissues. Optical imaging detects local absorbers such as blood, and the fluorescence of cellular and molecular components in tissue. MRI images soft tissues within the body, as well as blood flow. Additionally, injection of contrast agents can improve visualization of internal organs, blood vessels, and tissues. Both the higher-energy (gamma rays and X-rays) and lower-energy (microwaves and radio waves) ends of the EM spectrum can be used for cancer therapy by directly damaging DNA or increasing heat to kill cells, respectively.

Figure 2.6 shows EM radiation or energy travels in a wave form. Each wave is defined by specific qualities, including **amplitude, frequency, wavelength,** and **period**. **Amplitude** is the maximum distance a particle in a wave is displaced from the midpoint or rest point. **Frequency** is the number of repetitions of a unique point within a wave per unit time. **Wavelength** is the distance a unique point within a wave travels per repetition. A wave's **period**

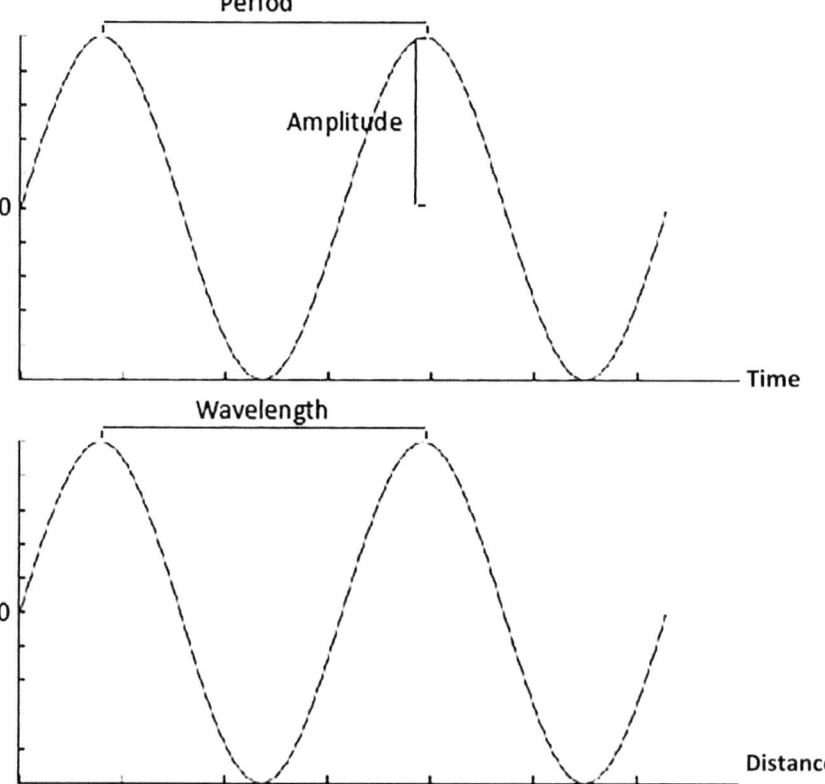

Figure 2.6

EM radiation or energy travels in a wave form. Each wave is defined by specific qualities, including amplitude, frequency, wavelength, and period. **Amplitude** is the maximum distance a particle in a wave is displaced from the midpoint or rest point. **Frequency** is the number of repetitions of a unique point within a wave per unit time. **Wavelength** is the distance a unique point within a wave travels per repetition. A wave's **period** is the amount of time for a particle within a wave to complete one cycle.

is the amount of time for a particle within a wave to complete one cycle. For medical imaging technologies, the types of EM radiation are mostly differentiated by the frequency of the periodic wave, or how many times a repeated point within the wave occurs per unit time. The energy of the wave is the potential energy stored by the electric and magnetic fields within the wave. Frequency is proportional to the **energy** of the wave; therefore, low-frequency waves are lower-energy waves and vice versa. The mathematical relationships between a wave's wavelength (λ) in nanometers (nm), frequency (n) in hertz (Hz), and energy (E) in joules (J) involve Planck's constant (h) in meter-kilogram-seconds (m^2 kg/s) and the speed of light (c) in meters per second (m/s) and are described by Equations 2.5 and 2.6:

$$E = h\upsilon, \tag{2.5}$$

$$E = h\frac{c}{\lambda}. \tag{2.6}$$

In general, the greater the density of a particular tissue type, the lower the EM wave penetrates into the tissue. The **penetration depth** of an EM wave is the distance the EM wave will travel into a material before losing $1/e$ or 63 percent of its energy (the number e, also known as **Euler's number**, is a constant approximately equal to 2.71828). The penetration depth of an EM wave within a material is dictated by the type of material and the amount of energy contained within the wave. Electromagnetic radiation can be either partially or completely reflected when an EM wave comes into contact with a surface. Some of the energy contained within the wave will be transferred into the material. Based on the material present and the energy of the EM wave, the EM wave will decay at different rates as it travels through the tissue. As a result, an EM wave may travel either long or short distances within the material, depending on the material properties. In general, the higher the amount of energy within the wave, the further into a material it will travel.

That being said, the energy of the radiation alone does not dictate penetration depth. As an EM wave moves through a heterogenous material, like tissues within the body, it encounters different types of structures and molecules. When the EM wave intercepts a structure or molecule, it can undergo one of two processes: absorption or scattering. If the molecule(s) does not absorb or scatter the light, the light will be transmitted through the sample. Figure 2.7 shows a simple illustration of absorption, scattering, and transmission. **Absorption** is the process of transferring energy from the EM wave into the molecule or structure. The energy transfer generally results in either heat or light being released by the molecule. **Scattering** is the process in which an EM wave undergoes a directional change after interacting with a molecule or structure. Both absorption and scattering can result in attenuation of the signal, which can in turn reduce **transmission** within an object.

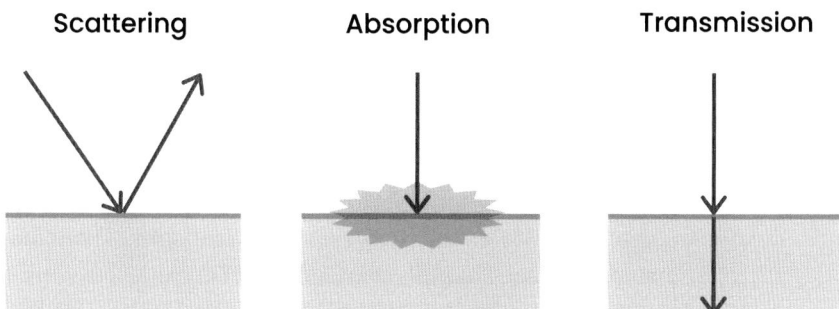

Figure 2.7 A simple illustration of absorption, scattering, and transmission. **Absorption** is the process of transferring energy from the EM wave into the molecule or structure. The energy transfer generally results in either heat or light being released by the molecule. **Scattering** is the process in which an EM wave undergoes a directional change after interacting with a molecule or structure. Both absorption and scattering can result in attenuation of the signal, which can in turn reduce **transmission** within an object.

As mentioned earlier, X-ray imaging of anatomical structures relies on absorption and scattering. Absorption and scattering can also provide functional information, most commonly blood content and/or flow. Leveraging multispectral imaging, where images are taken across different wavelengths of light, can allow for optical measurement of blood flow and content without an exogenous contrast agent (Bouchard et al., 2009), owing to the optical absorption of hemoglobin in the red blood cells (RBCs). Doppler ultrasound can be used to estimate the blood flow as a result of **scattering** from RBCs, which gives rise to echo signals from blood for **Doppler** applications. Point-of-care technologies (POCTs) based on optical and ultrasound imaging will be discussed in Chapter 5.

A phenomenon that is specific to the optical window of the EM spectrum is **fluorescence**. Fluorescence is the emission of light from a molecule that has absorbed light in the ultraviolet (UV) or visible part of the spectrum. The emitted light has a longer wavelength and therefore lower energy than the absorbed radiation. In general, the emission occurs in the visible region of the spectrum. Fluorescence can occur from naturally occurring molecules in tissue, the most common of which are electron carriers that reflect cellular metabolism, including reduced nicotinamide adenine dinucleotide (NADH) and flavin adenine dinucleotide (FAD), and structural proteins including collagen and elastin. An **electron carrier** is a molecule capable of accepting one or more electrons from another molecule, referred to as an **electron donor**. An electron carrier plays an important role in cellular metabolism. **Structural proteins** are responsible for cell shape and movement, providing support to major structures such as bones, cartilage, hair, and muscles, among other functions related to structure. This group includes proteins such as collagen, actin, myosin, and keratin.

Imaging systems can also provide functional information, most commonly blood content and/or flow, as discussed earlier. Blood content/flow can be monitored through a number of different imaging technologies, some of which require exogenous agents. Optical imaging can be used to measure movement of fluorescent agents such as indocyanine green (ICG) to measure blood flow rates (Nishigori et al., 2016). Alternatively, leveraging multispectral imaging, where images are taken across different wavelengths of light, can allow for optical measurement of blood flow and content without an exogenous contrast agent (Bouchard et al., 2009). Another example is Doppler ultrasound. While regular ultrasound uses sound waves to produce images, Doppler ultrasound can be used to estimate the blood flow through blood vessels by detecting high-frequency sound waves from circulating RBCs.

Example: How Much Higher Is the Energy in X-rays Over Optical Wavelengths?

Question: X-rays use EM waves with wavelengths around 10^{-10} m. Conversely, optical imaging uses wavelengths around 5×10^{-7} m. What is the ratio of the energy of an EM wave with a wavelength of 10^{-10} m (X-ray) to an EM wave with a wavelength of 5×10^{-7} m (optical)? What can you infer about their penetration depths based on the difference in energies?

Answer: Plugging into Equation 2.6 for the X-ray (10^{-10} m or 0.1 nm) and longest (5×10^{-7} m or 500 nm) wavelengths, we get:

$$E_{\text{X-ray}} = h \frac{c}{0.1 \text{ nm}},$$

$$E_{\text{Optical}} = h \frac{c}{500 \text{ nm}}.$$

To find the ratio, we divide the two energies:

$$\frac{E_{\text{X-ray}}}{E_{\text{Optical}}} = \frac{h \dfrac{c}{0.1 \text{ nm}}}{h \dfrac{c}{500 \text{ nm}}}.$$

Planck's constant and the speed of light show up in both the numerator and denominator and can be canceled out:

$$\frac{E_{\text{X-ray}}}{E_{\text{Optical}}} = \frac{\dfrac{1}{0.1 \text{ nm}}}{\dfrac{1}{500 \text{ nm}}}.$$

This simplifies to:

$$\frac{E_{380\text{nm}}}{E_{700\text{nm}}} = \frac{500 \text{ nm}}{0.1 \text{ nm}} = 5{,}000.$$

Through this example we found that X-rays contain about 5,000 times more energy than an EM wave in the optical range. Because X-rays have higher energy, they have a deeper penetration depth than optical light rays. As a result, X-rays are more useful for imaging structures deep within the body than are optical light rays.

Now that we have discussed some of the basic principles underlying imaging technologies, we will revisit the five major types of imaging technologies that are used in cancer control: X-ray (used for mammography and CT), ultrasound, optical imaging, MRI, and PET. The absorption and scattering features along with the penetration depth of EM radiation can highlight specific features within the human body. As a result, tissue features can be delineated by the degree to which they absorb or scatter waves. X-rays, optical imaging, and ultrasound imaging (although not considered EM radiation) all rely on differences in absorption and scattering to differentiate features within the body. For example, bones show up as white (low signal) on an X-ray film because they are extremely dense and do not permit X-rays to pass through them. Conversely, softer tissues (or air) show up as gray or even black (high signal) because X-rays pass through them easily. Ultrasound relies on scattering of sound waves when they are reflected from interfaces between substances. The sound waves either travel through the tissues of the body or they are reflected (echo). Increasing echo generated from tissue structures is visualized in grayscale, from black to white. Liquids, such as water or urine, have low scattering, whereas dense tissues, such as tumors, have high scattering.

Magnetic resonance imaging uses a fundamentally different type of contrast than X-rays, optical waves, or ultrasound. It uses radio frequencies to measure water content within the body. Large magnets are used to align hydrogen atoms within water molecules. Radio waves are then pulsed to disrupt the hydrogen alignment. After the pulse, the hydrogens return to alignment and emit a signal that the detector within the MRI captures. The emitted signals are then used to form an image based on the differences in water content.

Positron emission tomography imaging requires the use of an exogenous agent for contrast. It measures EM radiation emitted from a radioactive tracer that is injected into the body. The **radioactive tracer** is a chemical compound in which one or more atoms have been replaced by a **radioisotope**, an element with unstable nuclei emitting energy in the form of **ionizing radiation**. Because ionizing radiation consists of high-energy EM waves, there is little attenuation within the body, allowing for imaging of deep-seated regions. The most common type of radiotracer for PET imaging for cancer is **fluorodeoxyglucose PET** (FDG-PET), which uses a radioactive glucose analogue called FDG as the radioisotope (Reske and Kotzerke, 2001). In the case

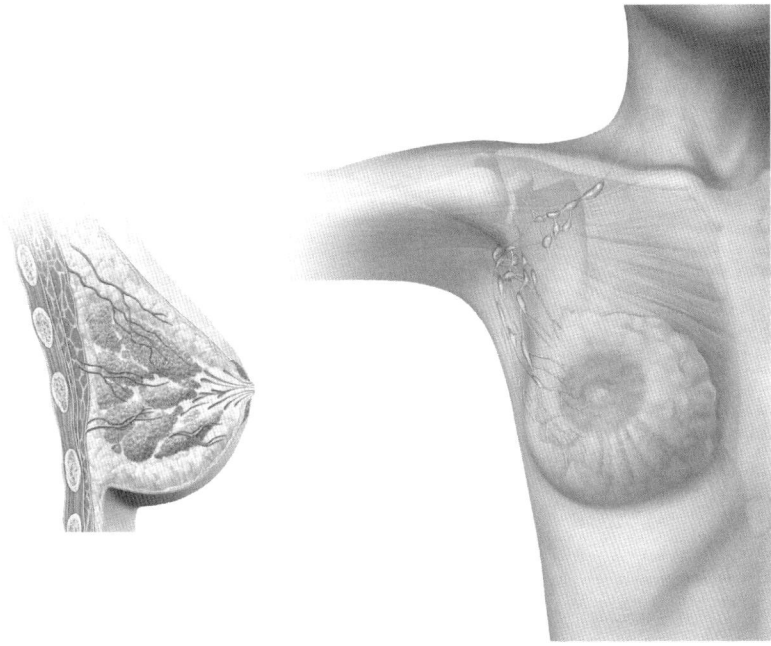

Figure 2.8 A visual representation of the lymph nodes (in white), which are located within the breast and the axilla, an area of the body near and underneath the armpit. The lymph nodes represent the path through which a breast cancer is likely to spread from the primary tumor. If and when the cancer spreads, it may appear in the **sentinel nodes**, which are the first set of nodes in the lymph node chain. The sentinel node is excised so that a pathologist can look at the tissue to determine whether there are cancerous cells present in the sentinel node.
Source: © Leonello Calvetti / Science Photo Library / Getty Images.

of FDG-PET imaging, contrast is developed by differences in glucose uptake levels between different tissue types. For example, the brain has high glucose uptake, whereas lungs have low glucose uptake. Tumors are known for their high uptake of glucose for growth, which helps develop contrast between tumors and surrounding healthy tissue.

As you learned earlier in the chapter, early spread of invasive breast cancer occurs through the lymphatic system within the breast to nearby lymph nodes. Figure 2.8 shows a visual representation of the lymph nodes (in white) which are located within the breast and the axilla, an area of the body near and underneath the armpit. The lymph nodes represent the path through which a breast cancer is likely to spread from the primary tumor. If and when a cancer spreads, it appears first in the **sentinel nodes**, which are the first set of nodes in the lymph node chain. The sentinel node is excised so that a pathologist can look at the tissue to determine whether there are cancerous cells present in the sentinel node. The **gamma probe** was developed as a simple and reliable technology to find the sentinel lymph node, similar to PET imaging but on a smaller scale. A gamma probe detects radiotracers that are injected into the lymphatic system surrounding the tumor (shown in white). Technetium-99m, the most commonly used radiotracer for sentinel node mapping, flows

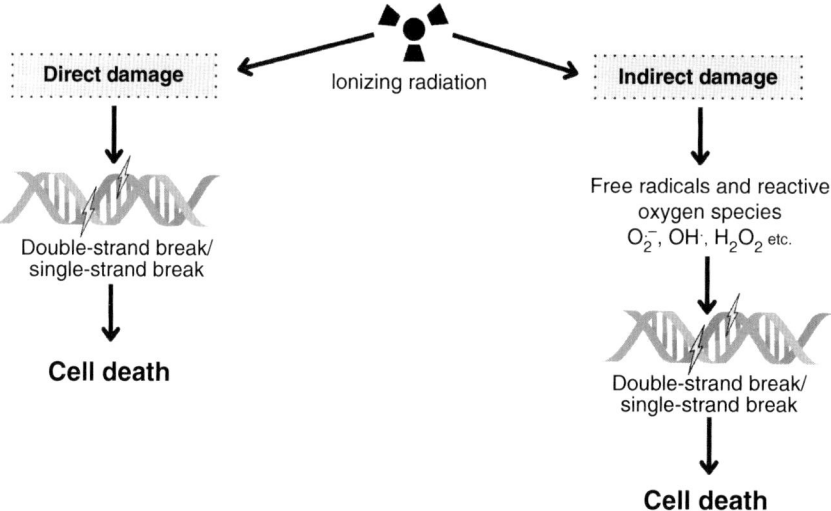

Figure 2.9 Ionizing radiation transmits energy to disrupt double-stranded DNA, which can cause cell death. Ionizing radiation can cause two different types of cell damage: direct and indirect. Ionizing radiation incites breaks within cellular DNA, which leads to cell death. Indirect damage is caused when ionizing radiation interacts with water molecules within the cell, which results in the formation of free radicals and reactive oxygen species which similarly damage DNA.

through the lymphatics, gathering in higher levels within the sentinel lymph node. The gamma probe is moved around the breast to determine where the sentinel node is located so that it can be excised for pathology.

Though we have described five imaging modalities separately, they are frequently used in combination to provide more refined insights. For example, fusing the molecular information from a tumor with anatomical or functional information can potentially improve both sensitivity and specificity by providing complementary information. Examples of these combinations are PET/MRI, PET/CT, and MRI/optical.

Beyond screening, identification, and assessment, how else can EM spectrum-based technologies be used in cancer care? Figure 2.5 shows that different parts of the EM spectrum can be harnessed by technologies for cancer treatment. The higher-energy end of the EM spectrum can create ionizing radiation in the form of X-rays and gamma rays for cancer treatment (Khan and Gibbons, 2014). As you can see in Figure 2.9, ionizing radiation transmits energy to disrupt double-stranded DNA, which can cause cell death. Ionizing radiation can cause two different types of cell damage: direct and indirect. Ionizing radiation incites breaks within cellular DNA, which leads to cell death. Indirect damage is caused when ionizing radiation interacts with water molecules within the cell, which results in the formation of free radicals and reactive oxygen species which similarly damage DNA. Although modern iterations of these technologies have increased precision and accuracy for targeting ionizing radiation primarily to the region containing the tumor, an unfortunate side effect of this therapy is cell death and subsequent damage to nearby noncancerous tissues (Hall, 2006). While ionizing radiation remains a mainstay for cancer therapy, other parts of the EM spectrum can be leveraged for treatment with fewer side effects.

Deeper Look: In Some Cases, EM Radiation Can Cause More Harm Than Good

Marie Curie is one of the most well-known names in science for her work in the fields of physics and chemistry. Earning the Nobel Prize in Physics in 1903 and in Chemistry in 1911, she developed methods to separate radioactive isotopes and used them to treat cancer. Marie and her husband, Pierre Curie, found radium, which was eventually used as a cancer treatment, in a sample of uraninite in 1898. However, one of the dangerous side effects from exposure to radium is anemia, which can be fatal. Marie Curie, and many others, would suffer from the side effects of radium.

With little to no regulation of radium, it was used in products including additives in toothpaste, "Revigator" (water with radium dissolved into it, marketed as a drink to cure ailments), and for painting clocks. Figure 2.10 shows women known as "radium girls" painting alarm clock faces at the Ingersoll factory in January 1932. The work involved using luminous radium paint to make the numbers on clocks, watches, and aeronautic dials glow in the dark. Hundreds of women worked in clock factories during World War I, where they painted watch and clock dials with glow-in-the-dark radium paint. It seemed a relatively safe job until women started developing serious symptoms such as anemia, radium jaw (deterioration of their jaw bones), and deadly cancerous tumors. Though some executives and scientists in the industry were increasingly aware and protected themselves, the women were not warned about the dangers and did not suspect problems until they had the symptoms.

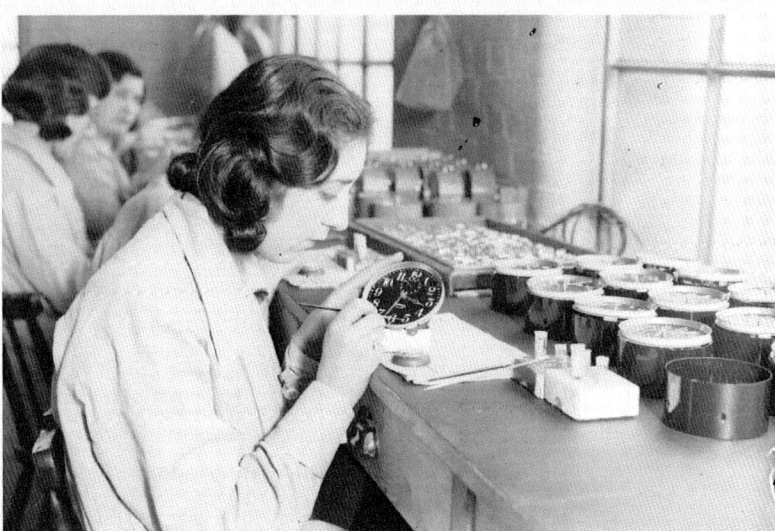

Figure 2.10
Women known as "radium girls" painting alarm clock faces at the Ingersoll factory in January 1932. The work involved using luminous radium paint to make the numbers on clocks, watches, and aeronautic dials glow in the dark.
Source: © Daily Herald Archive / Contributor / SSPL / Getty Images.

Tumor ablation, a minimally invasive therapy, can also use EM radiation; however, it depends on a less energetic EM wave, which induces necrosis within a tumor using thermal means. **Necrosis** is a nonspecific form of uncontrolled cellular death and can be caused by injury, radiation, or chemicals. Rather than relying on ionizing radiation, some methods of tumor ablation damage cancerous tissue through the generation of extreme temperatures (Chu and Dupuy, 2014). Ablation technologies treat a significantly smaller volume of tissue compared to ionizing radiation, and thus are used for local tumor treatment rather than systemic treatment (Knavel and Brace, 2013). Energy-based ablation techniques include radio frequency (RF), microwave (MW), laser, and high-intensity focused ultrasound (HIFU) systems. In addition to EM-based ablation methods, cryotherapy causes tissue damage through freezing, and chemical ablation disrupts cellular functions. We will examine tumor ablation in depth in Chapter 6.

Most of the technologies described above are complex and/or expensive, and are therefore located in hospitals to maximize the frequency of use, as well as to defray the cost of procurement and maintenance. Additionally, cancer diagnosis and treatment are also performed in specialized clinics or hospitals, as highly trained personnel are co-located with the equipment in those settings. Technology complexity, cost, and ease of access (i.e., primary care setting vs. hospital setting) are all inextricably linked. Complexity both drives up cost and requires highly trained professionals for technology operation and, in the case of diagnostic imaging technologies, image interpretation.

Molecular Testing, Omics, and Imaging

Up to this point we have primarily discussed general diagnostic testing strategies that provide a "yes/no" answer to the question "Is there a tumor present?" as well as tumor size for staging purposes. Recent advances in technology are ushering in a new era of diagnostic testing, referred to as molecular testing. **Molecular diagnostics** involves the process of identifying a disease by studying molecules – such as proteins, DNA, and RNA – in a tissue or fluid. Molecular testing holds the potential to provide greater precision and patient-specific treatments than previous technologies. Molecular tests can have clinical impacts on cancer patients in two areas: identification of heritable cancers and tumor treatment specificity. **Heritable cancers** are inherited cancers caused by a mutation in a gene that was present in the egg or sperm cell at the time of fertilization. These cancers make up a fraction of common cancers (e.g., breast, colon, and prostate cancer) as well as less common cancers such as pancreatic and ovarian cancer.

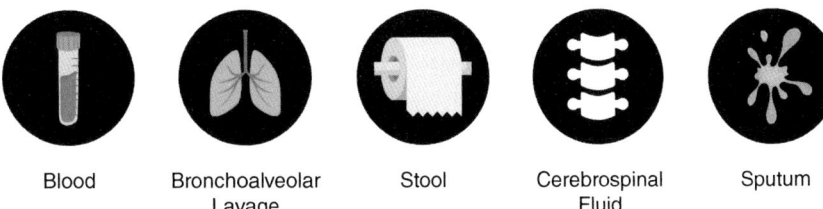

Figure 2.11 Different types of samples used for molecular testing. Molecular tests look for a particular sequence of DNA or different levels of protein expression in these samples. We will first look at methods for DNA detection.

Additional applications include monitoring of residual cancer following treatment and early tumor detection. Here, we show new insights provided by molecular testing, how molecular testing is performed, and how it can be used in combination with some of the imaging technologies described in the previous section to improve cancer diagnostics and prognostics. These techniques enable us to transition from "Is there a tumor present?" to "What type of tumor is present and how can we best treat it?"

What are the steps in molecular testing? Before any molecular testing can be performed, testing samples must be collected. Samples used for molecular testing are not limited to biopsies of the tumor itself. The different types of samples typically collected for molecular testing typically include blood, lavage, stool, cerebrospinal fluid, and sputum. Figure 2.11 shows the different types of samples used for molecular testing. Molecular tests look for a particular sequence of DNA or different levels of protein expression in these samples. We will first look at methods for DNA detection.

The development of modern clinical DNA testing is owed to the invention of the polymerase chain reaction (PCR) (Mullis and Faloona, 1987), a technique which is used to amplify multiple copies of a small amount of DNA taken from a biological sample to a large enough amount to evaluate genetically. Kary Mullis is credited with pioneering PCR, and received the Nobel Prize in Chemistry in 1993 for this discovery. Polymerase chain reaction techniques require relatively simple instrumentation and infrastructure, while using only minute amounts of biological material.

Figure 2.12 shows the general process for PCR, which includes the following steps: denaturation, annealing, and extension. **Denaturation** is the process of separating the two strands of DNA from each other using heat. In the **annealing** process, a primer is connected to the target DNA region following separation of the two strands of DNA. A primer is a small segment of DNA that is introduced to the segment of DNA that is being targeted. After annealing, the protein Taq polymerase is used to complete the new DNA strands. One cycle of this process will double the amount of DNA present – therefore, the PCR method for amplifying

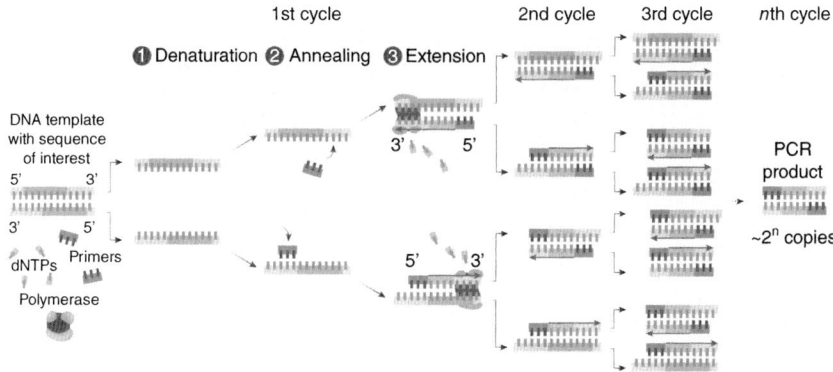

Figure 2.12 The general process for PCR includes the following steps: denaturation, annealing, and extension. Denaturation is the process of separating the two strands of DNA from each other using heat. In the annealing process, a primer is connected to the target DNA region following separation of the two strands of DNA. After annealing, a protein is introduced that completes the new DNA strands.
Image: Schematic mechanism of PCR created by "Enzoklop" on Wikimedia Commons. CC-BY-SA.

DNA can be repeated to provide exponential growth. Newer versions of PCR can incorporate a fluorophore into the DNA strands that can be measured by an optical detector to quantify the amount of DNA that has been amplified.

Other methods to identify gene expression include fluorescence in situ hybridization (FISH) and reverse transcription PCR (RT-PCR). FISH is a technique to locate a specific segment of DNA within a chromosome using a fluorescently modified strand of target DNA to quantify gene expression. Rather than amplifying DNA, FISH is typically performed directly on a tissue sample and imaged with a microscope. As a result, FISH can be performed more quickly than PCR because there are fewer steps. However, FISH is a less sensitive test than PCR, owing to the lack of amplification. RT-PCR is used to study RNA rather than DNA. RNA is downstream of DNA and can report on gene expression rather than gene presence. RT-PCR adds an initial step prior to DNA amplification, in which the RNA sample undergoes reverse transcription to produce a strand of DNA (the opposite of transcription, which creates a strand of RNA from DNA, hence the name "reverse transcription"). Once a strand of DNA has been derived via reverse transcription, PCR is used to amplify the RNA for testing. Each of these techniques (PCR, RT-PCR, and FISH) is routinely used in cancer control in the US.

Molecular testing informs breast cancer treatment. There are three main subtypes of breast cancer: estrogen receptor (ER+); those that express human epidermal growth factor receptor (HER2+); and triple-negative breast cancer, which does not have a specific receptor that characterizes it. Cancer cells expressing the estrogen receptor, just like normal breast cells, receive signals from estrogen that promote their growth (Yager and Davidson, 2006). When the estrogen receptor binds to estrogen, a signaling cascade is initiated resulting in cell growth and proliferation. HER2 is a protein encoded by the gene *ERBB2* and is overexpressed in a subset of breast cancers. Normal levels of *ERBB2* expression lead to appropriate growth of cells within the body; however, increased *ERBB2* expression can lead to uncontrolled cell growth. HER2 overexpression is typically an indicator of poor prognosis and highly aggressive tumors.

Polymerase chain reaction can be used to check a woman's risk level of developing breast cancer at some point in her lifetime by probing for mutations to a pair of genes called breast cancer 1 (*BRCA1*) and breast cancer 2 (*BRCA2*). When functioning normally, *BRCA1* and *BRCA2* actually protect against breast and other cancers. In a subset of women, however, either or both of the *BRCA* genes can be mutated. If they are mutated, a woman is at an increased risk of developing breast cancer at some point in her lifetime.

Figure 2.13 shows some of the classic features of a family with a deleterious *BRCA1* mutation across three generations, including affected family members with breast cancer or ovarian cancer and a young age at onset. The square corresponds to a male and the circle corresponds to a female. The filled circles and squares correspond to those affected by the trait. The crossed-off circles and squares correspond to diseased individuals. The numbers correspond to the age at the time of diagnosis (dx in the figure). *BRCA1* mutation can be transmitted through maternal or paternal lineages. For women who undergo genetic testing and learn that they have inherited a *BRCA1/2* mutation before they receive a breast cancer diagnosis, there are ways to reduce their risk of going on to develop the disease, such as mastectomy.

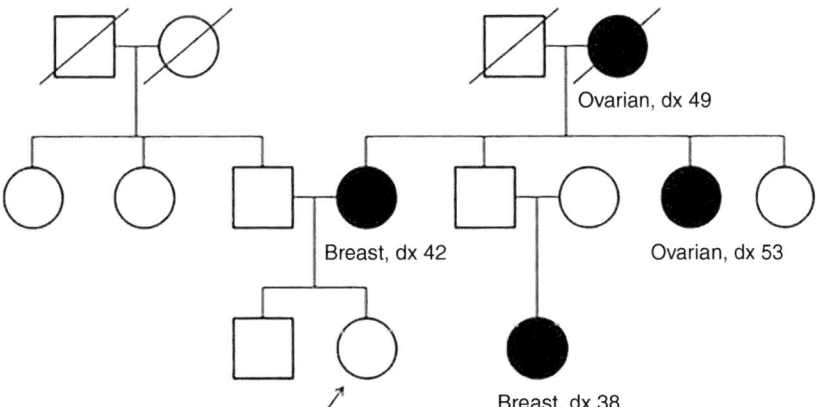

Figure 2.13 Classic features of a family with a deleterious *BRCA1* mutation across three generations, including affected family members with breast cancer or ovarian cancer and a young age at onset. The square corresponds to a male and the circle corresponds to a female. The filled circles and squares correspond to those affected by the trait. The crossed-off circles and squares correspond to diseased individuals. The numbers correspond to the age at the time of diagnosis (dx).
Source: National Cancer Institute.

Deeper Look: When Does a Preexisting Condition Become an Existing Condition?

The Genetic Information Nondiscrimination Act (GINA) widely prohibited discrimination based on genetic makeup by healthcare insurers and employers when it went into effect in 2008. However, this Act fell short of its promises. To name just a few examples, it did not prevent discrimination by life, disability, or long-term care, and only covered those who were asymptomatic.

Even if a consumer could secure an individual market policy, most states had no restrictions on what insurers could charge in monthly premiums. Thus, insurers were able to charge higher rates based on health status or medical history, demographic information (such as age and gender), and a person's occupation, among other factors.

The Affordable Care Act (ACA), introduced by the Obama Administration, banned these practices and established a community rating where the individual and small-group markets can vary based solely on four factors: family size, geographic location, age, and tobacco use. These reforms made coverage more affordable for many with preexisting conditions who could no longer be rated out of coverage entirely.

Table 2.1 compares insurance coverage for preexisting conditions with GINA and the ACA. GINA protections only apply to genetic information for previvors (unaffected carriers) who have not been diagnosed with the related disease. Manifest disease is not protected under GINA. Under the ACA, no one can be denied health insurance due to a preexisting condition. However, disability and life insurance are different; preexisting conditions are taken into consideration when issuing a policy. Lifting discrimination against preexisting conditions has significant implications. The Kaiser Family Foundation estimated that 27–65 percent of nonelderly adults have a preexisting condition that would make them uninsurable. The global pandemic COVID-19 could be considered a preexisting condition in the future, especially for those who face long-term effects of the virus.

Table 2.1 Comparison of insurance coverage for preexisting conditions under GINA and the ACA

GINA protections only apply to genetic information for previvors (unaffected carriers) who have not been diagnosed with the related disease. Manifest disease is not protected under GINA.

Federal/national	Affordable Care Act (ACA) Health insurance protections	Genetic Information Nondiscrimination Act (GINA) Health insurance protections	Life, long-term care, and disability insurance protections
Previvors	Yes	Yes	No
Survivors	Yes	No	No

Polymerase chain reaction, and more specifically quantitative PCR (qPCR), is useful for detecting gene expression levels. However, PCR cannot inform on protein expression levels, which are more indicative of functional changes in response to gene expression. While there are many ways to measure protein expression levels, two of the gold standard laboratory techniques for interrogating protein expression are immune-based assays that use basic immunology principles for target detection. Immune-based assays identify target antigens outside of the body using engineered antibodies. **Antibodies** are large proteins used by the immune system to recognize specific **antigens**, which are substances that elicit an immune response. The antibodies can be labeled fluorescently or using colorimetric indicators for detection with common laboratory equipment. **Enzyme-linked immunosorbent assays** (ELISA) is a method that provides information on levels of protein expression via direct measurement of extracted protein with an antibody and a plate reader that measures changes in absorption or fluorescence depending on the amount and type of antibody. Higher protein levels will result in greater amounts of antibody. A second type of assay for protein expression in **immunohistochemical staining** (**IHC**). This involves staining a tissue section using fluorescent or colorimetric antibodies within. Imaging of the IHC stained section is performed using a microscope.

Example: Can PCR of Circulation Cell DNA (ctDNA) Serve as an Alternative or Be Combined with FISH or IHC to Improve the Detection of HER2 Positive Breast Cancer Patients?

Question: HER2 amplification is routinely determined by IHC or FISH on tissue biopsy. Pathologists can use IHC analysis of a tumor biopsy to examine the expression levels of HER2 within a tumor. Additional testing must be performed to determine HER2 levels using FISH to probe expression levels of the gene *ERBB2*, which encodes HER2. While IHC and FISH are considered the gold standard, they are labor-intensive and require a biopsy. To detect HER2 amplification status, digital PCR (dPCR) is a promising candidate technology. Traditional quantitative PCR is only capable of relative quantification. dPCR, on the other hand, achieves absolute quantification. Moreover, performing dPCR on circulating DNA (ctDNA) is less invasive as it only requires a blood draw.

The table below shows the HER2 detection rate of ctDNA with dPCR and ICH/FISH in tissue for stage III breast cancer patients. What is the sensitivity, specificity, PPV, and NPV for each test? What would need to be true about the overlap in positive and negative results between the two tests in order for them to be useful in combination?

	Actually positive	Actually negative
Predicted positive	dPCR: 11 FISH/IHC: 26	dPCR: 3 FISH/IHC: 3
Predicted negative	dPCR: 20 FISH/IHC: 5	dPCR: 36 FISH/IHC: 36

Answer: To calculate the sensitivity, specificity, PPV, and NPV, we first must determine the number of true positives, true negatives, false positives, and false negatives. The number of true positives is the number that dPCR or FISH/IHC predicted positive that were actually positive (top left corner of the table); therefore, the number of true positives for dPCR and FISH/IHC are 11 and 26, respectively. The number of true negatives is the number that dPCR or FISH/IHC predicted negative that were actually negative (bottom right corner of the table); therefore, the number of true negatives for dPCR and FISH/IHC are 36 and 36, respectively. The number of false positives is the number that dPCR or FISH/IHC predicted positive that were actually negative (top right corner of the table); therefore, the number of false positives for dPCR and FISH/IHC are 3 and 3, respectively. The number of false negatives is the number that dPCR or FISH/IHC predicted negative that were actually positive (bottom left corner of the table); therefore, the number of false negatives for dPCR and FISH/IHC are 20 and 5, respectively. Now we can calculate the statistics using Equations 2.1–2.4 for each:

$$\text{Sensitivity}_{dPCR} = \frac{11}{11+20} \times 100 = 35\%,$$

$$\text{Sensitivity}_{IHC/FISH} = \frac{26}{26+5} \times 100 = 84\%,$$

$$\text{Specificity}_{dPCR} = \frac{36}{36+3} \times 100 = 92\%,$$

$$\text{Specificity}_{IHC/FISH} = \frac{36}{36+3} \times 100 = 92\%,$$

$$\text{PPV}_{dPCR} = \frac{11}{11+3} \times 100 = 79\%,$$

$$\text{PPV}_{IHC/FISH} = \frac{26}{26+3} \times 100 = 90\%,$$

$$\text{NPV}_{dPCR} = \frac{36}{20+36} \times 100 = 64\%$$

$$\text{NPV}_{IHC/FISH} = \frac{36}{5+36} \times 100 = 88\%.$$

For a combination of dPCR and IHC/FISH to be useful, there must not be complete overlap between the false positives and false negatives. In other words, the two tests need to make different mistakes.

Metabolomics:
Molecular study of cellular energy use

Proteomics:
Molecular study of protein expression

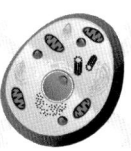

Genomics:
Molecular study of gene expression

Microbiomics:
Molecular study of bacteria in the body

Figure 2.14 Different "omics" techniques. Genomics provides complete sets of genes or heredity units that dictate some characteristic encoded by its DNA pattern. **Proteomics** provides collections of proteins that can be expressed from the genome. **Metabolomics** provides comprehensive counts of metabolites or by-products and products of energy production and consumption in an organism as they relate to cancer biology (Cho, 2010). More recently, **microbiomics** (the study of composition of bacteria making up an individual's gut flora) has been implicated in cancer biology (Schwabe and Jobin, 2013).

Building blocks – such as PCR, ELISA, and IHC – have led to advances in molecular testing defined broadly as "omics." Each "ome" contains millions of data points that collectively provide information on the biological activity of a tumor. As a result, "omics" investigations require intensive computational power. Figure 2.14 shows the different "omics" techniques. **Genomics** provides complete sets of genes or heredity units that dictate some characteristic encoded by its DNA pattern; **proteomics** provides collections of proteins that can be expressed from the genome; and **metabolomics** provides comprehensive counts of metabolites or by-products and products of energy production and consumption in an organism (Cho, 2010). More recently, **microbiomics** (the study of composition of bacteria making up an individual's gut flora) has been implicated in cancer biology (Schwabe and Jobin, 2013). Each "ome" provides unique insights into cancer development, progression, and response to therapy. It is important to note, however, that "omics" is not specific to cancer and is used in many other areas of medical research.

While PCR is useful for studying individual genes, studying a large number of genes, as is required for genomic analysis, requires capabilities that extend beyond PCR. **Next-generation sequencing** (NGS) (Schuster, 2008) is a massive parallel sequencing technology that offers ultra-high throughput, scalability, and speed. The technology is used to examine the expression levels of a large number of genes, requiring heavy computing infrastructure.

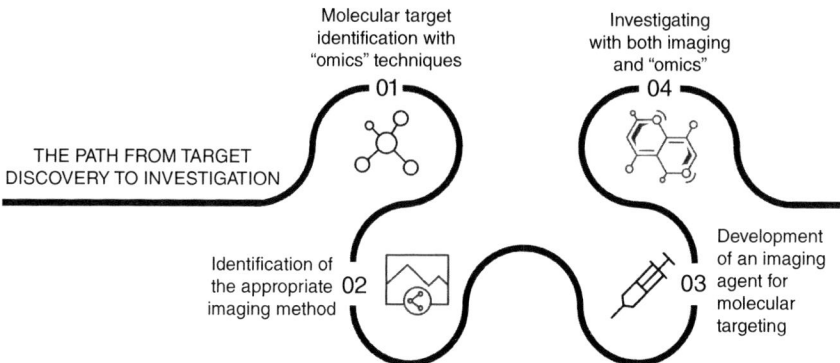

Figure 2.15 Molecular understanding of disease can be used to inform development of molecular imaging methodologies. For example, "omics" techniques can aid in development of new molecular diagnostic and therapeutic targets. Depending on the type of target, a particular imaging method (e.g., PET, MRI, etc.) can be selected and an imaging agent developed to image the molecular target.

These techniques are used for many genomic studies. Similar technologies have been developed for proteomics and metabolomics, such as **mass spectrometry**, an analytical tool useful for measuring the mass-to-charge ratio (m/z) of one or more molecules present in a sample. These measurements can be used to calculate the exact molecular weight of the sample components.

Molecular testing mechanisms have greatly increased our scientific understanding of cancer. Now that we have discussed many of the advantages of molecular testing and the methods for performing molecular testing, what are some of the limitations? We have already alluded to one of them, which is the requirement of major computational power. Though computers were conceived of in the early nineteenth century, it was not until the second half of the twentieth century that computational power reached a point where computers were ubiquitously adopted. As computational power has increased, more advanced analytical studies, such as "omics," have become possible. That being said, "omics" studies only became possible in recent decades and computers powerful enough for large-scale studies remain confined to a few institutions.

A second major limitation of molecular testing approaches is that they provide only a static glimpse of the cell or tissue at the exact time point during which they are harvested. For clinical applications this can be somewhat circumvented by collecting samples at multiple time points. However, multiple tissue and blood collections are not practical for patient care as the amount of tissue and blood needed would require multiple invasive procedures. This leaves many questions about tumor dynamics and longitudinal trends unanswered. Figure 2.15 shows how molecular understanding of disease can be used to inform development of molecular imaging methodologies. For example, "omics" techniques can aid in development of new molecular diagnostic and therapeutic targets. Depending on the type of target, a particular imaging method (e.g., PET, MRI, etc.) can then be selected and an imaging agent developed to image the molecular target.

Though multiple molecular imaging probes that work with optical, MRI, and ultrasound have been developed, PET was perhaps the first molecular imaging technology. As discussed earlier, FDG-PET directly images the uptake of glucose in organs within the body. Glucose plays an important role in tumor growth. Early investigations of cancer metabolism revealed increased glycolysis, reflecting a greater demand for glucose. Though healthy tissue can and does use glycolysis as a source of energy, particularly when oxygen is scarce, tumors regularly use glucose as a primary energy source even when oxygen is present (Macbeth and Bekesi, 1962; Dang, 2012). This aberrant metabolic signature was discovered by Otto Heinrich Warburg in the early twentieth century. He was awarded the Nobel Prize in Physiology or Medicine for this discovery in 1931. Though we now know that cancer metabolism is much more complex than glycolysis, modern-day PET imaging still uses the foundational work of Otto Warburg to probe the body for cancer. The increase in glucose uptake within the tumor compared to the surrounding tissue creates contrast between the tumor and healthy tissue on PET images.

Unlike molecular imaging, which is designed to have high specificity (e.g., those that bind to a specific receptor such as EGFR), PET imaging can suffer from background noise. For example, PET imaging is not effective for the detection of brain tumors because the brain itself has levels of glucose uptake. Conversely, water content provides contrast between healthy brain tissue and tumor tissue, naturally showing contrast on an MRI image. Magnetic resonance imaging has a high specificity (greater than 90 percent) and moderate sensitivity (72–90 percent) for detecting cancer (Yan et al., 2016), and reduces the number of unnecessary biopsies, which can cause swelling, bleeding, blood clot, and infection.

Staying with PET imaging, there are now molecular radiotracers that can address the contrast challenges associated with FDG-PET. For example, 16α-^{18}F-fluoroestradiol (^{18}F-FES) is an ER-targeting radiotracer with high sensitivity and specificity for detection of ER-positive tumors, which is highly expressed in 70–80 percent of breast cancers. Figure 2.16 shows imaging examples from two patients who underwent ^{18}F-FES and FDG scans. Patient A had mediastinal lesions on both ^{18}F-FES and FDG. Patient B had mediastinal disease clearly seen on FDG-PET but not visible on ^{18}F-FES. The core biopsy of a metastatic axillary lesion from Patient A showed ER-positive breast cancer, while that from a vertebral lesion in Patient B showed ER-negative breast cancer. ^{18}F-FES was FDA-approved on May 20, 2020 as a diagnostic agent for the detection of ER-positive lesions. ^{18}F-FES

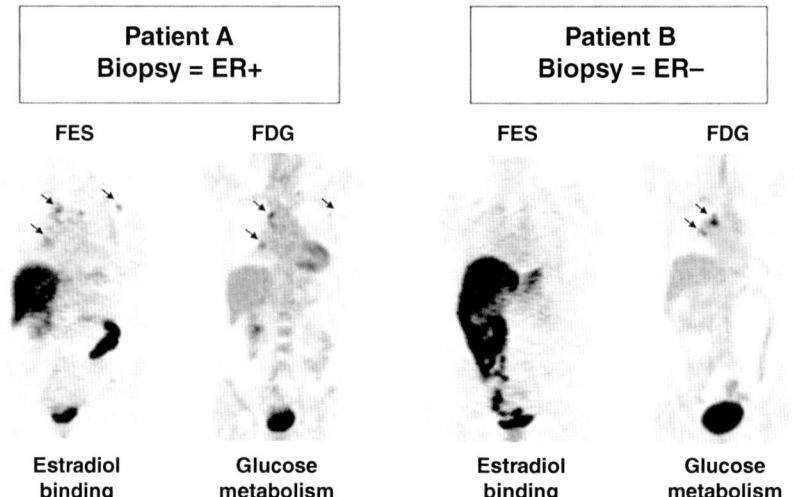

Figure 2.16 Imaging examples from two patients who underwent ^{18}F-FES and FDG scans. Patient A had mediastinal lesions on both ^{18}F-FES and FDG. Patient B had mediastinal disease clearly seen on FDG-PET but not visible on ^{18}F-FES. The core biopsy of a metastatic axillary lesion from Patient A showed ER-positive breast cancer while that from a vertebral lesion in Patient B showed ER-negative breast cancer.
Source: Copyright © 2013, World Molecular Imaging Society.

provides sensitive detection of ER-positive malignancy in several anatomic sites, including bone, lymph nodes, and in particular brain, which is problematic for FDG-PET imaging. Further, ER-positive breast cancers with low metabolic activity are not well visualized by FDG, and can be imaged with ER-specific molecular imaging.

Beyond glucose, the field of molecular imaging has expanded rapidly to incorporate an array of molecular agents that can be used with other imaging modalities, including optical, ultrasound, and MRI techniques. The molecular imaging agents can include metal ions, radioactive isotopes, microbubbles (bubbles that are 1–10 μm), antibodies, antigens, and enzymes (proteins used to catalyze chemical reactions), to name just a few examples. For applications in cancer, molecular imaging agents are employed to establish the presence or absence of a particular target. For example, molecular imaging agents could be used to identify whether or not a particular protein is expressed in a tumor that could be exploited with a particular therapy.

Classes of Systemic Therapies

Now that we have discussed how "omics" and molecular imaging technologies can be used to identify molecular targets for therapy, we will discuss how this has impacted the types of therapies available to treat cancer.

Classes of Systemic Therapies

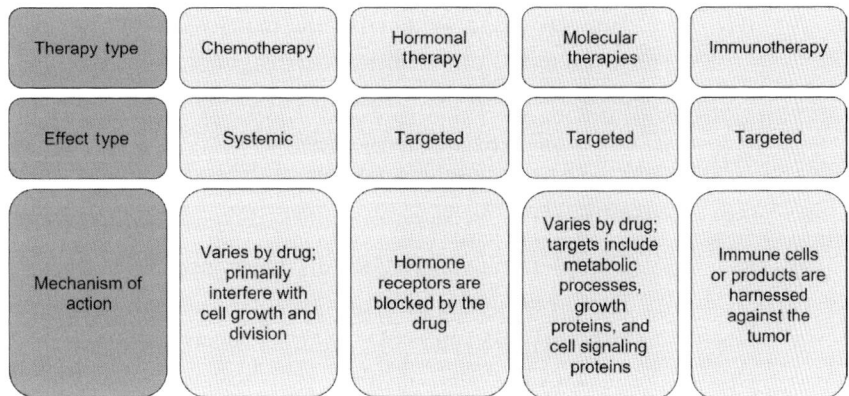

Figure 2.17 Different classes of drugs for cancer therapy. Cancer therapies can be broadly separated into four classes: chemotherapy, hormonal therapy, molecular therapy, or immunotherapy, though some drugs fit within more than one class.

Figure 2.17 shows different classes of drugs for cancer therapy. Cancer therapies can be broadly broken into four classes: chemotherapy, hormonal therapy, molecular therapy, or immunotherapy, though some drugs fit within more than one of these classes. In this section, we will delve into each type of therapy to explain whether it acts systemically or specifically targets cells within the body, as well as more specifically how each class of therapy works. We will also look at the benefits and limitations of each class of therapies. One of the most well-known and -regarded texts that chronicles the history of cancer is *The Emperor of All Maladies: A Biography of Cancer* (Mukherjee, 2010). In this text, Siddhartha Mukherjee covers the entire history of cancer, from its first appearances millennia ago through the development of treatments from the nineteenth century to the present day. Mukherjee explores the biology of tumors and how we have learned to treat them, using case studies to highlight the experiences of those who have fought (both won and lost) battles with cancer.

Chemotherapy, the earliest form of therapy for cancers, was first deployed in the early 1900s (DeVita and Chu, 2008). A variety of chemotherapy drugs are used today, and they remain the most common treatment for cancer. Chemotherapies work by targeting cellular machinery involved in cell proliferation. For example, cyclophosphamide, one of the most commonly available and widely used chemotherapies on the World Health Organization's (WHO) essential medicines list, belongs to a class of chemotherapies called alkylating agents, which bind to DNA and induce crosslinking to inhibit cell division, ultimately leading to cell death. Given their mechanisms of action, chemotherapies are lethal to any cell that is undergoing rapid division (i.e., proliferating cells). As a result, chemotherapies have a host of undesirable side effects due to their lack of molecular specificity to the tumor.

How do we know whether the therapy is working, and how is the benefit measured? In the short term, imaging can be used for early response to therapy. Some of the metrics used can be tumor size (anatomical imaging), reduction in angiogenesis (functional), or reduction in glucose uptake (molecular). The response criteria for anatomical assessment of tumors following treatment are:

Complete response (CR): disappearance of all target lesions.

Partial response (PR): at least a 30 percent decrease in the sum of the longest diameter (LD) of target lesions, taking as reference the baseline sum LD.

Stable disease: neither sufficient shrinkage to qualify for PR nor sufficient increase to qualify for PD, taking as reference the smallest sum LD since the treatment started.

Progressive disease (PD): at least a 20 percent increase in the sum of the LD of target lesions, taking as reference the smallest sum LD recorded since the treatment started or the appearance of one or more new lesions.

In addition to tumor size, pathologic tumor response to therapy is an important metric that is used for prognosis. **Pathologic complete response (pCR)** is defined as the lack of all signs of cancer in tissue samples removed during surgery or biopsy after treatment. The ultimate metric of the effectiveness of cancer therapy, however, is survival. There are three different metrics that are often reported. **Overall survival** (OS), **disease-free survival** (DFS), and **progression-free survival** (PFS). Overall survival is the percentage of people in a study or treatment group who are still alive for a certain period of time after they were diagnosed with or started treatment for a disease, and is often stated as a five-year survival rate. Disease-free survival is the length of time after the end of primary treatment that the patient survives without any signs or symptoms of that cancer. Progression-free survival is the length of time during and after treatment that a patient lives with the disease in which it is stable or does not progress.

The Kaplan–Meier estimate is one of the best options for measuring the fraction of subjects alive for a period of time after treatment. The effect of an intervention is assessed by measuring the number of subjects who survived or were saved over a certain period of time after that intervention. The survival probability at any particular time, S_t, is calculated using Equation 2.7, where N_{LS} is the number of subjects living at the start and N_D is the number of subjects who have died:

$$S_t = \frac{N_{LS} - N_D}{N_{LS}}. \qquad (2.7)$$

Example: Which Chemotherapy Is Better?

Question: A clinical trial is comparing two novel chemotherapies for patients with triple-negative breast cancer. There were 100 patients in each group at the beginning of the study. The number of patients who died each year for the first five years is shown in the table below. Calculate the cumulative survival probability for each drug for each year. How would your interpretation of the better-performing drug change if you looked at the cumulative survival probability at year 3 vs. year 5?

Year	1	2	3	4	5
Drug A deaths	5	5	3	2	0
Drug B deaths	3	3	3	3	3

Answer: To calculate the cumulative survival probability for each year, we first need to calculate the cumulative number of deaths each year, which is simply the sum of the deaths from all preceding years:

Year	1	2	3	4	5
Cumulative drug A deaths	5	10	13	15	15
Cumulative drug B deaths	3	6	9	12	15

The survival probability for each year can then be calculated using Equation 2.7:

Year	1	2	3	4	5
Cumulative drug A deaths	5	10	13	15	15
Survival probability drug A	(100 − 5)/100	(100 − 10)/100	(100 − 13)/100	(100 − 15)/100	(100 − 15)/100
Cumulative drug B deaths	3	6	9	12	15
Survival probability drug B	(100 − 3)/100	(100 − 6)/100	(100 − 9)/100	(100 − 12)/100	(100 − 15)/100

The numbers further simplify as shown below.

Year	1	2	3	4	5
Cumulative drug A deaths	5	10	13	15	15
Survival probability drug A	95%	90%	87%	85%	85%
Cumulative drug B deaths	3	6	9	12	15
Survival probability drug B	97%	94%	91%	88%	85%

At year 3, the survival probability is higher for drug B than for drug A (91 vs. 87 percent). At year 5, the survival probability for both drugs is the same (85 percent). As a result, looking at the survival probability at year 3 may falsely lead a researcher to believe that drug B works better than drug A.

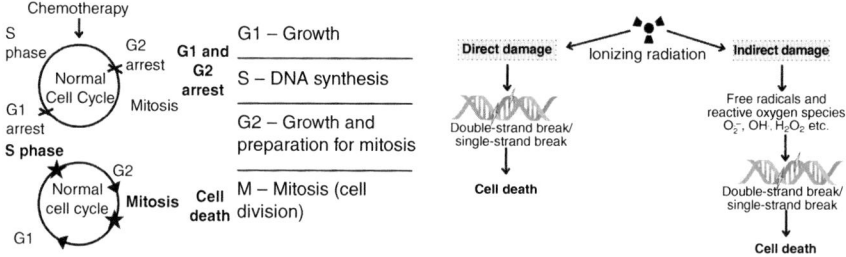

Figure 2.18 Mechanism of action for chemotherapy and radiation therapy. Most chemotherapies work by blocking cell division, with the idea being that cancer cells are rapidly dividing, leading to some level of specificity. However, in practice chemotherapy will kill any dividing cell, leading to off-target side effects.

When we think about cancer treatment, we frequently only talk about benefits such as improvement in survival time. Unfortunately, these benefits are not without side effects. It is important to understand both the risks and benefits of a particular therapy, something physicians discuss in detail with patients. Radiation therapy and chemotherapy are both mainstays in cancer treatment, despite being relatively old treatment methods. As shown in Figure 2.9, ionizing radiation transmits energy to disrupt double-stranded DNA, which can cause cell death. Figure 2.18 shows the mechanism of action for chemotherapy. Most chemotherapies work by blocking cell division, with the idea being that cancer cells are rapidly dividing, leading to some level of specificity. However, in practice chemotherapy will kill any dividing cell, leading to off-target side effects. As a result, chemotherapy has a number of undesirable side effects, including fatigue, nausea, vomiting, and hair loss.

With the "omics" revolution and improvements in imaging allowing for unprecedented discovery of the mechanisms underpinning tumor biology, more specific signaling nodes have been identified, which can be targeted by specific drugs. Two examples of drug classes enabled by the "omics" revolution are **hormonal therapy** and **molecular therapy**. These therapies are commonly used as **adjunct therapies** to chemotherapies, which are administered either before (**neoadjuvant therapy**) or after (**adjuvant therapy**) local therapy (surgery). Hormonal therapy is a treatment that targets a specific hormone. Molecular therapy is a treatment that targets a specific molecule. Adjuvant therapies are treatments used in addition to a primary treatment. This more holistic approach helps doctors and patients achieve greater efficacy in all treatments used. In the following paragraphs, we will explore examples of hormonal and molecular therapies.

Tamoxifen is an example of a hormonal therapy used to target estrogen receptor-positive (ER+) breast cancer (Buckley and Goa, 1989). Tamoxifen binds to the estrogen receptor to prevent estrogen from binding to the receptor without triggering cancer cell growth. Turning off this signaling cascade can eventually lead to cell death (Haran et al., 1994). Trastuzumab is an example of a molecular therapy used to treat HER2+ breast cancer (McKeage and Perry, 2002). Trastuzumab binds to HER2 and prevents HER2 signaling, leading to cell death. In a clinical trial, patients receiving chemotherapy plus trastuzumab showed increased DFS over patients receiving only chemotherapy.

Trastuzumab has a two-pronged effect. In the same way that tamoxifen prevents the estrogen receptor from binding to estrogen, trastuzumab blocks growth factors from binding to HER2. Blocking HER2 signaling eventually leads to cell death. At the same time, trastuzumab belongs to a class of drugs called monoclonal antibodies, which can signal the immune system to attack the cell to which the drug is attached (Scott et al., 2012). It is important to note, however, that not all molecular therapies are monoclonal antibodies. Molecular therapies such as trastuzumab also suffer from similar limitations to hormonal therapies – specifically, drug resistance.

Molecular therapies have an advantage over hormonal therapies with respect to drug resistance. Tamoxifen is the therapy for ER+ tumors, and if there is drug resistance the only alternative is chemotherapy. However, if there are changes in molecular profiles that makes a tumor nonresponsive to a molecular therapy, new avenues for molecular therapies can be pursued. Using trastuzumab as an example, if a tumor downregulates HER2 expression, which would render the tumor resistant to trastuzumab, it may upregulate another growth factor receptor, such as epidermal growth factor receptor (EGFR), providing another molecular target for treatment with a different molecular therapy.

Deeper Look: Should Patients Have Access to a Lifesaving Drug That Is Not FDA-Approved?

HER2 is a tyrosine kinase that plays a critical role in cell growth. The overexpression or gene amplification of HER2 has been found in about 20–30 percent of breast cancers, which is classified as the HER2-positive subtype (Vu and Claret, 2012). HER2-positive breast cancer has the second-poorest prognosis among breast cancer subtypes and is correlated with lower DFS and OS rates.

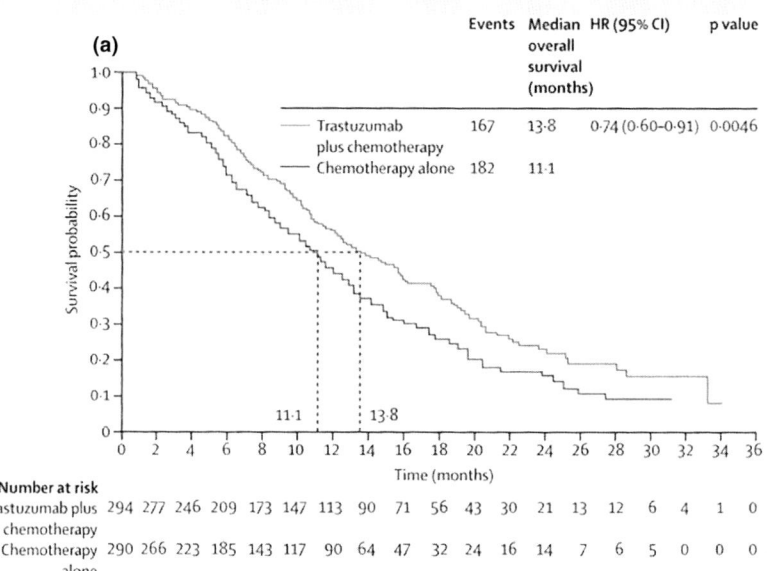
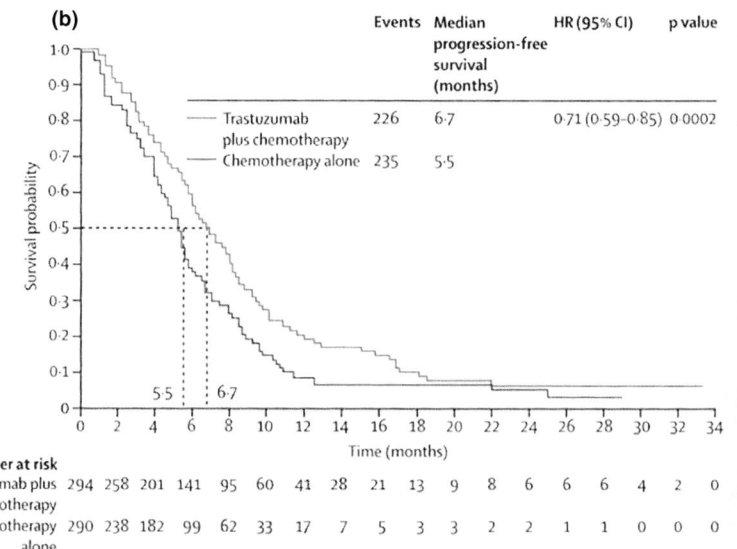

Figure 2.19 Mechanism of action of trastuzumab (a), and the survival benefit it provides to breast cancer patients (b),. A monoclonal antibody that is targeted at the extracellular domain of the HER2 protein, trastuzumab, when combined with chemotherapy, significantly improves DFS over the administration of chemotherapy alone. Source: (b) Copyright © 2010 Elsevier Ltd. All rights reserved.

> Dennis Slamon at the University of California Los Angeles is credited with discovering the role HER2 plays in breast cancers, as well as the development of the drug trastuzumab for treating HER2+ breast cancer patients. A clinical trial conducted by Genentech demonstrated unequivocally that trastuzumab provides a significant benefit to patients over standard of care. Figure 2.19 shows the mechanism of action of trastuzumab (a), and the survival benefit it provides to breast cancer patients (b). A monoclonal antibody that is targeted at the extracellular domain of the HER2 protein, trastuzumab, when combined with chemotherapy, significantly improves DFS over the administration of chemotherapy alone.
>
> At the time that the original trial was conducted, women who were not eligible to participate also wanted to receive the drug, hoping it could potentially help them (particularly those who had exhausted all other options). However, the drug had not yet been proven safe and effective for FDA approval. In addition, large-scale manufacturing of the drug itself was very complex, limiting the supply to patients within the trial. However, strong patient advocacy motivated the company to find an equitable solution. In 1995 Genentech worked with patient advocates to set up one of the first FDA-approved expanded access programs for a cancer medicine. It allowed certain people who weren't eligible for the trial to receive Herceptin before its approval.

Immunotherapies are the final treatment we will discuss. This class of therapies works entirely differently from chemotherapy, hormonal therapy, or molecular therapy. Recently, the immune system has come to the forefront of cancer therapy development. Activating the immune system to attack the tumor directly serves as an elegant approach to cancer therapy. As part of its normal function, the immune system, which consists of **innate immunity** and **adaptive immunity**, detects and destroys abnormal cells and most likely prevents or curbs the growth of many cancers (De Visser et al., 2006). Innate immunity is the process of nonspecifically identifying pathogens to prevent disease spread. Adaptive immunity is the process of specifically identifying pathogens based on an antigen to prevent disease spread.

Figure 2.20 shows the cells of the immune system. All cells within the immune system originate from the same type of precursor cell, called a **hematopoietic stem cell**. Based on different cues from within the body, the hematopoietic stem cell can differentiate (turn into) into different types of cells. The main cell types within the innate immune system include neutrophils, mast cells, basophils, eosinophils, macrophages, natural killer cells, and dendritic cells. The **dendritic cells** play a role in bridging the cells of the innate immune system with those of the adaptive immune system, which include different types of B cells (plasma cells, memory B cells) and T cells (cytotoxic T cell, helper T cell, and memory T cell). While the exact roles of each type of immune cell are still being investigated, the key players within

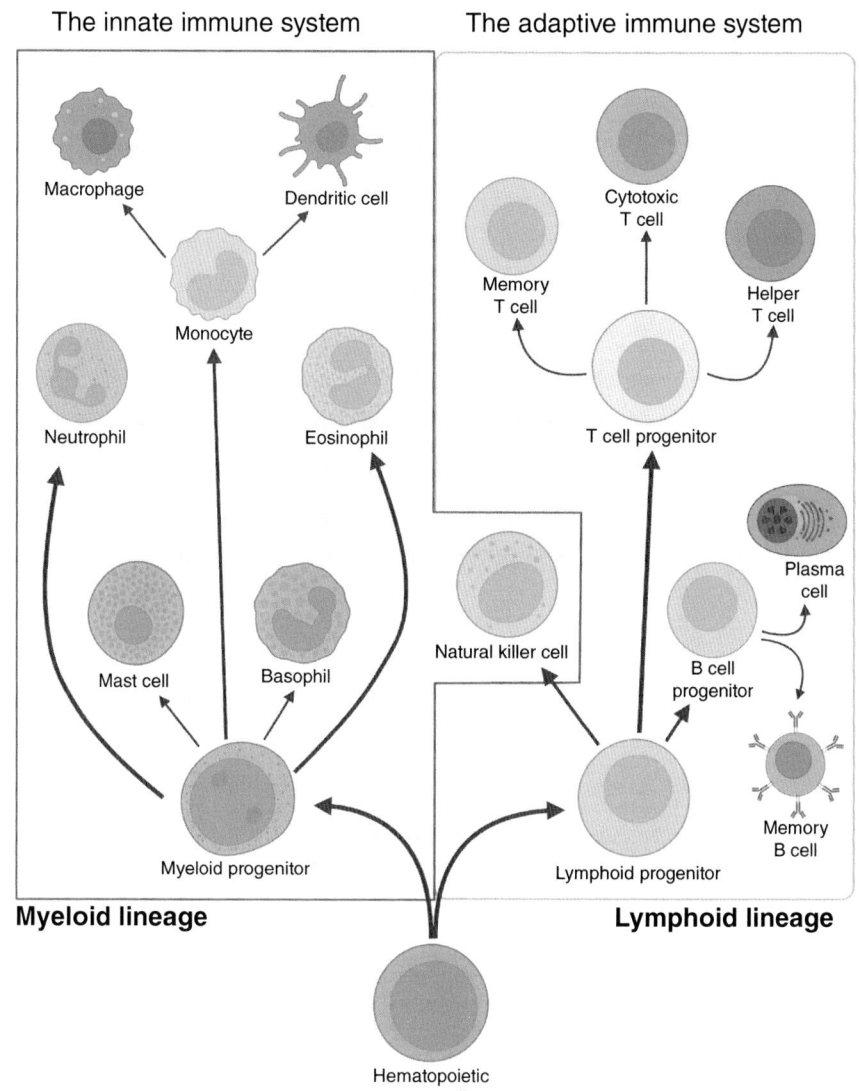

Figure 2.20
Cells of the immune system. All cells within the immune system originate from the same type of precursor cell, called a hematopoietic stem cell. Based on different cues from within the body, the hematopoietic stem cell can differentiate (turn into) into different types of cells. The main cell types within the innate immune system include neutrophils, mast cells, basophils, eosinophils, macrophages, natural killer cells, and dendritic cells. Image: Author image using Biorender.

the immune system for cancer are macrophages and dendritic cells from the innate immune system, along with T cells (both cytotoxic and helper) from the adaptive immune system.

Innate immunity staves off infection long enough for the adaptive immune system to kick in and fully remove the pathogen. Through the innate immune response, dendritic cells collect cellular debris, which frequently contains antigens that the immune system can use to learn to recognize the foreign entity (Steinman and Hemmi, 2006). In the case of cancer, these antigens are referred to as **tumor antigens**. The dendritic cells then present the antigen to **T cells** and **B cells**, the two main cell types involved in adaptive immunity (Bonilla and Oettgen, 2010). The process of antigen selection and presentation followed by clonal expansion of highly specific T cells and B cells, trained to recognize the antigen, takes time; however, cells of the adaptive immune system are much more adept at eliminating foreign pathogens than are innate cells. Adaptive immunity also has the ability to form **memory T cells** and **memory B cells**, which can quickly become reactivated when the antigen is present again, promoting lasting immunity and reducing the incidence of reinfection (Crotty and Ahmed, 2004).

What role does the immune system play in cancer? **Tumor-infiltrating lymphocytes** (TILs) are immune cells that can migrate from the lymphatic system into a tumor. If TILs are present within a tumor, they serve as an indication that the immune system is responding to the tumor. Frequently, patients whose tumors contain higher levels of TILs have better treatment outcomes (Clemente et al., 1996). Unfortunately, even though the immune system can naturally prevent or slow cancer growth due to TIL activity, cancer cells find ways to evade the immune system. Below we will examine how tumors evade the immune system and how immunotherapies can prevent immune evasion.

Immune checkpoints are signaling pathways that reduce immune system activity. Immune checkpoints normally function to maintain the checks and balances of the immune system. These checkpoints can be hijacked by cancers, allowing the tumor to shield itself from the immune system (Pardoll, 2012). Checkpoints typically altered by cancers are those that involve a major component of the immune system: T cells. Drugs called **immune checkpoint inhibitors** are used to block immune checkpoints in order to boost the immune response against cancer. The two most commonly targeted immune checkpoints for cancer therapy involve PD-1 and CTLA-4. Each of these checkpoints plays a role in reducing immune cell activation and, in some cases, can lead to immune cell senescence and death. James Allison, an immunologist at MD Anderson Cancer Center, and Tasuku Honjo, a Japanese physician scientist and immunologist, were awarded the Nobel Prize for Physiology or Medicine in 2018 for their discoveries that the immune checkpoints could be inhibited, therefore activating the immune system as a form of cancer treatment.

Other methods of activating the immune system outside of immune checkpoints are areas of active investigation. Monoclonal antibodies are immune system proteins that can be designed to target cancer cells, making them visible to the immune system. Another approach to boost the immune response is to harvest immune cells from a patient, grow them to large numbers in a lab, then reinject them into the patient to elicit a larger immune response against the tumor than the original population (Yamaguchi et al., 2003). In another approach, called chimeric antigen receptor T cell therapy (CAR T cell therapy), patients' T cells are extracted from their blood and modified so they can bind to a certain protein on the patient's cancer cells and then introduced back into the patient's bloodstream (Maude et al., 2014). These CAR T cells then attack the tumor with a high level of specificity. It is possible that these approaches can be combined with immune checkpoint inhibitors to improve overall response to immunotherapies.

Looking Ahead

The last 100 years have seen incredible strides in cancer innovations. A number of technological innovations have led to breakthroughs in the ways cancer is screened, diagnosed, and treated – one noteworthy example being targeted immunotherapies. In fact, by understanding tumor characteristics through an ensemble of technologies as described in this chapter, treatment can be truly personalized, thereby improving the safety and efficacy of cancer treatment. It is certain that technological advances will continue to promote new and better diagnostic and therapeutic technologies, with the continued caveat that costs will rise as well, potentially increasing the gap between what is available and what can be afforded.

The benefits of improvements in cancer technologies are not shared across the globe. The WHO projects that cancer-related deaths will increase at a much faster rate in LMICs compared to HICs. Cancer is the second leading cause of deaths globally, accounting for an estimated 9.6 million deaths in 2018. In countries where health systems are strong, survival rates for many types of cancers are improving, owing to accessible early detection, treatment, and survivor care. Many health systems in LMICs, however, are least prepared to manage this burden, and large numbers of cancer patients globally do not have access to timely diagnosis and treatment. The global cancer burden is expected to increase to 28.4 million cases in 2040, a 47 percent rise from 2020, with a larger increase in LMICs (64–95 percent) vs. HICs (32–56 percent).

In the next chapter we will examine some of the ways in which improvements in medical technologies and tests have left LMICs behind, using cervical cancer as a case study. These challenges have paved the way for transformative innovations for screening, diagnosis, and treatment that are now translatable to these underserved communities, thereby breaking down geographical barriers. These new technologies comprise molecular tests, imaging devices, and therapies based on ablation, which will be discussed in greater detail in Chapters 4–6, respectively. All of these technologies are described by a key set of features, including the ability to be translated out of a specialized setting to a local clinical setting where patients may come for primary care, affordable such that they can be scaled broadly, and effective in that they do not compromise quality over standard of care methods used in wealthy countries such as the US.

SUMMARY

In this chapter we have explored how cancer control has evolved in the US throughout the course of the twentieth century. Generally, cancer control paradigms include three main steps: screening for cancer using a test that has a high specificity (i.e., low false positive rate); diagnosis for cancer using a test that is highly sensitive (i.e., low false negative rate); and treatment, informed by pathology. As was illustrated for breast cancer, tests with high specificity for cancer are preferable for screening because they help prevent overdiagnosis of benign conditions as cancer, and reduced sensitivity can be overcome by frequent surveillance. In contrast, diagnostic tests need to have high sensitivity to avoid missing cancers.

Electromagnetic waves are frequently leveraged throughout cancer control paradigms, from screening through treatment. Electromagnetic waves vary in wavelength and energy, providing different opportunities for use in cancer control. They can be used in a host of imaging technologies, including PET, X-ray (including X-ray CT), optical, and MRI. High-energy EM radiation in the form of gamma rays can be used to induce DNA damage as a form of cancer treatment, called radiation therapy. On the lower end of the energy spectrum, microwaves and radio waves can be used for highly precise thermal ablation of tumors.

Without additional innovation, EM-based imaging is primarily limited to answering questions such as "Is there a tumor present, how big is it, and where is it located?" The "omics" revolution, allowed in large part by the ability to amplify small amounts of DNA for study using PCR, opened up new areas of inquiry into molecular testing, permitting researchers to ask more interesting questions using imaging in combination with "omics," such as "What type of tumor is present and how can we best treat it?" The advent of molecular testing ushered in a new era of therapy development.

Over the course of the twentieth century, four major spheres of cancer therapy have emerged: chemotherapy, hormonal therapy, molecular therapy, and immunotherapies. Chemotherapy is a mainstay in cancer treatment which continues to be augmented by more and more sophisticated therapies. Hormonal therapies first emerged as a method to treat cancers with a particular hormone dependence (e.g., ER+ breast cancers). Similarly, molecular therapies such as trastuzumab gained popularity due to their ability to treat specific drivers of cancer growth, such as HER2+ breast cancers. However, tumors in a subset of patients can develop resistance to hormonal or molecular therapies over time. Immunotherapies activate the body's immune system to attack the tumor directly. Discovery of immune checkpoints, which suppress immune responses, has led to immune checkpoint inhibitors, which are at the forefront of modern cancer therapy.

PROBLEMS

Cancer Control in the US

1. What is the difference in populations that go for breast cancer screening vs. breast cancer diagnostic biopsy?
2. What is the reason for screening to have high specificity and diagnosis to have high sensitivity?
3. At what point in the evolution of breast cancer is ductal carcinoma in situ (DCIS) considered invasive cancer?
4. What is the criterion for defining breast cancer as metastatic?
5. The sensitivity and specificity of a novel mammogram technique are 92 and 90 percent, respectively. Calculate the positive and negative predictive values for the new mammogram if the prevalence of disease is 8/100,000.

Imaging Technologies for Screening, Diagnosis, and Treatment of Cancer

6. What is the shortest wavelength of the electromagnetic spectrum and the corresponding energy in electron volts? What imaging or therapeutic technology is it used in? Do the same for the longest wavelength in the electromagnetic spectrum. What imaging or therapeutic technology is it used in?
7. What is the difference in the ways surgery and ablation therapy control tumors?
8. What range of the EM spectrum is visible to the eye for use in light microscopy? What are the different types of interactions between light and tissue and what types of diagnostic information can they provide?
9. What is a basic characteristic of the interaction between EM radiation and tissue that affects the penetration depth?
10. Blood content/flow provides functional information through imaging. What are the technologies that can detect blood? What part(s) of the EM spectrum do they rely on?

Molecular Testing, Omics, and Molecular Imaging

11. What types of molecular tests are used for DNA analysis and what test is used for measuring protein expression?
12. FISH provides a readout related to the expression of the *HER2* oncogene. In IHC, a light microscope is used to image a slide of a tissue section stained for HER2 and the number of cells that show expression of the HER2 protein are counted across the image. What are two reasons IHC could be less accurate than FISH? What are the consequences of a molecular test incorrectly reporting that a patient has the *HER2* oncogene when she does not or vice versa?

13. Techniques such as CT and MRI are used to look at the size of the tumor following therapy to evaluate therapy response. What type of tumor characteristic is imaged with PET? As the tumor shrinks, would you expect to see PET imaging signal increase or decrease? Why?

Classes of Systemic Therapies

14. Why are chemotherapy and radiation therapy toxic to normal parts of the body? Why is hair loss a common side effect of chemotherapy?
15. If the five-year survival probability for a patient with stage I breast cancer is 90 percent if they receive a lumpectomy plus radiation therapy and 80 percent if they only receive a lumpectomy, how many more patients would be alive after five years in the lumpectomy plus radiation therapy group if 500 patients were treated with each therapy regimen?
16. What are three similarities and three differences between a hormonal therapy and a molecular therapy?
17. What is drug resistance and how can molecular therapy be modified to overcome it?
18. Is the adaptive or innate immune response involved in preventing cancer recurrence? Explain your reasoning.
19. What is the primary mechanism of action for an immune checkpoint inhibitor? If a tumor is immunologically cold (i.e., there are very few immune cells within the tumor), would an immune checkpoint inhibitor be an effective therapy? Why or why not?
20. Ulcerative colitis is a disease caused by overactivation of the immune system. Humira® is a form of antibody therapy that helps reduce this overactivity. What type of immune cell is upregulated to suppress the overactive immune system? Is this same cell population increased or decreased if a tumor is undetectable by the immune system?

REFERENCES

Bonilla, F. A., & Oettgen, H. C. 2010. Adaptive immunity. *Journal of Allergy and Clinical Immunology*, 125, S33–S40.

Bouchard, M. B., Chen, B. R., Burgess, S. A., & Hillman, E. M. 2009. Ultra-fast multispectral optical imaging of cortical oxygenation, blood flow, and intracellular calcium dynamics. *Optics Express*, 17, 15670–15678.

Buckley, M. M.-T., & Goa, K. L. 1989. Tamoxifen. *Drugs*, 37, 451–490.

Bushberg, J. T., & Boone, J. M. 2011. *The Essential Physics of Medical Imaging*, Lippincott Williams & Wilkins, Philadelphia, PA.

Buzug, T. M. 2011. Computed tomography. In Kramme, R., Hoffmann, K.-P., & Pozos, R. (eds), *Springer Handbook of Medical Technology*. Springer, New York.

Cho, W. C. 2010. *Omics Approaches in Cancer Research: An Omics Perspective on Cancer Research*. Springer, New York.

Chu, K. F., & Dupuy, D. E. 2014. Thermal ablation of tumours: biological mechanisms and advances in therapy. *Nature Reviews Cancer*, 14, 199–208.

Clemente, C. G., Mihm Jr, M. C., Bufalino, R., et al. 1996. Prognostic value of tumor infiltrating lymphocytes in the vertical growth phase of primary cutaneous melanoma. *Cancer: Interdisciplinary International Journal of the American Cancer Society*, 77, 1303–1310.

Crotty, S., & Ahmed, R. 2004. Immunological memory in humans. *Seminars in Immunology*, 16, 197–203.

Dagenais, G. R., Leong, D. P., Rangarajan, S., et al. 2020. Variations in common diseases, hospital admissions, and deaths in middle-aged adults in 21 countries from five continents (PURE): a prospective cohort study. *The Lancet*, 395, 785–794.

Dang, C. V. 2012. Links between metabolism and cancer. *Genes and Development*, 26, 877–890.

De Visser, K. E., Eichten, A., & Coussens, L. M. 2006. Paradoxical roles of the immune system during cancer development. *Nature Reviews Cancer*, 6, 24–37.

DeVita, V. T., & Chu, E. 2008. A history of cancer chemotherapy. *Cancer Research*, 68, 8643–8653.

Fisher, B. A., Bryant, J., Margoleserg, D. M., Fisherer, J. J., & Wolmark, N. 2002. Twenty-year follow-up of a randomized trial comparing total mastectomy, lumpectomy, and lumpectomy plus irradiation for the treatment of invasive breast cancer. *New England Journal of Medicine*, 347, 1233–1241.

Habib, S. H. & Saha, S. 2010. Burden of non-communicable disease: global overview. *Diabetes & Metabolic Syndrome: Clinical Research & Reviews*, 4, 41–47.

Hall, E. J. 2006. Intensity-modulated radiation therapy, protons, and the risk of second cancers. *International Journal of Radiation Oncology, Biology and Physics*, 65, 1–7.

Haran, E. F., Maretzek, A., Goldberg, I., Horowitz, A., & Degani, H. 1994. Tamoxifen enhances cell death in implanted MCF7 breast cancer by inhibiting endothelium growth. *Cancer Research*, 54, 5511–5514.

Hesselink, J. R., Edelman, R. R., & Zlatkin, M. 1990. *Clinical Magnetic Resonance Imaging*, Saunders, Philadelphia, PA.

Khan, F. M., & Gibbons, J. P. 2014. *Khan's The Physics of Radiation Therapy*, Lippincott Williams & Wilkins, Philadelphia, PA.

Knavel, E. M., & Brace, C. L. 2013. Tumor ablation: common modalities and general practices. *Techniques in Vascular and Interventional Radiology*, 16, 192–200.

Macbeth, R. A. L., & Bekesi, J. G. 1962. Oxygen consumption and anaerobic glycolysis of human malignant and normal tissue. *Cancer Research*, 22, 244–248.

Maude, S. L., Frey, N., Shaw, P. A., et al. 2014. Chimeric antigen receptor T cells for sustained remissions in leukemia. *New England Journal of Medicine*, 371, 1507–1517.

Mckeage, K., & Perry, C. M. 2002. Trastuzumab. *Drugs*, 62, 209–243.

Mukherjee, S. 2010. *The Emperor of All Maladies: A Biography of Cancer*. Simon and Schuster, New York.

Mullis, K. B., & Faloona, F. A. 1987. Specific synthesis of DNA in vitro via a polymerase-catalyzed chain reaction. *Methods in Enzymology*, 155, 335–350.

Nishigori, N., Koyama, F., Nakagawa, T., et al. 2016. Visualization of lymph/blood flow in laparoscopic colorectal cancer surgery by ICG fluorescence imaging (Lap-IGFI). *Annals of Surgical Oncology*, 23, 266–274.

Pardoll, D. M. 2012. The blockade of immune checkpoints in cancer immunotherapy. *Nature Reviews Cancer*, 12, 252–264.

Reske, S. N., & Kotzerke, J. 2001. FDG-PET for clinical use. *European Journal of Nuclear Medicine*, 28, 1707–1723.

Schuster, S. C. 2008. Next-generation sequencing transforms today's biology. *Nature Methods*, 5, 16–18.

Schwabe, R. F., & Jobin, C. 2013. The microbiome and cancer. *Nature Reviews Cancer*, 13, 800–812.

Scott, A. M., Allison, J. P., & Wolchok, J. D. 2012. Monoclonal antibodies in cancer therapy. *Cancer Immunity Archive*, 2012, 12.

Steinman, R. M., & Hemmi, H. 2006. Dendritic cells: translating innate to adaptive immunity. In Pulendran, B., & Ahmed, R. (eds), *From Innate Immunity to Immunological Memory*. Springer, New York.

Vu, T. & Claret, F. X., 2012. Trastuzumab: updated mechanisms of action and resistance in breast cancer. *Frontiers in Oncology*, 2, 62.

Yager, J. D., & Davidson, N. E. 2006. Estrogen carcinogenesis in breast cancer. *New England Journal of Medicine*, 354, 270–282.

Yamaguchi, Y., Ohshita, A., Kawabuchi, Y., et al. 2003. Adoptive immunotherapy of cancer using activated autologous lymphocytes: current status and new strategies. *Human Cell*, 16, 183–189.

Yan, P.-F., Yan, L., Zhang, Z., et al. 2016. Accuracy of conventional MRI for preoperative diagnosis of intracranial tumors: a retrospective cohort study of 762 cases. *International Journal of Surgery*, 36, 109–117.

3 Cervical Cancer: The Face of Inequity

Public health measures in the US to reduce smoking, such as banning TV ads, the Nonsmokers' Rights Movement, and large "sin taxes," have been significant factors in reducing the rates of lung cancer incidence in the twentieth century (Centers for Disease Control and Prevention, 1999; Siegel et al., 2020). For cervical cancer, much of the decline in mortality can be primarily attributed to medical innovations. In fact, the incidence and mortality of cervical cancer decreased more than 10-fold over the latter part of the twentieth century, largely due to well-organized screening and treatment programs that were born out of key medical advances (Safaeian et al., 2007). Cervical cancer prevention is an exemplar of how a cancer that was deadly 100 years ago is close to elimination in Western society today.

Cervical cancer was a devastating disease in the middle of the twentieth century. The book *The Immortal Life of Henrietta Lacks* (Skloot, 2010) introduces an African American woman who lived in Baltimore in the early 1900s. Figure 3.1 shows a photograph of Henrietta Lacks and the HeLa cells from her cervical cancer. When Henrietta was diagnosed with cervical cancer at the Johns Hopkins School of Medicine, her cancer was already advanced and her symptoms painful. She died when she was 31 years old, leaving five young children behind. Henrietta became famous after her death because of her cervical cancer cells, which were harvested during one of her treatments. Her cells went on to revolutionize medicine through important discoveries. It is important to note, however, that she was not informed or asked permission to use her cells for research. Modern-day clinical research requires patients to provide informed consent prior to undergoing any research study activity, which will be discussed later in this chapter.

In this chapter, we will learn about the role that technology played in achieving the major milestones in reducing cervical cancer mortality. The types of advances that have been developed are based on molecular testing and imaging innovations, which inform the appropriate type of treatment. In spite of the success in preventing cervical cancer in wealthy countries, the disease continues to kill hundreds of thousands of women annually, many in the prime of their lives, in low- and middle-income

Cervical Cancer: The Face of Inequity

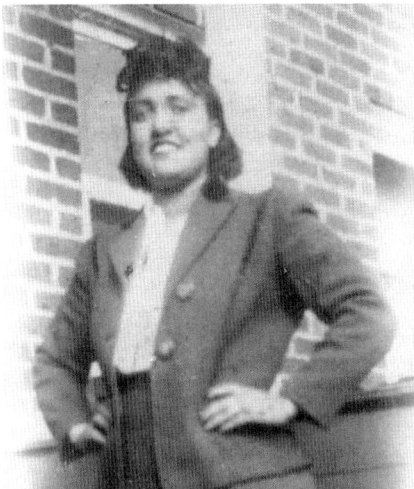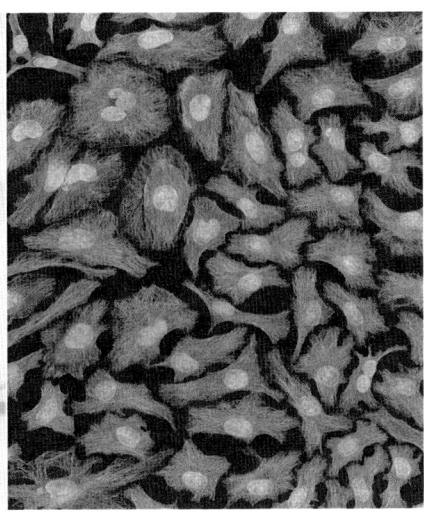

Figure 3.1 A photograph of Henrietta Lacks and the HeLa cells from her cervical cancer. The book *The Immortal Life of Henrietta Lacks* (Skloot, 2010) introduces an African American woman who lived in Baltimore in the early 1900s. When Henrietta was diagnosed with cervical cancer at the Johns Hopkins School of Medicine, her cancer was already advanced and her symptoms painful. She died when she was 31 years old, leaving five young children behind.
Source: (a) Credit: Lacks Family, via The Henrietta Lacks Foundation; (b) © National Institutes of Health/Stocktrek Images/Getty Images.

(LMICs) countries. The good news is that a new set of medical advances that are appropriate, affordable, and accessible are making headway in directly addressing this inequity.

LEARNING OBJECTIVES

The Cervix and Cervical Cancer
- The anatomy of the cervix and the progression of cervical cancer;
- the relationship between the human papilloma virus (HPV) and cervical cancer;
- the natural history of cervical cancer and how it informs cervical cancer prevention.

The Evolution of Modern Gynecology
- The screening and treatment program for cervical cancer prevention in the US;
- key innovations that have dramatically reduced cervical cancer mortality in Western countries and the innovators who created them;
- the clinical decision-making model from the time of screening to the time of treatment.

The Virus That Has Revolutionized Screening
- The strains of the HPV virus that cause cervical cancer;
- how the HPV virus has led to primary (vaccination) and secondary (HPV testing) prevention of cervical cancer;
- the advantages of HPV testing over the Pap smear.

Cervical Cancer Is a Disease of Health Disparities

- The incidence and mortality of cervical cancer and the resulting inequities that are reflected by the significant disparities;
- the resource-stratified WHO guidelines and tools recommended for cervical cancer elimination by 2099;
- calculation of the disability-adjusted life years lost to calculate the overall burden of disease.

The Cervix and Cervical Cancer

A basic understanding of the anatomy of the cervix and the progression of cervical precancer to cancer will provide a foundation for examining the development of technologies for cervical cancer screening, diagnosis, and treatment. Figure 3.2 shows the anatomy of the cervix and cancer progression. The cervix comprises the **os** and the **epithelium**, which is referred to as columnar if on the **endocervix** or squamous if on the **ectocervix**.

The **cervix** is the lowest portion of the uterus and opens into the vagina. It is a little over one inch long and only about one inch wide. The **cervical os** is the narrow opening of the cervix connecting the uterus to the vagina. Made up largely of muscle tissue, it plays a major role during pregnancy and delivery. Specifically, the os dilates (opens up) as the cervix effaces (gets thinner) during childbirth. The cervix is essentially the portal to life, as this is where

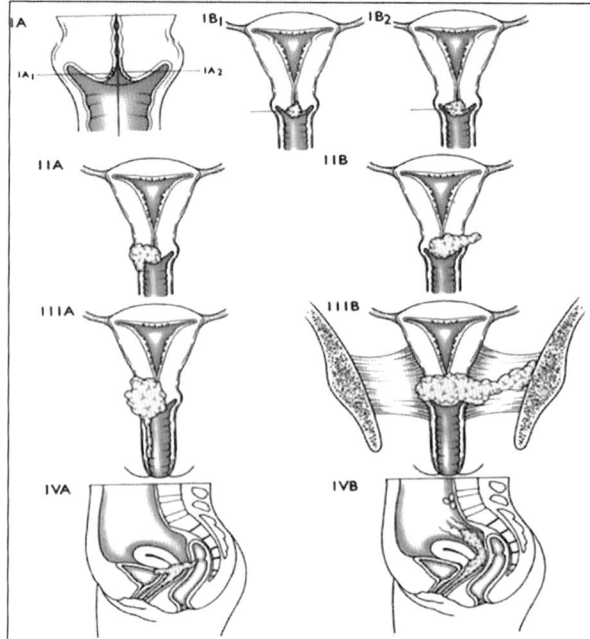

Figure 3.2

The anatomy of the cervix and cancer progression. The cervix comprises the **os** and the **epithelium**, which is referred to as columnar if on the **endocervix** or squamous if on the **ectocervix**. Source: Edna Maite Mohuba, Tebogo Maria Mothiba, and Livhuwani Muthelo. Licensed under a CC BY 4.0 license.

The Cervix and Cervical Cancer

a baby moves from its mother's uterus out through the vaginal canal and into the world. The cervix also undergoes changes during the menstrual cycle. Menstrual blood flows from the sloughing uterine wall through the cervix to outside of the body through the vaginal canal.

There are three parts of the cervix: The **ectocervix** is the lowest part of the cervix, which is visible through the vagina. The **endocervix**, also called the endocervical canal, is the innermost part of the cervix and is the passage between the ectocervix and the uterus. The **transformation zone** is the region of the cervix where the cell type changes from columnar to squamous. The **epithelium** that covers the ectocervix is referred to as squamous, and that covering the endocervix is referred to as columnar or column-like.

The stage before precancer develops into cancer is referred to as **carcinoma in situ**, meaning it has not become invasive. As it invades the cervix, it becomes **stage I**. With increasing spread, the staging for cervical cancer increases until it leaves the cervix, at which point it is considered **stage IV**. As stage increases, **five-year survival rates** decrease from 100 percent for stage 0 to 7 percent for stage IV. In the US, the majority of patients are diagnosed with cervical precancer, which is stage 0 cervical cancer. This is equivalent to ductal carcinoma in situ (DCIS), which is confined to the ducts in the breast. When caught at the precancer stage, cervical cancer is curable, with a 100 percent five-year survival rate. Unfortunately, when left untreated cervical precancer can progress to more advanced stages with much lower five-year survival rates.

Figure 3.3 shown the process by which the human papilloma virus (HPV) initiates carcinogenesis. A sexually transmitted infection, the HPV virus

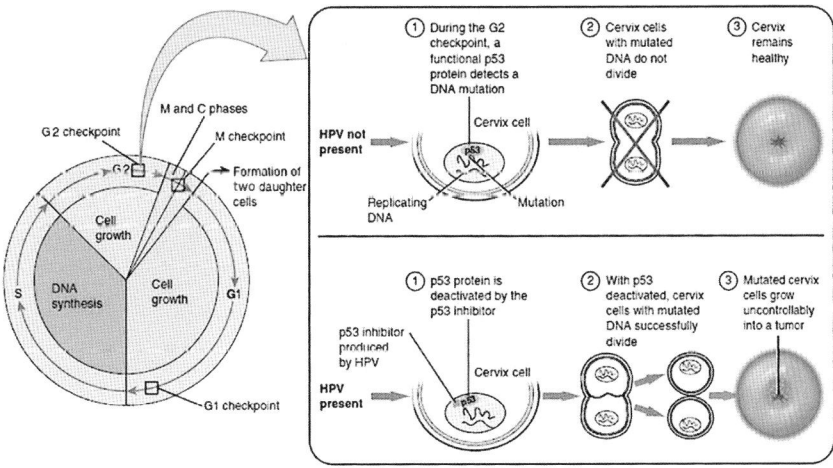

Figure 3.3 The process by which HPV initiates carcinogenesis. A sexually transmitted infection, the HPV virus inhibits a protein called p53, whose main function is to block the G2 checkpoint of the cell cycle if DNA mutations that lead to aberrant cell division are detected. These DNA mutations will go unnoticed if p53 is inhibited.
Source: OpenStax, under a CC BY 3.0 license.

inhibits a protein called p53, whose main function is to block the **G2 checkpoint of the cell cycle** if DNA mutations that lead to aberrant cell division are detected. These DNA mutations will go unnoticed if p53 is inhibited. During normal activity, cells go through four distinct stages, referred to as the cell cycle. This cycle is: increase in cell size (gap 1, or G1, stage); generation of DNA copies (synthesis, or S, stage); preparation for cell division (gap 2, or G2, stage); and finally, cell division (mitosis, or M, stage).

Example: How Can Expanding Access to Cervical Cancer Save Lives?

Question: How many women diagnosed with stage I cervical cancer this year could be saved in the course of the next five years if half of them received access to cervical cancer screening while they had precancer? Assume 500,000 women are diagnosed with some form of cervical cancer this year, 47 percent of women diagnosed have stage 1 cervical cancer, and the five-year survival rate for stage 1 cervical cancer is 85%.

Answer: We can see that 47 percent of women diagnosed with cervical cancer are diagnosed at stage I. Therefore, each year 47 percent of the 500,000 women are diagnosed with stage I cervical cancer:

$$0.47 \times 500,000 = 235,000 \text{ women with stage I cervical cancer per year.}$$

We can also see that the five-year survival rate for stage I cancer is 85 percent. Therefore, 15 percent of the women diagnosed with stage I cervical cancer will die within five years:

$$0.15 \times 235,000 = 35,250 \text{ deaths within five years.}$$

Finally, the survival rate for stage 0 cervical cancer (i.e., cervical precancer) is 100 percent. Therefore, half of the women who died would have lived if they had access to cervical cancer screening while they had cervical precancer:

$$0.5 \times 35,250 = 17,625 \text{ women saved.}$$

As you can see from this example, expanding access to earlier screening would save nearly 18,000 lives over the course of five years.

Figure 3.4 shows the different stages of cervical intraepithelial neoplasia (CIN), an indicator of disease extent. Cervical intraepithelial neoplasia is defined as the abnormal growth of cells on the surface of the cervix, which are dividing at a much greater rate than normal cells. Following a prolonged HPV infection, abnormal-appearing epithelial cells divide at a much greater rate than normal cells. On a histopathology slide, CIN can be divided into CIN I, II, and III, which correspond to the thickness within the epithelium that the

The Cervix and Cervical Cancer

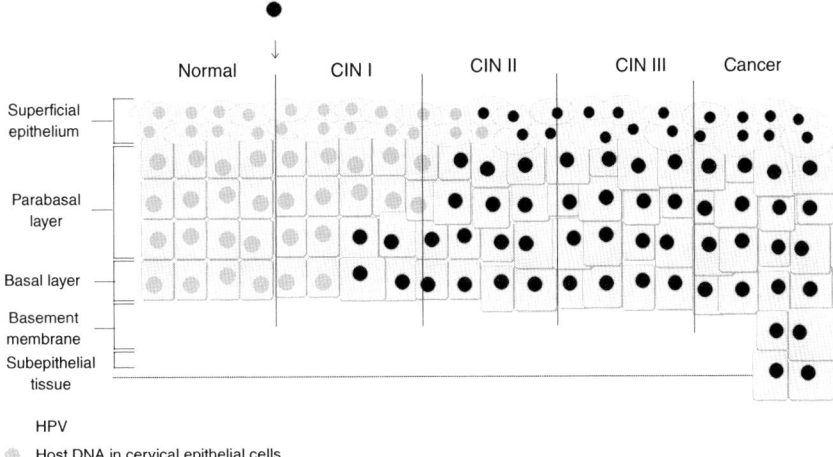

Figure 3.4 The different stages of CIN, an indicator of disease extent. Following a prolonged HPV infection, abnormally appearing epithelial cells divide at a much greater rate than normal cells. On a histopathology slide, CIN can be divided into CIN I, II, and III, which correspond to the thickness within the epithelium that the abnormal cells occupy.

abnormal cells occupy. The top third of the epithelial layer being occupied by these cells is referred to as CIN I; two-thirds as CIN II; and the full thickness as CIN III. These lesions are not cancerous, but if left untreated they can turn into cancer and metastasize or spread to other parts of the body and become deadly. This is the nomenclature pathologists use to define the extent of precancerous disease within the epithelium.

Figure 3.5 shown the natural history of cervical cancer. The development of cervical cancer following HPV infection is a very slow process, taking

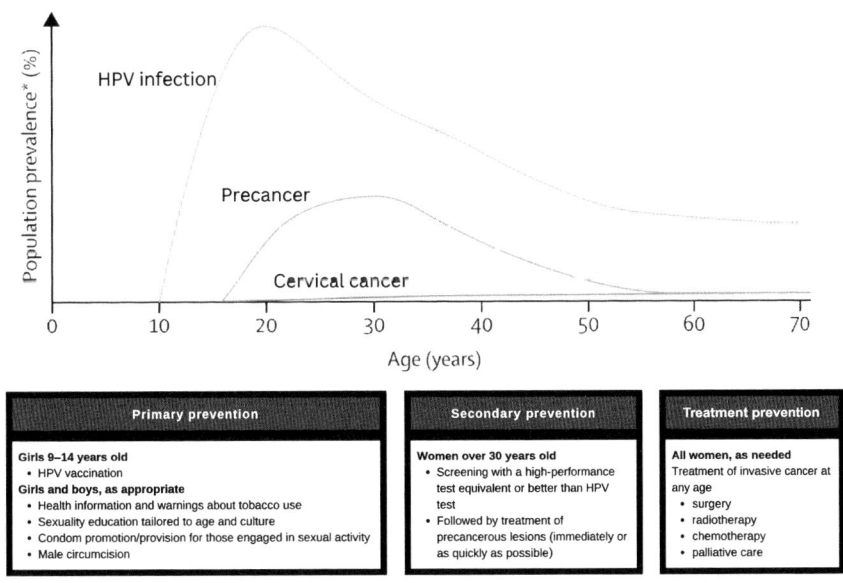

Figure 3.5 The natural history of cervical cancer. The development of cervical cancer following HPV infection is a very slow process, taking anywhere from 15–20 years, with several signposts along its course for early preventive interventions. Source: Wentzensen and Schiffman (2018). © 2017 The Author(s). Published by Elsevier Ltd.

anywhere from 15–20 years, with several signposts along its course for early preventive interventions. Due to its slow-growing nature, screening and treatment at early stages are both essential and extremely successful at reducing the number of cervical cancer cases (Lees et al., 2016). HPV infections will naturally clear within a few months to a few years following initial infection; therefore, most HPV infections will never lead to cervical precancer or cancer. That being said, women with weakened immune systems from HIV or other immunosuppressive diseases can develop cervical precancer more quickly following HPV infection than women with normal intact immune systems. The WHO guidelines for cervical cancer prevention are informed by the natural history of the disease, and include vaccination of adolescents, secondary prevention for women older than 30 years, and tertiary prevention for women who have cancer at any age.

Deeper Look: HeLa Cells and Informed Consent for Biospecimens

---

The **Common Rule** was established in the 1990s to protect patients who volunteer for federally funded research studies. Under this rule, research protocols must be reviewed and approved by an **institutional review board** (IRB) to ensure that the rights of the research subjects are protected. This includes both the requirement for informed consent and the protection of patient privacy. The informed consent process includes an explanation of the purpose of the research, a description of the research procedures, and a description of the risks and benefits of the research, among other things.

The book *The Immortal Life of Henrietta Lacks* brought to the forefront ethical issues around the use of biospecimens without informed consent and patient confidentiality, both of which were not in place at the time the HeLa cells were obtained. In 2011 the Common Rule was modified to include stringent regulations on the use of biospecimens for research, which immediately became a controversial issue in the scientific community. The Common Rule defined human subject research to include not only studies that obtain data from a patient for current research, but also those using biospecimens from prior research. The major argument was that with this stipulation, it would be an administrative nightmare to access the enormous databases of archived patient data for scientific discoveries.

In response to these concerns, the definition of human subject research was yet again modified in the revised Common Rule in 2018. Figure 3.6 shows the flowchart for the updated Common Rule of January 19, 2018. Informed consent is required if biospecimens are used for research they were originally intended for, but not for secondary research if the patient information is not identifiable. In the case of identifiable information, the research would either undergo full IRB or limited IRB review if the former was waived. If Henrietta Lacks was alive today, an investigator would need to obtain informed consent in order to use the HeLa cells directly for primary research and would also need to ensure her confidentiality. However, if her sample was already stored IRB consent would not be required unless there was identifiable information.

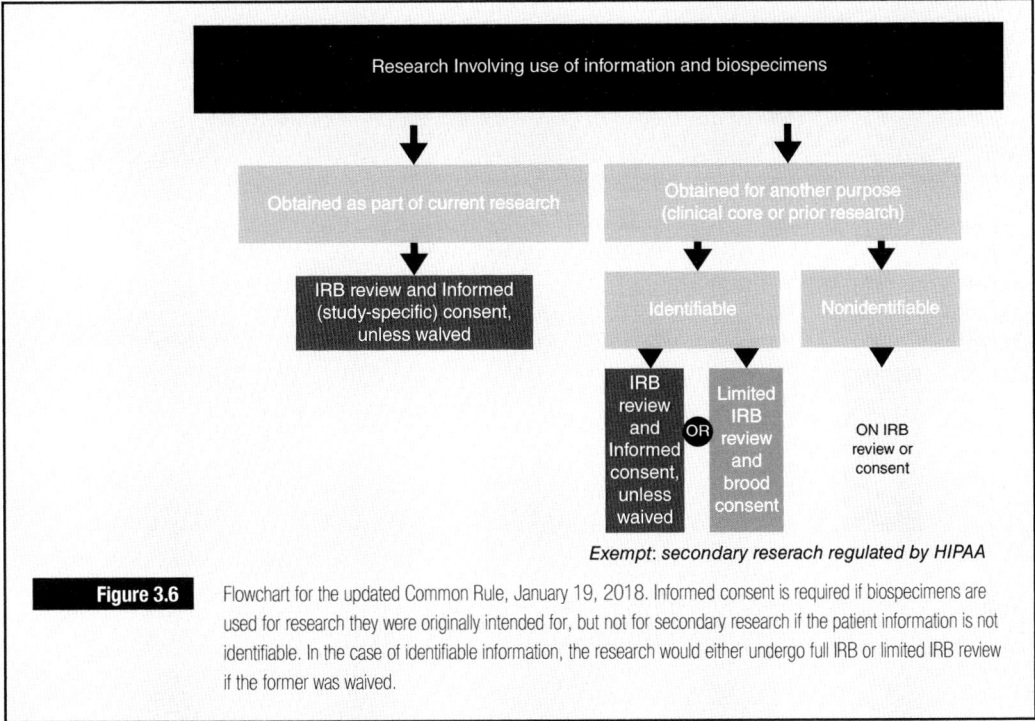

Figure 3.6 Flowchart for the updated Common Rule, January 19, 2018. Informed consent is required if biospecimens are used for research they were originally intended for, but not for secondary research if the patient information is not identifiable. In the case of identifiable information, the research would either undergo full IRB or limited IRB review if the former was waived.

The Evolution of Modern Gynecology

Today, in the US and other high-income countries (HICs), cervical cancer has an extremely low incidence rate compared to what it was in the early part of the twentieth century. This is, in large part, due to technological innovations that played a significant role in evidence-based and subsequently precision diagnostics based on the causality of the disease. Three key innovations have drastically improved cervical cancer screening and diagnosis. **Pap smear**, the **colposcope**, and the **speculum** have led to the way cervical cancer prevention is organized. A **Pap smear** is a screening test for cervical cancer in which a sample of cells is collected from the cervix for cytology testing. A **colposcope** is a large, low-magnification microscope used to view the cervix from outside the body. A **speculum** is an instrument that is used by gynecologists to visualize the cervix through the vagina. The treatment procedure commonly used for removal of precancerous lesions is called the **loop electro excision procedure** (LEEP). Figure 3.7 shows the current screening, diagnosis, and treatment paradigm.

During a Pap smear, a sample of cells is taken from the cervix and placed onto a slide for viewing under a microscope. The slide is examined for the presence of abnormal cells that may indicate the presence of cervical precancer or cancer. If the slide has abnormal cells present, the result of the Pap smear is

82 Cervical Cancer: The Face of Inequity

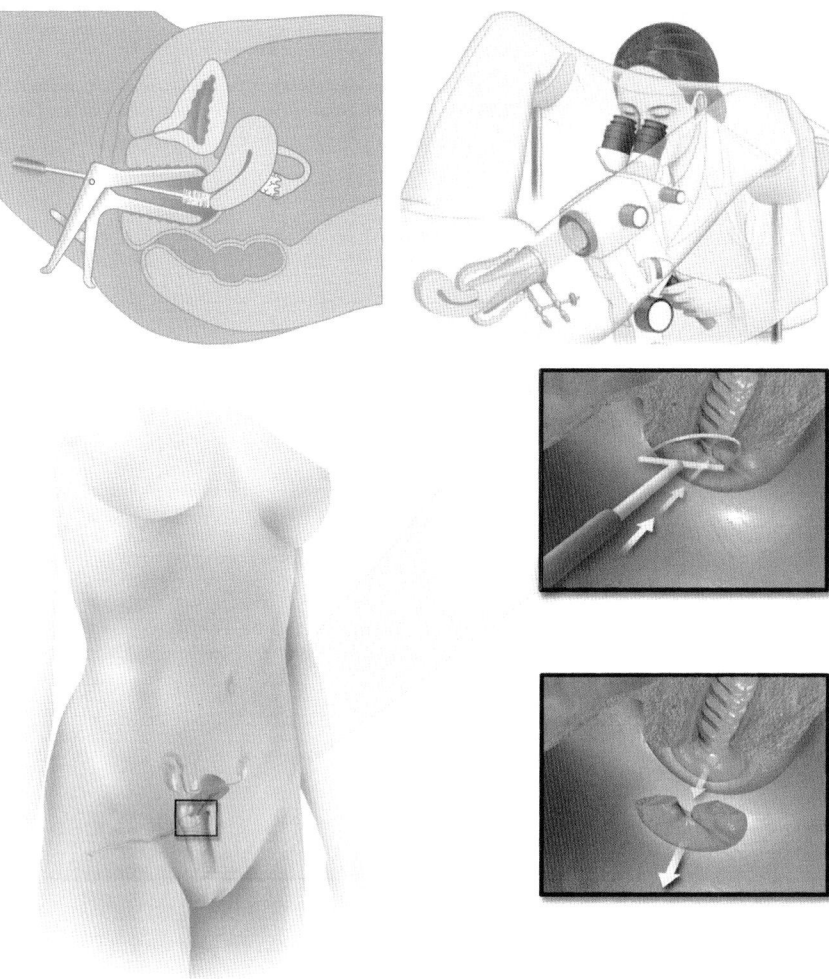

Figure 3.7 The current screening, diagnosis, and treatment paradigm. A Pap smear is a screening test for cervical cancer in which a sample of cells is collected from the cervix for cytology testing. A colposcope is a large, low-magnification microscope used to view the cervix from outside the body. A speculum is an instrument that is used by gynecologists to visualize the cervix through the vagina. Biopsies obtained during colposcopy are used to make a decision to treat the patient. The treatment procedure commonly used for removal of precancerous lesions is called the loop electro excision procedure.
Source: (a) © Dorling Kindersley / Dorling Kindersley RF / Getty Images; (b) Kobara et al. (2021); (c) Authored by 'BruceBlaus' under a CC-BY-SA license; (d) © Dorling Kindersley / Dorling Kindersley RF / Getty Images.

considered "positive" and additional testing is needed. If no abnormal cells are present, the result is considered negative and no additional testing is performed.

Figure 3.8 shows the creations of the founders of modern gynecology. **George Papanicalou** invented the Pap smear, **Hans Hinselmann** designed the first colposcope, and **James Marion Sims** the speculum. Each of these inventions, in their own way, helped transition cervical cancer screening from intuitive to evidence-based medicine. We will take a closer look at the

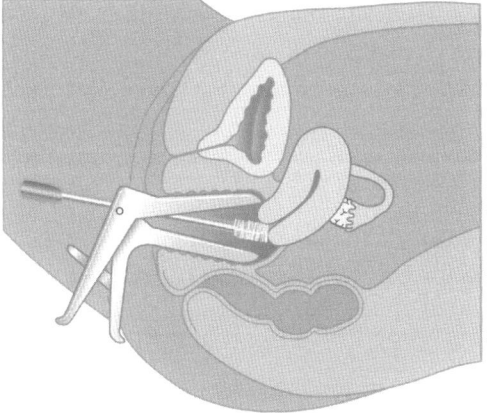
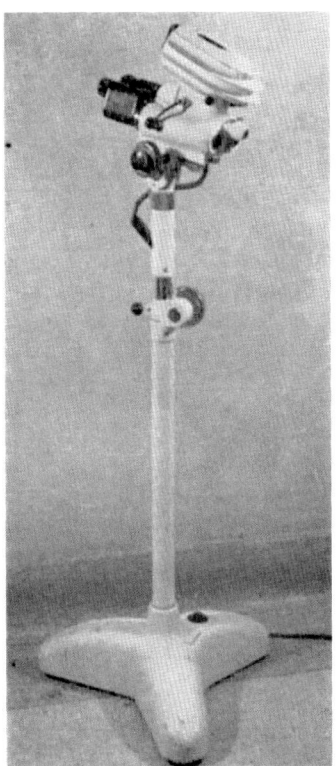

Figure 3.8

The creations of the founders of modern gynecology. George Papanicalou invented the Pap smear, Hans Hinselmann designed the first colposcope, and James Marion Sims the speculum.

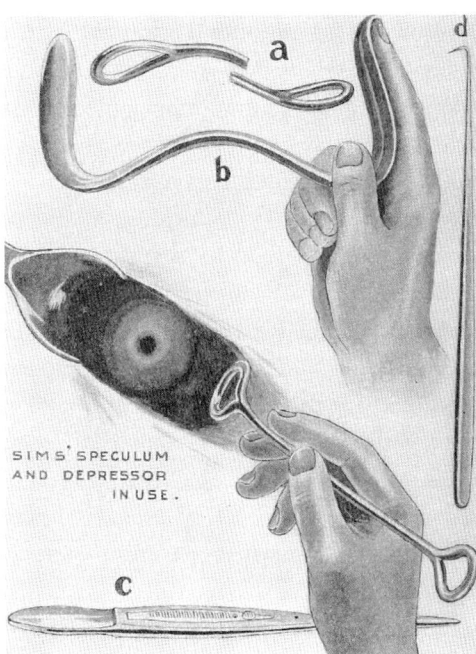

development of each of these innovations and their respective inventors in this section. It is interesting to note that all three inventors were men and the inventions, though important, were designed in a way that was functional but not necessarily comfortable for the patient.

The first invention that transitioned the diagnosis of cervical cancer from intuitive to empirical medicine was the Pap smear (Lees et al., 2016). Invented by Greek physician George Papanicolaou, the dramatic decrease in the incidence of cervical cancer over the second half of the twentieth century is attributed to the Pap smear. Papanicolaou immigrated to the US in 1913, at the age of 30, after receiving his medical degree. Within a year, he was working at both the New York University Department of Pathology and the

Cornell University Medical College (now Weill Cornell Graduate School of Medical Sciences) Department of Anatomy. Initially inspired by his work on the reproductive cycle of guinea pigs, Papanicolaou transitioned his work to the study of human reproductive anatomy and discovered the utility of vaginal smears in diagnosing uterine cancer. In 1943, with Dr. Herbert F. Traut, he published a clinical study correlating the vaginal smear with uterine cancer. Figure 3.9 shows the impact of Pap smear screening on the incidence of cervical cancer in the US. The Pap smear has reduced the incidence of cervical cancer from 40 to 10 per 100,000 women in the US.

A contemporary of George Papanicolaou, Hans Hinselmann, invented a second revolutionary device in the screening and treatment cascade of cervical cancer: the colposcope. Colposcopes are low-power microscopes used to visualize the cervix from outside the body. Colposcopes are typically involved in cervical cancer diagnosis, where they are used to guide a physician to take a biopsy of any suspicious regions on the surface of the cervix. The biopsy will then be evaluated for the presence of cervical precancer or cancer by another highly trained healthcare provider, called a pathologist.

In 1924, Hinselmann was tasked with writing about cervical cancer. With no simple way of viewing the cervix, he was struck with the idea of using some type of magnification. Hinselmann began working on the concept of the colposcope, to allow a magnified view of the cervix to aid in identifying any abnormal areas for biopsy in patients with a positive Pap smear. Although the device had the potential to revolutionize cervical imaging, physicians were slow to adopt it for a variety of reasons, including its unusually large size. It was not until the 1970s that the colposcope became a routine part of gynecological practice in the US (MacLean, 1979; Fusco et al., 2008).

Both the Pap smear and colposcopy procedures require the use of a mechanism to spread apart the vaginal walls to provide access to the cervix. The Sims

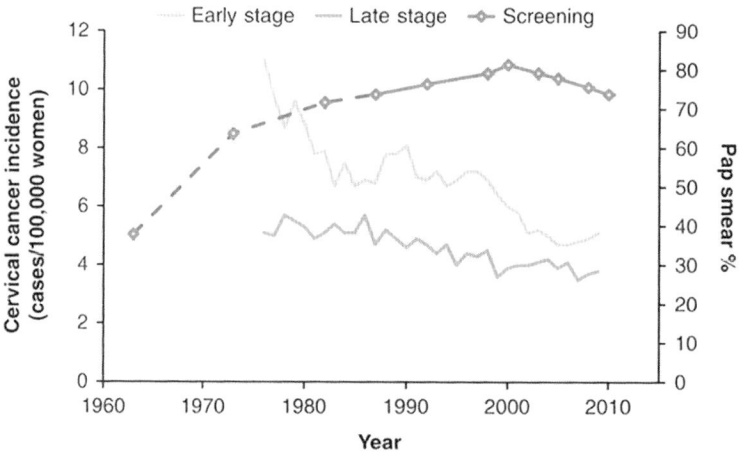

Figure 3.9 Impact of Pap smear screening on the incidence of cervical cancer in the US. The Pap smear has decreased the incidence of cervical cancer from 40 to 10 per 100,000 women in the US. Source: Yang, Davis, Gross, and Yu (2018).

speculum and its modern-day successor the duckbill speculum, expand the vaginal walls, allowing the cervix to be seen from outside the body. Without the speculum, procedures like the Pap smear and colposcopy would not be possible. Almost a century before the inventions of Hinselmann and Papanicolaou, American physician James Marion Sims invented a crude version of the modern speculum. Like most physicians in the nineteenth-century South, Sims had little interest in treating female patients – and no specific gynecological training. However, like most inventions, the speculum was born of a need – the need to treat a wealthy woman who suffered from pelvic and back pain after falling off a horse. To treat these injuries, Sims realized he needed to look directly into her vagina. This is what inspired him to develop the precursor to the modern speculum: the bent handle of a pewter spoon.

Deeper Look: The Women Behind Medical Advances

J. Marion Sims used his access to enslaved people to test many medical procedures, including highly invasive and painful surgeries, without their consent. He used his relationship with a wealthy enslaver to test the speculum on young women working on his property (Kenny et al., 1999). Figure 3.10 shows an illustration of Sims preparing to examine an enslaved girl called Lucy. Almost all of the procedures were performed without anesthesia, as Black

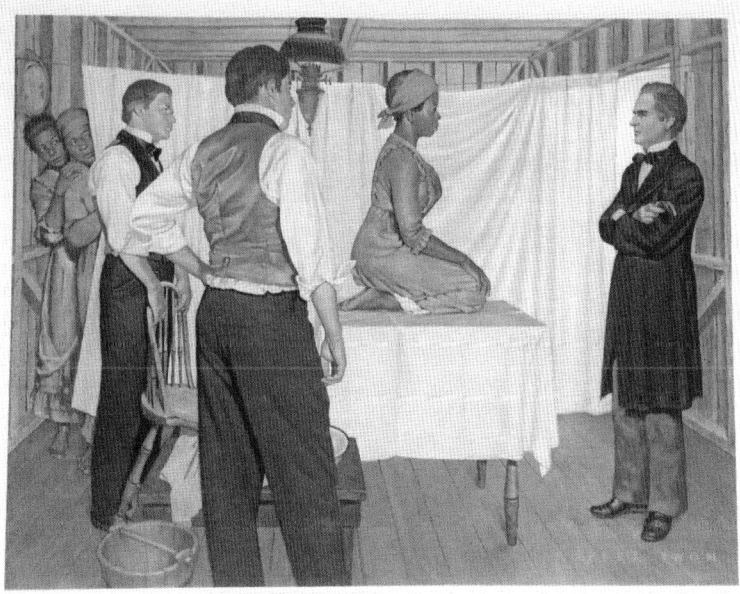

Figure 3.10

Illustration of Sims preparing to examine an enslaved girl called Lucy. Almost all of the procedures were performed without anesthesia, as Black women were thought to be immune to pain. Source: Robert J. Thom, Marion Sims: Gynecologic Surgeon (Alabama, 1845). Courtesy of University of Michigan.

women were thought to be immune to pain. Because the slave trade was banned in the early 1700s, the only means of procuring new slaves was to birth them in the US. As a result, Black female reproductive health became important to enslavers to ensure their own economic future. J. Marion Sims operated on one Black female slave, Anarcha, without anesthesia or her consent approximately 30 times in a five-year period, using experimental procedures to try to remedy her fistula. His final surgery was successful and earned him great recognition in the medical community for his method to repair vaginal fistulas. While physicians like Sims are remembered and praised for their contributions to the medical field, and in Sims' case his contributions to gynecology, the Black women they experimented on are frequently left unacknowledged. The statue honoring Dr. J. Marion Sims at a perimeter wall of New York City's Central Park was removed on April 17, 2018, where protesters demanded it be taken down. The Public Design Commission voted unanimously to do so. The following day, the Parks Department removed it, and it has been relocated to Sims' burial site in Green-Wood Cemetery in Brooklyn.

The Pap smear test involves the sampling of cells scraped from the entire cervix. These cells are processed to create a cytology slide. A cytologist, a laboratory professional, uses a microscope to examine slides for suspicious cells under a microscope. Although the Pap smear can be performed in a primary care clinic, samples often need to be shipped to specialized laboratories for testing.

Colposcopy involves the excision of biopsies from abnormal areas. The biopsied tissues are processed into thin tissue sections on a slide for review by another specialized provider, called a pathologist. A **pathologist** is a physician who investigates the cause and effect of diseases or injuries. Anatomical pathologists perform visual, microscopic, and molecular analyses of tissues, as is the case with cervical biopsies. Diagnosis of the pathology slide is considered the gold standard, or the ground truth. Colposcopy informs whether to treat the patient or not. If the pathology diagnosis is positive, the patient will return to the health facility for a third visit. During this visit, the individual will undergo a LEEP (Wright Jr et al., 1992), the primary treatment for cervical precancer. Histopathology slides of the LEEP specimen also undergo a review by a pathologist to ensure the edges of the specimen (margin) do not have residual disease.

If the pathology slide shows that the biopsied area has cancer rather than precancer, the patient will undergo a different treatment scheme, which frequently includes surgery, radiation, and/or administration of systemic drugs, depending on the cancer stage. Nearly all cervical cancer therapy regimens involve surgery. Depending on the stage and severity of the cancer, the gynecologist will remove appropriate portions of the tumor and surrounding normal tissue to ensure the complete removal of cancerous cells.

Figure 3.11 shows a cytology slide of a negative and positive Pap smear and a pathology slide of normal tissue, and CIN I, II, and III. A Pap smear has high specificity but low sensitivity for detecting cancer cells owing to the fact that sampling error can lead to collection of a small number of positive cells within a larger population of negative cells. This is acceptable when the prevalence of disease is low, as is the case in the general population in the US. Pathology has a high sensitivity rate and a low specificity rate. This ensures that any suspicious areas are biopsied, with the understanding that the majority will be negative.

Innovators are always thinking of new ways to improve previous inventions. As mentioned earlier, the colposcope was large and unwieldy. Its design is largely attributed to the earlier invention of the speculum; Hinselmann's colposcope was developed to be used in conjunction with the widely used speculum. This low-power microscope, unlike other

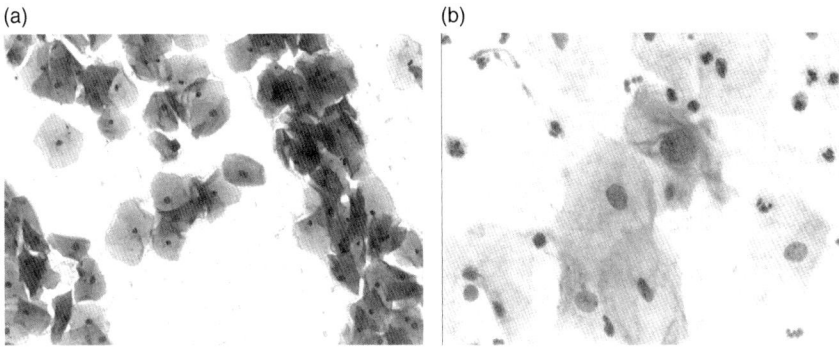
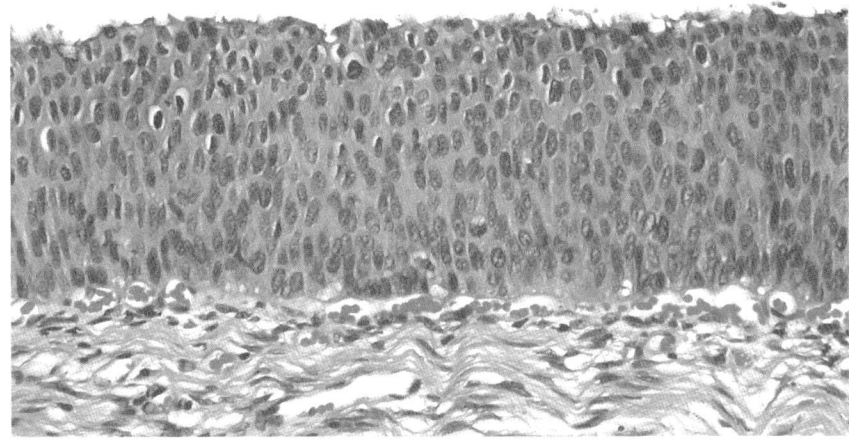

Figure 3.11 Cytology of a (a) negative and (b) positive Pap smear and (c) histopathology section of normal tissue, and (d–f) CIN I, II, and III. A Pap smear has high specificity but low sensitivity for detecting cancer cells owing to the fact that sampling error can lead to collection of a small number of positive cells within a larger population of negative cells. Source: (a) Department of Pathology, Calicut Medical College under a CC BY-SA 4.0 license; (b) Authored by "Alex-brollo" under a CC BY-SA 3.0 license; (c–f) Ed Uthman under a CC BY 2.0 license.

Figure 3.11 (cont.)

(d)
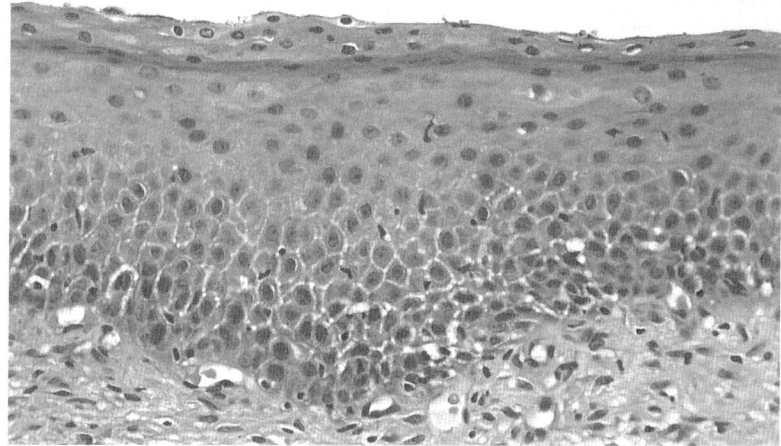

(e)
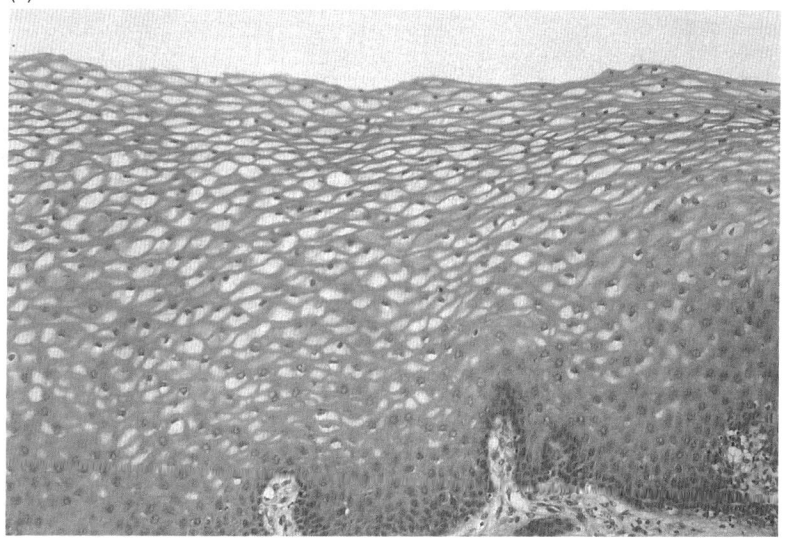

(f)
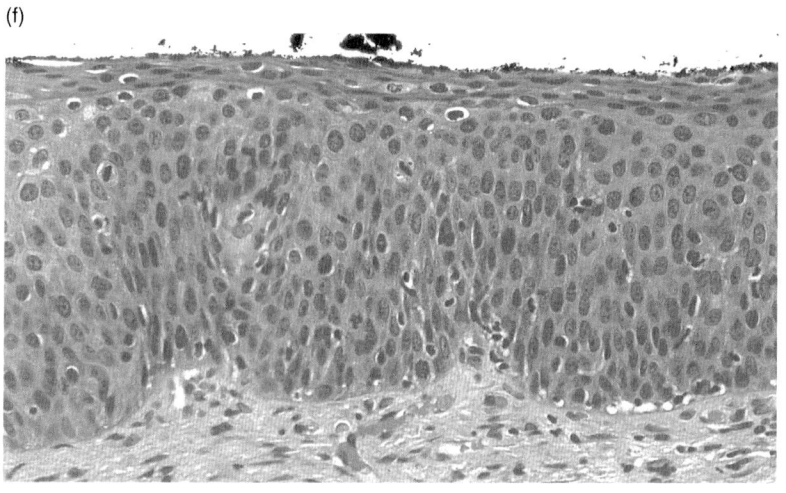

conventional microscopes, has to magnify the cervix from a distance of at least 30 cm. Hinselmann's colposcope was a new innovation that built on an existing invention, the speculum, to create new functionality. An advantage of this approach is that the new invention can easily be integrated into current practices. One disadvantage, however, is that its design is significantly constrained by the prior invention. One might speculate what the form factor of the colposcope might have been, had the speculum not existed. One might wonder whether the colposcope could have been developed such that it was much closer to the cervix and, consequently, less complex and expensive? This will be discussed in Chapter 5.

Example: How Screening Rates Affect Cervical Cancer Survival

Question: Compare the mortality rate for cervical cancer between a high-income country where the prevalence of disease is low (2 per 100,000 people with cervices), and a low-income country where the prevalence of disease is high (40 per 100,000 people with cervices). Assume the following: 90 percent of people receive screening in the high-income country, 30 percent of people receive screening in the low-income country; the sensitivity of the Pap smear is approximately 50 percent; 100 percent of patients who receive treatment (i.e., screen positive) do not develop invasive cervical cancer (ICC); 40 percent of patients who do not receive treatment for their cervical precancer develop ICC; and there is a 50 percent mortality rate from ICC.

Answer: It is easiest to perform the necessary calculations using a decision tree (Figure 3.12). Let us begin with the HIC case, where the incidence rate is 2 per 100,000 people. The first branches separate out people who receive screening from those who do not. Since 90 percent receive screening, 10 percent do not. Looking at the left set of branches, of the 10 percent who do not receive screening, we assume that 40 percent will develop ICC and 60 percent will not. Of the 40 percent with ICC, 50 percent will die, which totals to 0.04/100,000. Going to the right branches, of the 90 percent who receive screening, 50 percent will screen positive (true positive) and 50 percent will screen

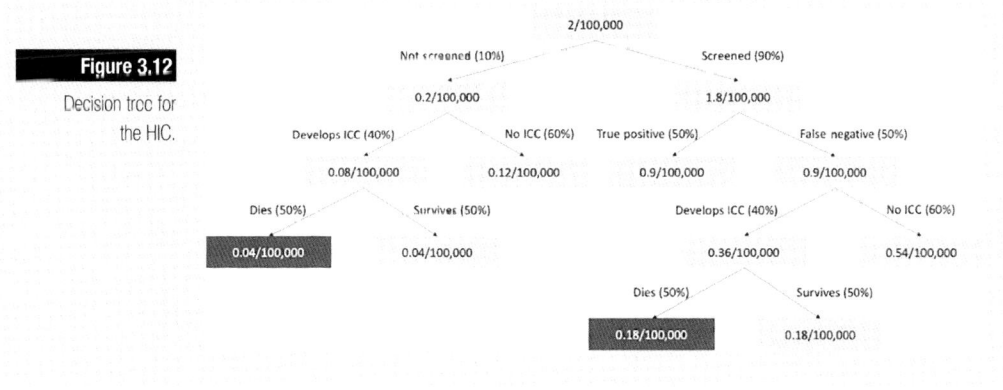

Figure 3.12 Decision tree for the HIC.

negative (false negative), because the sensitivity of the screening test is 50 percent. Of the 50 percent who screen negative, 40 percent will develop ICC, and 50 percent of those will die, which totals to 0.18/100,000. Adding the two together gives 0.22/100,000 as the mortality rate in the high-income country.

The same methodology can be applied to a low-income country (LIC) with the change in disease prevalence and screening rate. As you can see in the decision tree in Figure 3.13, 6/100,000 die from lack of screening and 1/100,000 women who are screened die, bringing the mortality rate to 7/100,000.

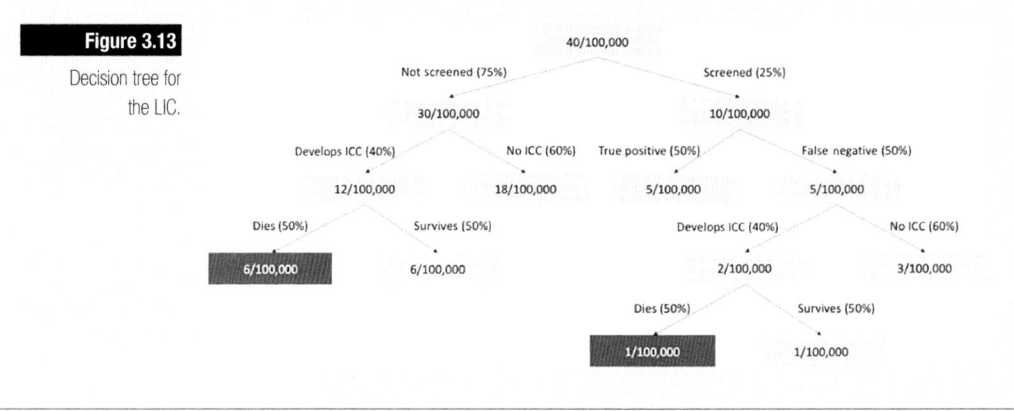

Figure 3.13 Decision tree for the LIC.

The Virus That Causes Cervical Cancer Has Revolutionized Primary and Secondary Prevention

In the US, the majority of cervical cancer cases are diagnosed during the precancerous stage as a result of a highly organized screening approach. Unfortunately, women in LMICs typically receive a cervical cancer diagnosis after it has progressed to the later stages, where mortality rates are high. In the next section, we will take a closer look at one innovation that has the potential to dramatically reduce cervical cancer deaths in LMICs.

The Pap smear and the colposcope are examples of inventions from evidence-based medicine, each resulting from medical knowledge regarding the disease. The underlying cause of cervical cancer, however, was still elusive at the time these innovations were conceptualized. Nearly all cervical cancer cases are a result of HPV, which is sexually transmitted. It can be prevented by vaccinating adolescents who have previously not been sexually active. In 1985, the *New York Times* reported that the HPV virus was linked to cancer, particularly cancers of the cervix and vulva. Figure 3.14 shows Dr. Harald zur Hausen, the Nobel laureate who discovered the HPV virus, and a Western blot showing the virus. In 1983, Dr. zur Hausen demonstrated the

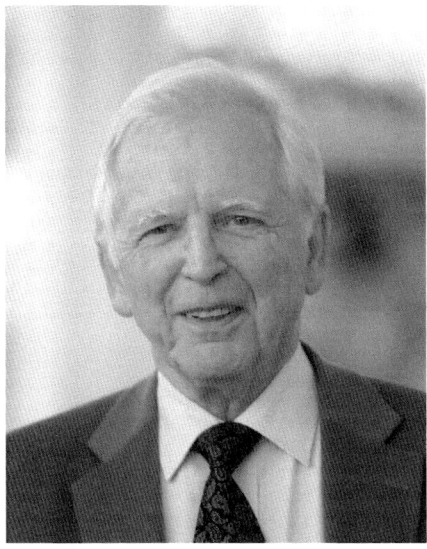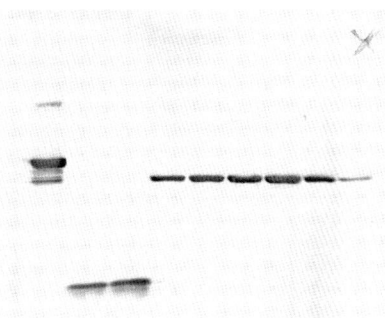

Figure 3.14 Dr. Harald zur Hausen, the Nobel laureate who discovered the HPV virus, and a Western blot showing the virus. In 1983, Dr. zur Hausen demonstrated the link between cervical cancer and HPV 16 and 18 (Dürst et al., 1983). He received the Nobel Prize in Physiology or Medicine for his work in 2008.
Source: (a) Armin Kuebelbeck under a CC BY-SA 3.0 license; (b) Magnus Manske under a CC BY-SA 3.0 license.

link between cervical cancer and HPV 16 and 18, which are responsible for more than 70 percent of cervical cancers (Dürst et al., 1983). He received the Nobel Prize in Physiology or Medicine for his work in 2008.

There are more than a dozen strains of HPV that can cause cervical cancer. However, **HPV 16** and **HPV 18** cause about 70 percent of cancers, with 17.2 percent of those caused by HPV 18. This seminal discovery about the most prevalent HPV strains in cervical cancer led to the development and introduction of the HPV vaccine, Gardasil, which protects against HPV 16 and HPV 18, as well as two strains of the HPV virus that cause genital warts. A nearly identical vaccine, Cervarix, developed by a different pharmaceutical company, protects against the same strains of HPV. A later version of the Gardasil vaccine, Gardasil 9, protects against more strains of HPV. Table 3.1 shows different types of HPV vaccines, the types of HPV they protect against, and the recommended gender and age range for use. The Centers for Disease Control and Prevention (CDC) does not recommend HPV vaccination for anyone 26 years of age or above. The primary reasons the CDC cites for this is the high likelihood that adults over 26 have already been exposed to HPV, and reduced efficacy of the HPV vaccine in people older than 26. The HPV vaccine is the second "anticancer" vaccine to be developed for the purpose of preventing cancer. The first is the hepatitis B vaccine, which prevents chronic hepatitis B infections, thereby preventing liver cancer caused by the hepatitis B virus (Blumberg, 1997).

Table 3.1 Different types of HPV vaccines, the types of HPV they protect against, and the recommended gender and age range for use

The Centers for Disease Control and Prevention (CDC) does not recommend HPV vaccination for anyone 26 years of age or above. The primary reasons the CDC cites for not vaccinating this age group is the high likelihood that adults over 26 have already been exposed to HPV and reduced efficacy of the HPV vaccine in people above 26.

Vaccine	Coverage (HPV types)	Gender and age range
Cervarix (bivalent HPV vaccine)	HPV 16 and 18	Females, 9–25 years
Gardasil (quadrivalent HPV vaccine)	HPV 6, 11 (genital warts), 16, and 18	Males and females, 9–26 years
Gardasil 9 (9-valent HPV vaccine)	HPV 6, 11 (genital warts), 16, 18, 31, 33, 45, 52, and 58	Males and females, 9–26 years

The CDC now recommends all adolescents be vaccinated against HPV as a way to prevent HPV infection to begin with, thereby greatly reducing the risk of developing cervical cancer. Even though vaccination is generally covered by insurance in the US, vaccination rates are shockingly low in young adolescents. According to a 2019 study, only 16 percent of US adolescents are vaccinated by the age of 13 (Bednarczyk et al., 2019), even though the CDC recommends vaccination at the age of 11 or 12. Barriers to vaccination include "weak and inconsistent provider recommendations" and "low parental demand for HPV vaccination" (National Vaccine Advisory Committee, 2016). National-scale vaccination and full coverage is not an instantaneous process. By implementing national immunization programs, nations will be making an investment in their population, but will not see the full effect until years down the road.

If a vaccine exists that can prevent more than 90 percent of cervical cancers, and monitoring strategies are highly successful at detecting early signs of the disease, why are an estimated 311,000 women still dying of the disease annually (Arbyn et al., 2020)? There are three main shortcomings. First, the HPV vaccine is not effective in individuals who are already infected with the virus. This means that the vaccine is not effective for nearly the entire adult population of the world, which makes screening still paramount for the adult population. Second, the current supply of vaccines does not meet global demand. There are multinational pushes for implementation of national HPV vaccine programs; however, many struggle to acquire the vaccine. Finally, the HPV vaccine is not affordable to scale (the process of increasing accessibility of a product by bringing it to new markets) in many

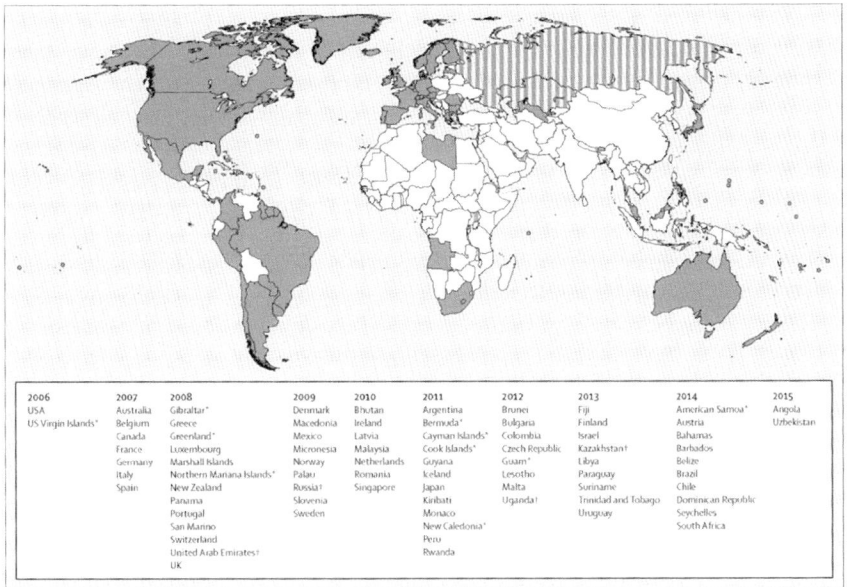

Figure 3.15 Countries with an established HPV vaccination program. The countries in gray have established HPV vaccination programs beginning in 2006 and beyond. Many countries in Africa, Asia, and Central America still did not have HPV vaccination programs as of 2014.
Source: Bruni et al. (2016). © 2016 The Author(s). Published by Elsevier Ltd. DOI: https://doi.org/10.1016/S2214-109X(16)30099-7. Licensed under a CC BY 4.0 agreement.

LMICs, particularly middle-income countries that have phased out of being eligible for a subsidized price provided by the Global Alliance for Vaccines and Immunization (GAVI).

It is estimated that only 1.4 percent of all women globally have been vaccinated against the virus (Bruni et al., 2016). In fact, the demand is so great that, in 2019, the WHO called for a temporary suspension of the vaccination of males until all females in need of the HPV vaccine receive it (Arie, 2019). Figure 3.15 shows the countries with an established HPV vaccination program. The countries in gray have established HPV vaccination programs beginning in 2006 and beyond. Many countries in Africa, Asia, and Central America still did not have HPV vaccination programs as of 2014.

Deeper Look: Supply and Demand of HPV Vaccines

As of 2020, 22 of 78 LICs and LMICs have introduced the HPV vaccine. This is lagging behind the 50 of 57 HICs and 35 of 59 upper-middle-income countries (UMICs) that have introduced HPV vaccination. The HPV vaccines can cost up to $168 in HICs. In 2011, GAVI and UNICEF were able to negotiate the price of vaccines down to as little as $4.50 per dose for LICs. While this makes the vaccines affordable, access to them has been affected by the limited supply, largely due to the fact that increasing global demand has outpaced production capacity. UNICEF continues to project that demand for HPV vaccines will outstrip supply in the short term.

Another challenge is that GAVI bases eligibility on national income. Countries become eligible for support if their average **gross national income** per capita is less than or equal to $1,630 over a three-year period. Once a country crosses the eligibility threshold, it phases out of GAVI's financial support. In this case, the cost of HPV vaccines is about three times the price of HPV vaccines for GAVI-eligible countries, creating financial barriers for middle-income countries (MICs) to procure and introduce HPV vaccines.

Knowledge about the connection between the HPV virus and cervical cancer would pave the way for a molecular HPV screening test. Unlike a Pap smear, the HPV test does not detect precancerous or cancerous cells. Instead, it identifies the presence of strains of the virus that could cause cancer in a patient. There are different HPV tests on the market today that use similar types of technologies. They test either DNA or RNA. In general, DNA testing had higher sensitivity and specificity than RNA testing; however, there is some variability with each test type.

Figure 3.16(a) shows the five-year cumulative incidence rate of high-grade precancer or moderate CIN (CIN II+) for women who have a negative Pap smear or a negative HPV test and (b) stratified by HPV strain. Women with a negative HPV test have a 10-fold lower long-term risk of developing cancer compared to those with a negative cytology test. Further, HPV 16 is high-risk, HPV 18/45 are medium-risk, and all other HPVs are considered low-risk. The implications here are that Pap smears needed to be repeated at regular intervals as at least 10 percent of the population with a negative Pap smear can still develop CIN. On the other hand, women can have a single or twice-lifetime HPV screens for cervical cancer. However, not all CIN II+ lesions have the same likelihood of developing cancer. With the availability of up to 14 oncogenic HPV types, long-term risk of advanced precancers or cancers can be stratified, which can be important in the management of women with a positive HPV test.

The HPV test is a molecular test, and is more precise test than the Pap smear. The Pap smear has been reported to have a sensitivity of only 55.4 percent, while an HPV (DNA) test has a sensitivity of greater than 90 percent (Kripke, 2008). Since HPV affects both the cervix and vagina, the cells do not need to be directly sampled from the cervix, providing the option for a self-test. Evidence demonstrates that HPV self-sampling is comparable to clinician-collected samples. Furthermore, provider acceptance of HPV self-testing is high and normally hard-to-reach women have overwhelmingly positive attitudes toward self-sampling (Gupta et al., 2018).

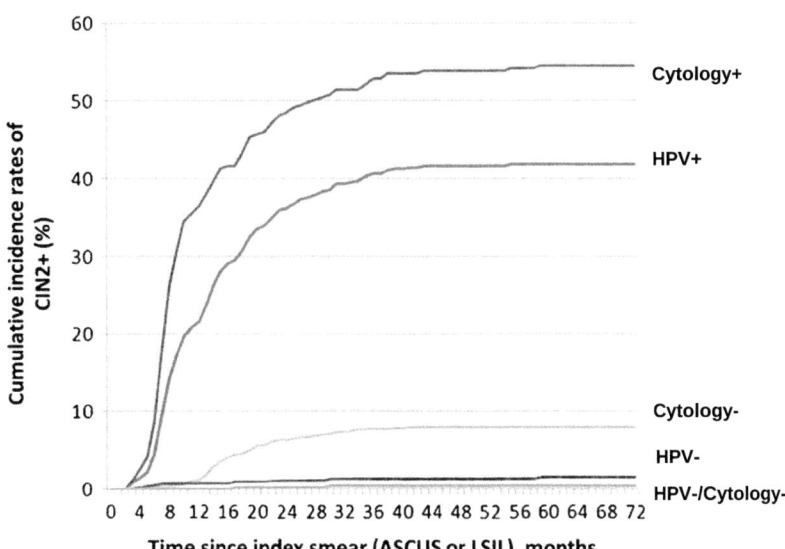
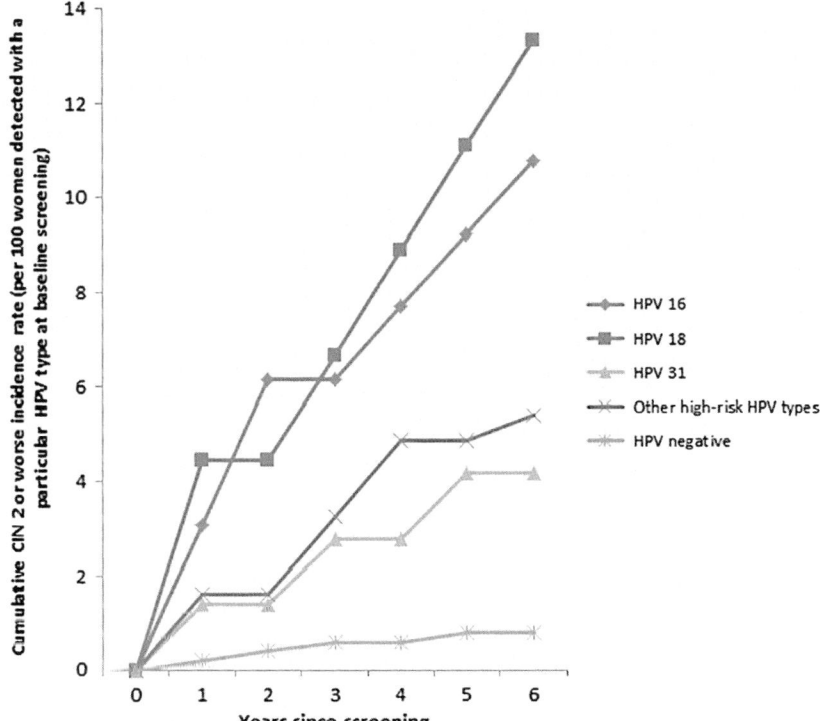

Figure 3.16 (a) The five-year cumulative incidence rate of high-grade precancer or moderate CIN (CIN II+) for women who have a negative Pap smear or a negative HPV test; (b) stratified by HPV strain. Women with a negative HPV test have a 10-fold lower long-term risk of developing cancer compared to those with a negative cytology test. Further, HPV 16 is high-risk, HPV18/45 are medium-risk, and all other HPVs are considered low-risk. Source: (a) Cancer Medicine 2014; 3(1): 182–189; (b) Joshi et al. (2019).

Table 3.2 compares the Pap and HPV tests. The HPV tests are more accurate and quantitative and, from a patient's perspective, increases the interval between screenings and provides the option for a self-test. The development of HPV testing as a method of screening for cervical cancer illustrates an

Table 3.2 A comparison of the Pap and HPV tests

HPV tests are more accurate and quantitative and, from a patient's perspective, increases the interval between screenings and provides the option for a self-test.

Features	Pap smear	HPV test
Accuracy	Sensitivity 50%	Sensitivity >90%
Interpretability	Read by a provider	Precise – read by a machine
Frequency of screening	Every 2–3 years	Once or twice in a lifetime
Accessibility	Requires a provider	Can be a clinic or self-test

important shift in cervical cancer care from evidence-based medicine to precision medicine. In spite of the advantages of the HPV test over the Pap smear, however, the majority of HPV tests are performed by clinical providers, though self-testing is gaining traction in LMICs. HPV self-testing will hopefully be accessible to the still large number of hard-to-reach women, and in doing so, will drive down the incidence of cervical cancer.

In the previous section we explored through an example how differences in disease prevalence and screening rates affect the cervical cancer mortality rate; however, there was one assumption that is potentially flawed – people are only screened once in their lives. Additional screening can help reduce the incidence of cervical cancer by catching people who may have received a false negative result during the first round. This is why the Pap smear has been so effective at reducing cervical cancer rates in the US even though it only has a sensitivity of 55.4 percent. In the US, physicians recommend regularly screening for cervical cancer with a Pap smear for women of average risk of developing cervical cancer. Because the process of developing cervical cancer from an HPV infection is slow, taking 10–20 years, regular screening intervals can increase the likelihood of detecting suspicious cells before they become invasive cancer. The high specificity of the Pap smear reduces the number of false positives that would require further evaluation in a population that has a low prevalence of the disease. Unfortunately, one of the problems in LMICs is that patients do not return to follow-up screening, which is another reason that the Pap smear may not be the best screening tool in all settings.

Example: Effect of Screening Frequency or Cervical Cancer Mortality

Question: Compare the mortality rates for cervical cancer between two LICs where the prevalence of disease is high (40 per 100,000 people with cervices), but one of the countries has implemented a screening campaign that has increased the lifetime screening from one to three. Assume the following:

- The sensitivity of the Pap smear is 50 percent.
- 100 percent of patients who receive treatment (i.e., screen positive) do not develop ICC.
- 40 percent of patients who do not receive treatment for their cervical precancer develop ICC, and 50 percent of them die from the ICC.

Answer: Using a decision tree is once again helpful for answering this question. In this case, we are assuming that all people are screened once in country 1 and all people are screened three times in country 2. Let us start with the case for country 1 (Figure 3.17): 50 percent will screen positive (true positive) and 50 percent will screen negative (false

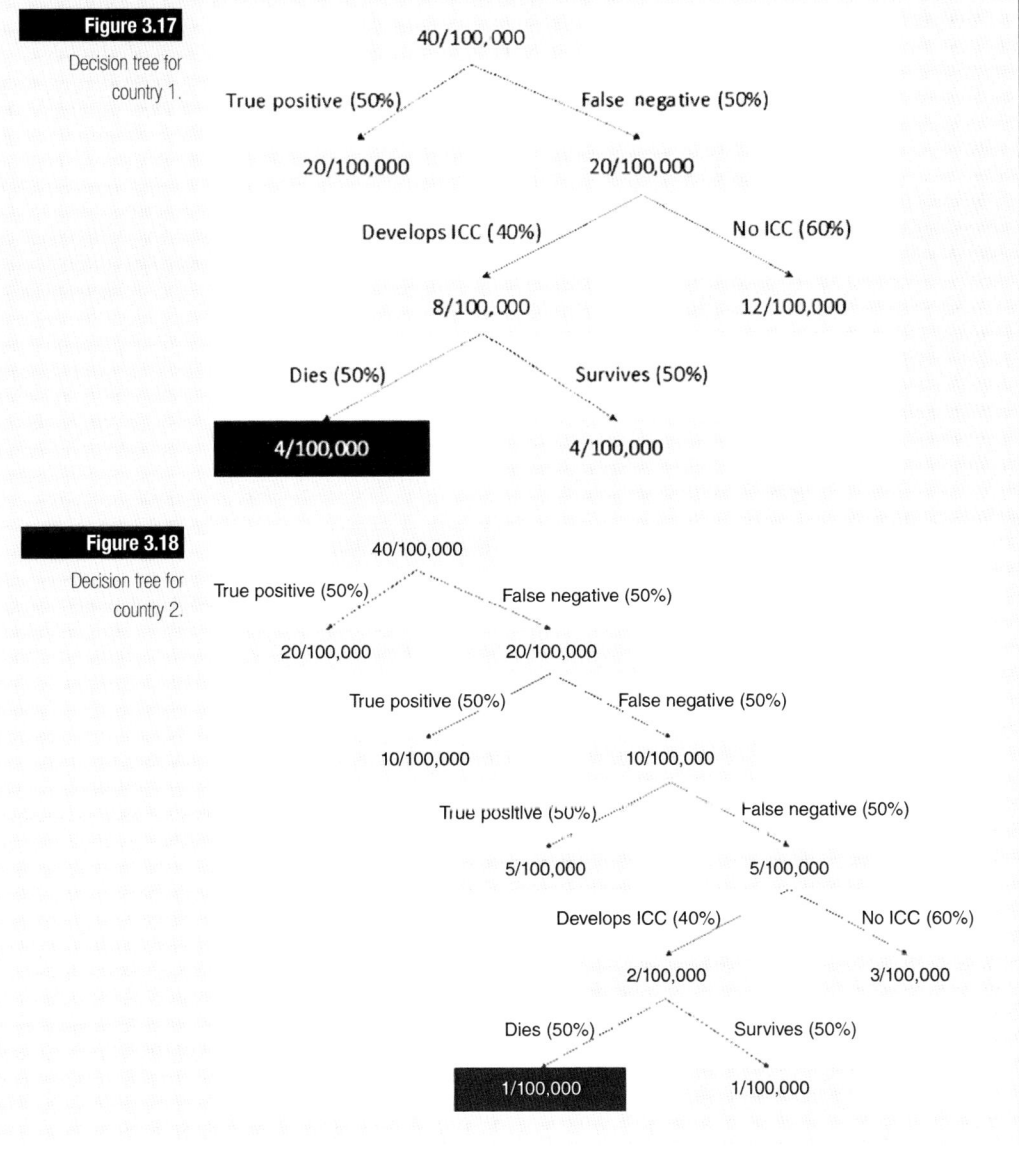

Figure 3.17 Decision tree for country 1.

Figure 3.18 Decision tree for country 2.

negative), because the sensitivity of the screening test is 50 percent. Of the 50 percent who screen negative, 40 percent will develop ICC and 50 percent of those will die, which totals to 4/100,000.

Now let us look at the case for country 2 (Figure 3.18). The decision tree needs to be modified, as instead of all false negatives resulting in lack of treatment, women return for follow-up screening two more times. This adds two more layers to the decision tree, providing additional opportunities for women to be triaged. As a result, the mortality rate in country 2 drops to 1/100,000 simply by adding two additional screenings.

Figure 3.19 shows the HPV detection and cervical cancer prevention schema. We already have all the tools to prevent the transition from cervical precancer to cancer, beginning with effective HPV vaccines to prevent cancer in future generations, and frequent screening with the Pap smear and/or HPV test to prevent cancer in the current generation. Of the numerous HPV strains, only a subset of these can lead to cervical cancer, with types 16 and 18 accounting for around 70 percent of cervical cancers. The two most prominent vaccines, Gardasil 9 and Cervarix, cover nearly all of the HPV types that can cause cancer. Screening tests for those who were not vaccinated can use either or both Pap smears to detect abnormal cells and HPV testing for the high-risk HPV types that cause cervical cancer.

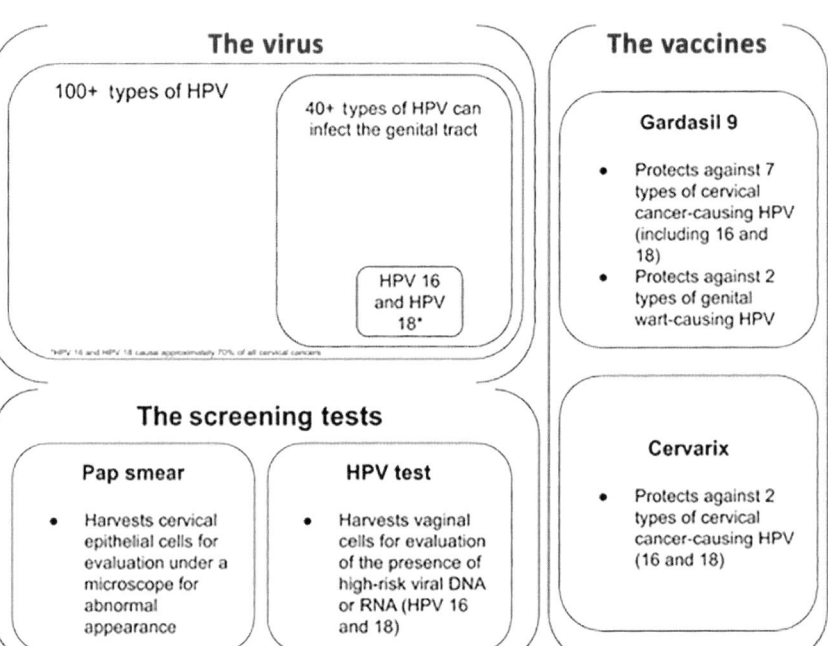

Figure 3.19 The HPV detection and cervical cancer prevention schema. We already have all the tools to prevent the transition from cervical precancer to cancer, beginning with effective HPV vaccines to prevent cancer in future generations, and frequent screening with the Pap smear and/or HPV test to prevent cancer in the current generation.

Cervical Cancer Is a Disease of Health Disparities

It is conceivable that the introduction of the HPV vaccine, options for HPV and Pap smear screening, coupled with technologies for early diagnosis and treatment would lead to cervical cancer elimination in the foreseeable feature. In other words, the link between causality and manifestation of disease has been established and this has been leveraged for precision diagnostics (HPV test). However, this is not the case. Cervical cancer outcomes vary with factors including race, socioeconomic status, and region (Yu et al., 2019). For example, Black and Hispanic women in the US have higher incidence and mortality rates and lower survival rates than white women (Yu et al., 2019). Today, cervical cancer affects the lives of more than 500,000 women globally, 85 percent of whom live in LMICs (Randall and Ghebre, 2016). More than half of these women die of the disease.

Cervical cancer continues to be a global public health crisis. Figure 3.20 shows the global incidence and mortality from cervical cancer. The map shows the geographical distribution of world age-standardized mortality of cervical cancer by country, estimated for 2018. In the US, incidence rates of cervical cancer are less than 6 per 100,000 women. Contrast that with countries in Africa, which have incidence rates of 40–80 per 100,000 women, a more than six-fold higher incidence rate. The mortality rate statistics are even more humbling. In the US, mortality from cervical cancer is nearly 10-fold lower than in LMICs. These disparities will only continue to worsen if there is not a commitment to eliminating cervical cancer globally.

The disproportionate cervical cancer deaths in LMICs reflects a major health disparity. Strategies to address cervical cancer elimination strive to achieve health equity. **Health disparity** and **health equity** are often used interchangeably, yet they are distinct. When defining metrics to close the gaps in disparities or inequity, it is important to understand the difference between the two. Health disparity is a quantity that separates a group from a reference point on a particular measure of health that is expressed in terms of a rate, proportion, mean, or some other quantitative measure. Disparities are measured from the most favorable group rate (preference for raising health among unhealthy groups). A health disparity refers to a higher burden of illness, injury, disability, or mortality experienced by one group relative to another.

Figure 3.21 shows the structural and institutional component of health equity. **Health inequities** lead to health disparities. Therefore, health disparity is a way to measure the health inequity gap. Health disparities can emerge owing to lack of equity of resources in the physical environment (first bracket), clinical care (second bracket), health behavior (third bracket), and social and economic factors (fourth bracket). A reduction in health disparities (in absolute and relative terms) is evidence that we are moving toward greater health equity. Relating this to the case of cervical cancer, the inequities that exist can be attributed in part to access and quality of care (second bracket in Figure 3.21). Developing and deploying solutions to improve both clinical care and clinical systems will reduce health disparities, thereby promoting health equity.

The next question is: What is the difference between health equity and health equality? Health equity is sometimes used interchangeably with the related term health equality. Equality is considered to exist when all individuals and groups of people are given equal treatment, regardless of need or outcome, whereas an equitable approach focuses on more equal outcomes, recognizing that disadvantaged groups may need more support or resources in order to achieve the same health outcomes as more advantaged groups. Figure 3.22 shows the conceptual difference between health equity and health inequality: The tallest person can reach the fruit, but the short person

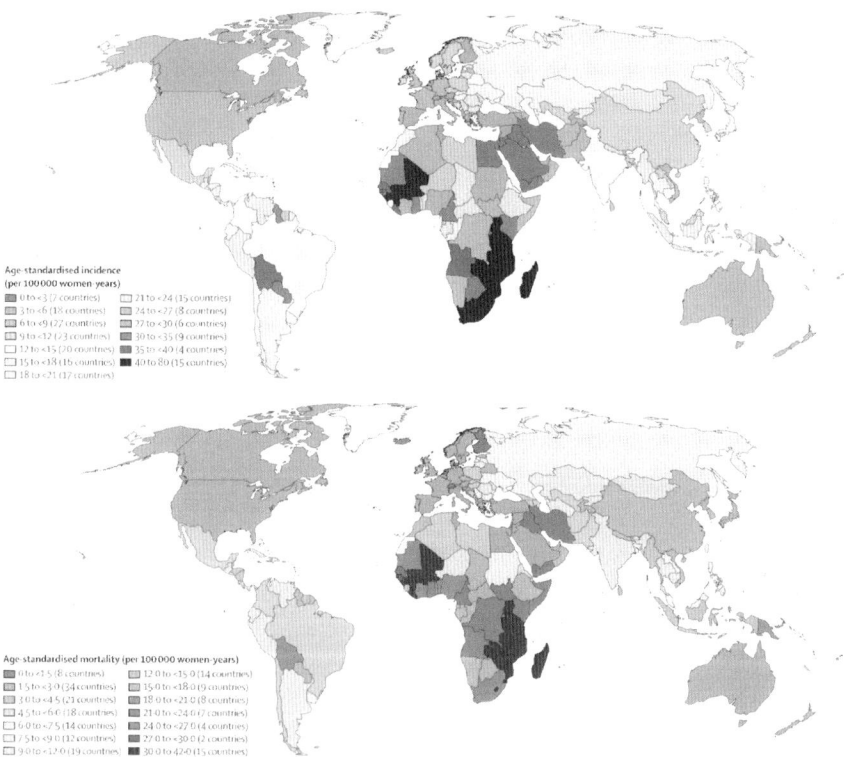

Figure 3.20 Global incidence and mortality from cervical cancer. The map shows the geographical distribution of world age-standardized mortality from cervical cancer by country, estimated for 2018. Looking at the US, incidence rates of cervical cancer are less than 6 per 100,000 women. Contrast that with countries in Africa, which have incidence rates of 40–80 per 100,000 women, a more than six-fold higher incidence rate. The mortality rate statistics are even more humbling. In the US, mortality from cervical cancer is nearly 10-fold lower than in LMICs.

Source: Estimates of incidence and mortality of cervical cancer in 2018: a worldwide analysis. Marc Arbyn, Elisabete Weiderpass, Laia Bruni, Silvia de Sanjosé, Mona Saraiya, Jacques Ferlay, Freddie Bray. The Lancet Global Health. © 2019 The Author(s). Published. www.thelancet.com/journals/langlo/article/PIIS2214-109X(19)30482-6/fulltext#figures.

Cervical Cancer Is a Disease of Health Disparities

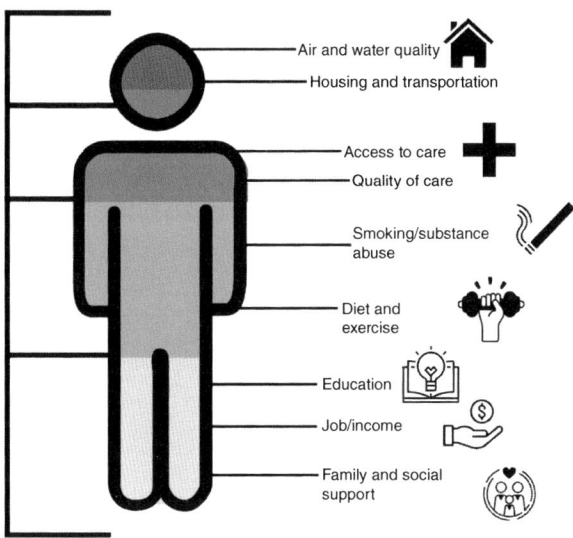

Figure 3.21 The structural and institutional component of health equity. Health inequities lead to health disparities. Health disparities can emerge owing to lack of equity of resources in the physical environment (first bracket), clinical care (second bracket), health behavior (third bracket), and social and economic factors (fourth bracket). A reduction in health disparities (in absolute and relative terms) is evidence that we are moving toward greater health equity.
Source: Adapted from The Greenlining Institute's image in AMN Healthcare's blog DEI Awareness: COVID-19 and Healthcare Disparities by Maisam Ileiwi.

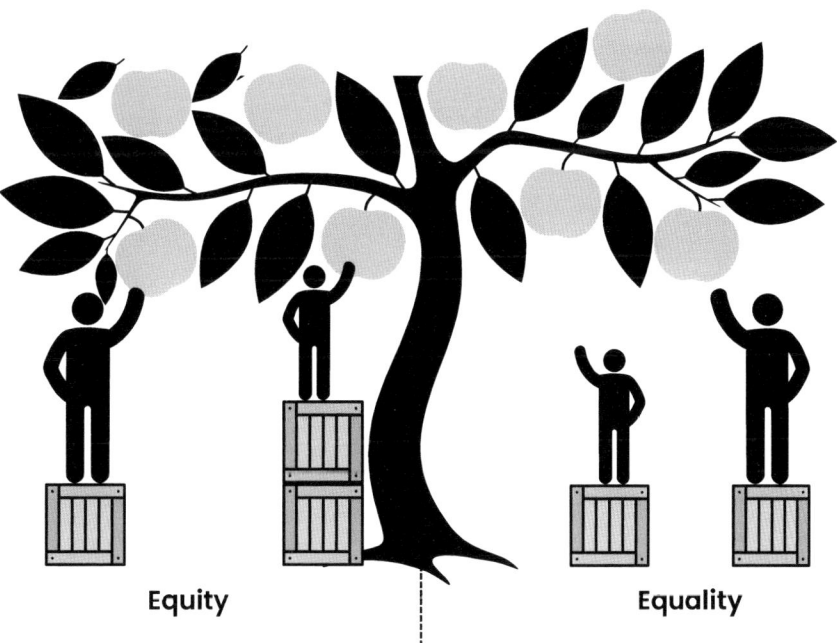

Figure 3.22. Conceptual difference between health equity and health inequality. The tallest person can reach the fruit, but the short person cannot. The resources provided are equal, but the outcome is different. When the height of the box is adjusted for the height of the person, all individuals can reach the fruit. This solution is equitable.

cannot. The resource provided are equal, but the outcome is different. When the height of the box is adjusted for the height of the person, all individuals can reach the fruit. This solution is equitable.

In an effort to close the inequity gap in cervical cancer, the director of the WHO, Dr. Tedros Adhanom Ghebreyesus, made a bold call to action in 2018 for all countries to eliminate cervical cancer by 2099. He underscored the fact that all the tools exist to prevent cervical cancer, and therefore creative strategies should be put into place to help break down structural and social barriers to elimination of this disease. In other words, even if all of the tools used in countries like the US were made available, thereby making all things equal, the difference in structural and social patterns in different environments would not necessarily lead to health equity. The WHO's call to action led to a recommendation for intensive HPV vaccination initiatives and screening programs to occur in tandem to rapidly reach the target of fewer than 4 deaths per 100,000 by 2099.

Figure 3.23 shows the modeling projections for the incidence of cervical cancer per 100,000 women. With a combination of intensive screening programs and vaccination campaigns, we are poised to eliminate cervical cancer within the next century. The WHO has now set short-term metrics to be achieved by 2030 in order to set the stage for the next century of efforts, as enumerated below:

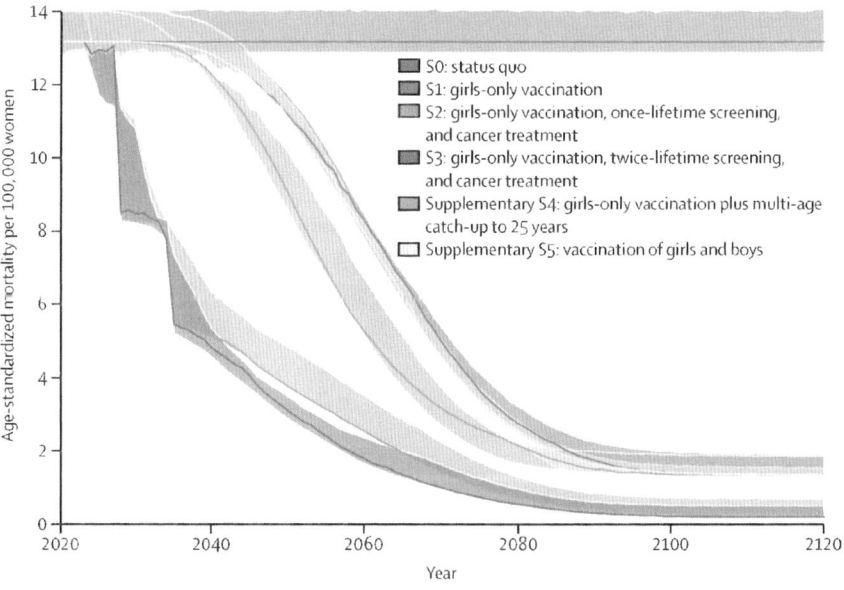

Figure 3.23 Modeling projections for incidence of cervical cancer per 100,000 women. With a combination of intensive screening programs and vaccination campaigns, we are poised to eliminate cervical cancer within the next century.
Source: Mortality impact of achieving WHO cervical cancer elimination targets: a comparative modelling analysis in 78 low-income and lower-middle-income countries. Karen Canfell, Jane J Kim, Marc Brisson, Adam Keane, Kate T Simms, Michael Caruana, Emily ABurger, Dave Martin, Diep T N Nguyen, Élodie Bénard, Stephen Sy, Catherine Regan, MélanieDrolet, Guillaume Gingras, Jean-Francois Laprise, Julie Torode, Megan A Smith et al. © 2020 The Author(s). Published by Elsevier Ltd. DOI: https://doi.org/10.1016/S0140-6736(20)30157-4. Licensed by under CC BY-NC-ND 4.0.

- 90 percent of girls fully vaccinated with HPV vaccine by 15 years of age;
- 70 percent of women screened using a high-performance test by 35 and 45 years of age;
- 90 percent of women identified with cervical disease are treated.

Given these important goals, it is essential to understand the current status of cervical cancer screening programs in many LMICs. Given the advantages of HPV testing over the Pap smear, it has been recommended as the primary screening tool. However, it is not widely available and, when available, a secondary test is required to provide specificity in order to prevent large numbers of women from being unnecessarily referred for confirmatory testing or treatment. Approximately 50 percent of women who are HPV-positive do not have any disease. Colposcopy with biopsy is the gold standard diagnostic test in HICs. Unfortunately, colposcopes are expensive and large, requiring housing in high-level healthcare facilities that remain beyond the reach of many women in LMICs. Therefore alternative methods are required.

Colposcopy coupled with biopsy is the standard diagnostic method in HICs (Figure 3.24). **Visual inspection with acetic acid (VIA)** is an alternative to colposcopy in LMICs, using visualization with the unaided eye. Though VIA is inexpensive, lack of magnification and provider variability makes it a

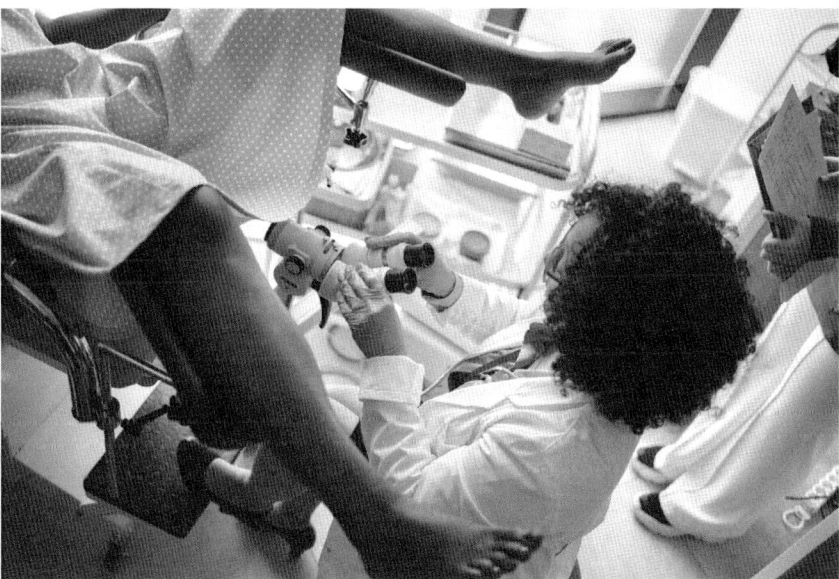

Figure 3.24 Colposcopy coupled with biopsy is the standard diagnostic method in HICs. Visual inspection with acetic acid is an alternative to colposcopy in LMICs, using visualization with the unaided eye. Though VIA is inexpensive, lack of magnification and provider variability makes it a poor screening or secondary test. In addition, standard colposcopes have additional features, such as using green light for image enhancement of blood vessels (a diagnostic feature), which is not possible with VIA.
Source: © Anchiy / E+ / Getty Images.

poor screening or secondary test. Also, standard colposcopes have additional features, such as using green light for image enhancement of blood vessels (a diagnostic feature), which is not possible with VIA.

Undoubtedly, HPV screening would be far more precise than VIA. There is yet another advantage – HPV screening can be performed as a self-test to avoid the duckbill speculum at the time of screening. The speculum is a barrier to cervical cancer screening. It can cause anxiety, fear, discomfort, pain, embarrassment, and/or vulnerability during the procedure (Lyimo and Beran, 2012). The speculum is also a cause of discomfort for women with vaginismus, which involves involuntary tightening of the vagina, often due to sexual abuse (Crowley, 2012); LMICs typically have the highest sexual violence rates worldwide, leading to higher incidence of vaginismus in these vulnerable populations (Garcia-Moreno et al., 2006; Williams et al., 2008; IARC, 2012). A number of countries have incorporated self-testing for HPV into their national guidelines; however, these tests remain unaffordable. Many of the HPV tests are made by wealthy countries and need to be significantly subsidized to be affordable in LMICs.

As mentioned previously, LEEP is the frontline treatment for cervical precancer and cancer in the US. Unfortunately, high cost, reliable access to electricity, and the need for highly trained operators preclude the widespread adoption of LEEP in LMICs. A low-cost therapeutic alternative to LEEP is ablation. Figure 3.25 shows two types of ablation therapies that are currently used in LMICs. **Cryotherapy** is an ablative method in which compressed gas (CO_2) and a metal probe are used to freeze abnormal tissue (Santesso et al., 2012). **Thermocoagulation** uses heat to destroy cervical tissue, and is gaining popularity for treatment of cervical abnormalities. Unlike cryotherapy, which requires hard-to-supply compressed gas tanks, the thermocoagulator does not require any consumables, making this method of ablation more attractive. However, not all women are eligible for ablation. According to the WHO, women are eligible for cryotherapy or thermal ablation only if the entire lesion and squamocolumnar junction are visible, and if the lesion does not cover >75 percent of the ectocervix.

In describing the disparities in cervical cancer treatment, much of the previous section has focused on cervical cancer deaths. A focus on mortality, however, does not account for the suffering that diseases cause to those living with them. Given that access to cervical cancer treatment may not be widely available, women may suffer for extended periods of time before they get better or ultimately succumb to the disease. Accounting for mortality *and* morbidity provides a more encompassing view on health outcomes. Figure 3.26 shows a visual representation of **disability-adjusted life years** (DALYs); this is the sum of both years living with disability (YLD), a measure of morbidity, and years of life lost (YLL), a measure of mortality. DALY is a standardized metric that allows for direct comparison of different disease burdens across

Cervical Cancer Is a Disease of Health Disparities

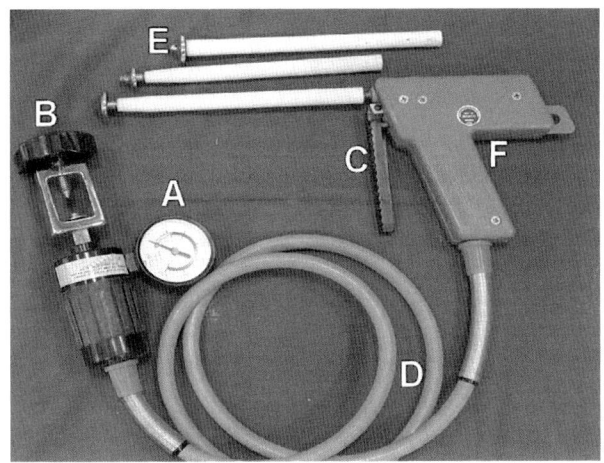

Figure 3.25

Two types of ablation therapies that are currently used in LMICs. Cryotherapy is an ablative method in which compressed gas (CO_2) and a metal probe are used to freeze abnormal tissue (Santesso et al., 2012). Thermocoagulation is an ablative method in which heat is used to destroy cervical tissue, and is gaining popularity for treatment of cervical abnormalities.
Source: (a) International Agency for Research on Cancer/World Health Organization. Atlas of Colposcopy: Principles and Practice; (b) International Agency for Research on Cancer/World Health Organization.

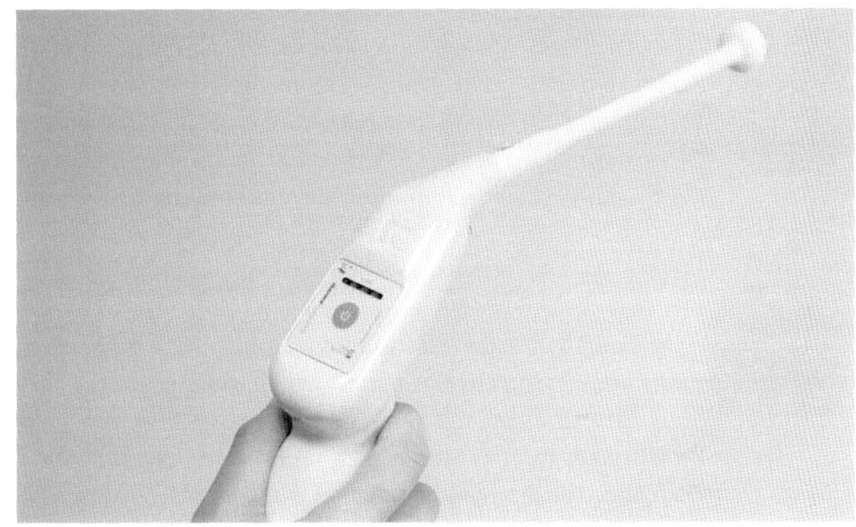

Figure 3.26

A visual representation of disability-adjusted life years (DALYs). This is the sum of years living with disability (YLD), a measure of morbidity, and years of life lost (YLL), a measure of mortality. DALY is a standardized metric that allows for direct comparison of different disease burdens across countries, between different populations, and over time. In short, DALYs measure health gaps over life expectancies.
Source: Original: Planemad Vector: Radio89 under a CC BY-SA 3.0 license.

countries, between different populations, and over time. In short, DALYs measure health gaps over life expectancies. Calculating the burden of disease using DALYs gives important information for policymakers.

Conceptually, one DALY is the equivalent of losing one year in good health because of either premature death *or* disease or disability. The DALY measures the difference between a current situation and an ideal situation where everyone lives to standard life expectancy in perfect health. Based on life tables, the standard life expectancy at birth is set at 80 years for men and 82.5 years for women, according to numbers from Japan, where men and women have the longest life expectancies. However, it is more relevant to use a country-specific life expectancy from the life tables. The calculations to determine DALY are shown below, where the equations do not use age weighting. The incorporation of this parameter makes the equations for DALY considerably more complex. Age weighting assigns greater weight to young adults than to those of older age or infants.

The basic equation for YLL is shown in Equation 3.1, where N is the number of deaths and L is the standard life expectancy in years at age of death (i.e., total life expectancy minus age at death). The basic equation for YDL is shown in Equation 3.2, where I is the number of incident cases, DW is the disability weight, and L is the average duration of disability in years:

$$YLL = N \times L, \qquad (3.1)$$

$$YDL = I \times DW \times L. \qquad (3.2)$$

For DALYs, the scale used to measure health state is converted to a "severity scale," whereby 0 is perfect health and 1 is death. A discounting function is used to assess the value of health gains now versus those in the future, reflecting the fact that people prefer a healthy life now rather than in the future. The discounting function is shown in Equation 3.3, where e is Euler's number (~2.71), r is the discount rate (usually 3 or 5 percent), and L is either the standard life expectancy in years at age of death (for a YLL calculation) or the average duration of disability in years (for YDL calculation):

$$\text{Discounting function} = e^{-rL}. \qquad (3.3)$$

Modifying Equations 3.1 and 3.2 to include the discounting function gives the final equations for YLL and YDL, as shown in Equations 3.4 and 3.5, respectively:

$$YLL = N \times \frac{1 - e^{-rL}}{r}, \qquad (3.4)$$

$$YDL = I \times DW \times \frac{1 - e^{-rL}}{r}. \qquad (3.5)$$

To calculate the DALY, you simply add YLL and YDL together, as shown in Equation 3.6. Note that the value of r can be the same or different for YLL and YDL:

$$DALY = N \times \frac{1-e^{-rL}}{r} + I \times DW \times \frac{1-e^{-rL}}{r}. \qquad (3.6)$$

Table 3.3 shows examples of disability weights used in YDL calculations. Disability weights reflect how much a medical condition affects a person. Cancers at the terminal stage have the highest disability weights.

Table 3.3 Examples of disability weights used in YDL calculations

Disability weights reflect how much a medical condition affects a person. Cancers at the terminal stage have the highest disability weights.

Disease or sequelae	Mean disability weight (untreated form)	Mean disability weight (treated form)
AIDS	0.50	0.50
Infertility	0.18	0.18
Diarrhea disease, episodes	0.11	0.11
Measles, episode	0.15	0.15
Tuberculosis	0.27	0.27
Malaria, episodes	0.20	0.20
Trachoma, blindness	0.60	0.49
Trachoma, low vision	0.24	0.24
Lower respiratory tract infection, episodes	0.28	0.28
Lower respiratory tract infection, chronic sequelae	0.01	0.01
Cancers, terminal stage	0.81	0.81
Diabetes mellitus cases (uncomplicated)	0.01	0.03
Unipolar major depression, episodes	0.60	0.30
Alcohol dependence syndrome	0.18	0.18
Parkinson disease cases	0.39	0.32
Alzheimer disease cases	0.64	0.64
Post-traumatic stress disorder	0.11	0.11
Angina pectoris	0.23	0.10

Table 3.3 (cont.)

Disease or sequelae	Mean disability weight (untreated form)	Mean disability weight (treated form)
Congestive heart failure	0.32	0.17
Chronic obstructive lung disease, symptomatic cases	0.43	0.39
Asthma, cases	0.10	0.06
Deafness	0.22	0.17
Benign prostatic hypertrophy	0.04	0.04
Osteoarthritis, symptomatic hip or knee	0.16	0.11
Brain injury, long-term sequelae	0.41	0.35
Spinal cord injury	0.73	0.73
Sprains	0.06	0.06
Burns (>60%), long term	0.25	0.25

Adapted from Murray and Lopez (1996).

Example: What Is the DALY for Terminal Cervical Cancer in Kenya?

Question: Calculate the annual DALYs for terminal cervical cancer in Kenya. Assume the following about Kenya:

- Average age at diagnosis for cervical cancer is 50.
- Average age at death from cervical cancer is 59.
- Number of people diagnosed with cervical cancer per year is 4,000.
- Number of people who die from cervical cancer each year is 2,000.
- The discount rate is 3 percent.

Answer: To calculate the DALYs, we need to first figure out the appropriate values for N, L, r, I, and DW. N is the number of deaths, which is given as 2,000. L is the time with disease, which is $59 - 50 = 9$. r is the discount rate, which is 0.03. The parameter I represents the incidence, which is given as 4,000. The DW can be looked up in Table 3.3, and is 0.81. Plugging all of this into Equation 3.6 gives:

$$DALY = 2{,}000 \times \frac{1 - e^{-0.03 * 9}}{0.03} + 4{,}000 \times 0.81 \times \frac{1 - e^{-0.03 * 9}}{0.03}$$
$$= 41{,}329.7$$

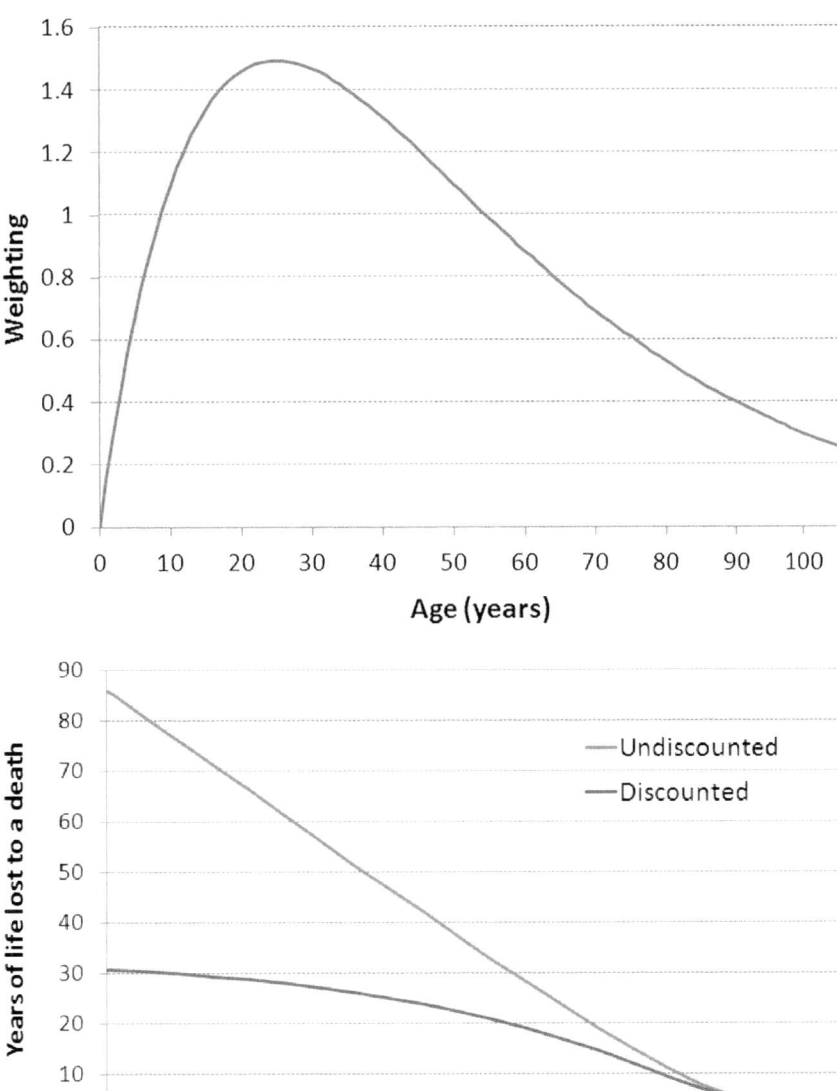

Figure 3.27

Illustration of discounted and undiscounted DALYs by age. The disability weight is higher for 20–40 years of age than those who are greater than 60 years of age or children under 10 years. Source: PAPP104 - S05: Measuring the burden of disease. UNFPA. Licensed under CC BY-SA 3.0.

An important part of the calculation of DALYs is the weighting by age. Figure 3.27 shows an illustration of discounted and undiscounted DALYs by age. The disability weight is higher for 20–40 years of age than those who are greater than 60 years of age or children under 10 years. The rationale for this weighting is that these individuals make the smallest contributions to the economy. Modifying the undiscounted graph by the weights results in almost a factor of three decrease for a child 10 years of age and decrease of 30 percent for someone who is 60 years of age, reducing the overall DALYs for these age groups.

> **Deeper Look: The DALY Dilemma**
>
> The calculation of DALYs is based on a societal construct of what is valued the most. Though it is widely used, it is not ideal. The first scenario relates to age. The DALY discounts future health gains and losses in children and the elderly. This assumption may not be true in all cultures. For example, in certain countries with a cash economy, children and elderly may in fact contribute to the workforce far more than the same population would in HICs. Another example would be the DALYs for two individuals, one who was born disabled and otherwise healthy, and the other who has a disability owing to an illness. Should a disabled person without an illness be valued less than a person who is disabled because of an illness? To tie this all together, consider the final scenario. Assume that a policymaker is able to invest in only one of two health initiatives. The first option will extend the life of one million healthy people for one year. The second will extend the life of one million people with cancer for one year. In either case the individuals will die at the end of one year. Which option should the policymaker pick? Based on the measure of DALYs it would be option two.

Looking Ahead

What we have learned in this chapter is that it is possible to develop accessible and affordable solutions that can bring screening and prevention of cervical cancer to the patient, rather than the other way around. This is in stark contrast to many of the solutions described in Chapter 2, where the cancer care continuum requires multiple touch points, different types of specialized technologies, and experts to interpret the results. Not only does the new cervical cancer prevention paradigm described in this chapter reduce the number of visits, it is less labor-intensive than standard-of-care methods. For example, the HPV test is quantitative (detects different HPV genotypes) and can be processed by a PCR machine. However, Pap smears require a centralized lab, extensive sample processing protocols, and a trained cytotechnologist who needs to find a few abnormal cells amid thousands of normal cells.

One challenge is that not all technologies are like the HPV test. Many affordable solutions will not be able to capture all of the attributes or surpass those of traditional devices and treatments. However, by concentrating on the core functionalities that present the highest amount of benefit to the end user, technologies can be developed to do a few things well. An illustrative example of the core functionalities criterion is the General Electric Vscan portable ultrasound machine (portable ultrasound will be discussed in greater detail in Chapter 5). The Vscan costs several thousand dollars rather than the hundreds of thousands for a bench-top ultrasound machine with all the bells and whistles. Even though it has a smaller field of view and penetration depth compared to bench-top ultrasounds, the portability and affordability of the Vscan can aid physical exams in rural communities to optimize treatment decisions.

There are different classes of technologies and/or services that can be disruptive in nature and transform healthcare access and outcomes. This can include technologies that have been repurposed from the applications they were originally intended for. An excellent example is the use of cell phones as both imaging technologies and as tools to facilitate new service delivery models. The second class of technologies uses the same principles as those designed for traditional equipment using lower-cost components to redesign them for context-specific use – the Vscan is a representative example. A third group of technologies is ones that result from transformative research efforts that reimagine solutions based on scientific advances. The next three chapters will describe these different types of technologies, beginning with molecular testing, progressing to imaging, and finally treatment.

SUMMARY

The cervix is seated at the lower end of the uterus, connecting the uterus to the vagina. Cervical precancer forms on the ectocervix, which can be viewed from outside the body. About 90 percent of cervical precancers are caused by persistent HPV infection, which over the course of 15–20 years can lead to the development of cervical precancer and cancer. This long time window provides ample opportunity for screening and early intervention to reduce incidence and mortality from cervical cancer.

The modern cervical cancer prevention paradigm is made up of three distinct stages: screening, diagnosis, and treatment. At each stage a decision is made as to whether the patient needs further care. The tools used in modern gynecological practice have been shaped primarily by three founders: George Papanicolaou, Hans Hinselmann, and James Marion Sims, who invented the Pap smear, colposcope, and speculum, respectively. Each of these innovations remain mainstays of cervical cancer prevention today. The Pap smear, despite its low sensitivity (high false negative rate) for detecting cervical precancer, has dramatically reduced mortality from cervical cancer through early and multiple screenings. The decision to move a patient through each stage of the three-visit process is based on cytology and pathology. Cytology involves the identification of a few positive or abnormal-looking cells in an otherwise large population of normal cells. Pathology provides a transverse section of the tissue and helps assess the stage of the disease by assessing the location and morphology of the abnormal cells.

The discovery of the link between HPV infection and cervical cancer allowed for new innovations in the cervical cancer prevention paradigm. The development of vaccines against HPV 16 and HPV 18, the two strains of HPV responsible for over 70 percent of cervical cancers, provides us with a new tool in our arsenal for preventing cervical cancer. The vaccine is given prior to any sexual activity that causes infection with the HPV virus. HPV testing is critical for those who have already matured out of the eligibility for the vaccine. The HPV test is not only quantitative; it has a much higher sensitivity than the Pap smear. It also allows for self-collection, after which the sample is processed in a lab. This has also shaped new guidelines for cervical cancer screening. HPV self-tests are allowing more women in LMICs, who have traditionally been hard to reach, to be screened for cervical precancer.

Unfortunately, despite numerous technical innovations aimed at reducing incidence of cervical cancer, it continues to persist today, with glaring disparities between wealthy and poor nations. This is in large part due to lack of access to the HPV vaccine, screening modalities, and therapy. The WHO's call to action has put global cervical cancer prevention on the international stage and clear metrics have been established against which to measure progress. New innovations are now in place to prevent cervical cancer mortality for the more than 500,000 women diagnosed with this devastating disease each year. Disability-adjusted life years is a useful metric for determining allocation of resources to put these programs in place. This system includes both a mortality and morbidity term to reflect the global burden of disease. Mortality alone does not account for the poor quality of life that cancer causes and the devastating impact on families and communities.

PROBLEMS

The Cervix and Cervical Cancer

1. What are the main features of the reproductive anatomy, and what role does each feature play?
2. If a pathologist is examining a slide of a transverse section of cervical tissue and observes a high density of cells in the epithelium, what feature will indicate whether the patient has precancer or cancer?
3. What protein does the HPV virus inhibit and what is the result of this? What is the normal function of the protein? If the HPV virus infection does not resolve and initiates the development of cervical precancer, approximately how long will it take for the individual to develop cancer?
4. Screening is needed for different populations – for example, one in which the cervical cancer prevalence is extremely low at 4 cases per 100,000, and another

in which the prevalence is extremely high at 40 per 100,000. Assuming that the Pap smear has a sensitivity of 50 percent and specificity of 95 percent, how many potential cancers could be missed in each population during a single screening event?

5. Increasing the rate of screening can decrease the incidence of cervical cancer and, as a result, cervical cancer mortality. Assuming the time from developing a low-grade cervical precancer (i.e., CIN I) to ICC is 15 years, anyone treated for cervical precancer during that 15-year period will not develop ICC, and everyone is screened five times during that period using a Pap smear, how would the number of women with ICC compare to that in question 4?

The Evolution of Modern Gynecology

6. What single invention led to a dramatic decline in cervical cancer in the US?
7. What strategy makes the Pap smear effective even though it has a low sensitivity? What is the difference between a cytology section and a pathology section? Which sample provides information on the stage of the disease?
8. Assume the Pap smear has a sensitivity and specificity of approximately 50 percent and 95 percent, respectively. Assume that the prevalence of cervical precancer is approximately 2 percent (200 for every 10,000 women screened). In a population of 100,000 women, how many true positives will the Pap smear detect? How many false positives will the Pap smear detect? Assuming the cost for each Pap smear is $5, what is the cost per positive detected?
9. For women who screen positive (true positives and false positives), colposcopy is performed. Assume colposcopy with biopsy has a sensitivity of 95 percent and a specificity of 50 percent. For the number of women who screen positive, how many true positives and false positives will colposcopy and biopsy detect? Assuming that the cost of colposcopy per patient is $300, what is the cost per positive detected?
10. Assuming that all patients who have precancer are treated and the treatment is successful, how many lives are saved? Assume 2 lives saved for every 100 women screened. What is the cost for each life saved based on the total cost of the Pap smear, colposcopy, and biopsy?

The Virus That Has Revolutionized Screening

11. Which two strains of HPV account for more than half of cervical cancer cases? For these two strains, which is most likely to lead to cancer and what will be the incidence rate of high-grade precancer (CIN II+) at five years follow-up for this particular HPV strain?

12. What is the reason for restricting the HPV vaccine to those who have not yet had sexual intercourse? Which region of the world has had the highest vaccination rate? Which region has had the lowest vaccination rate? What is one reason for this disparity?
13. Screening is needed for different populations – for example, one in which the cervical cancer prevalence is extremely low at 4 cases per 100,000, and another in which the prevalence is extremely high at 40 per 100,000. Which screening test is best suited for the low- and high-prevalence populations?
14. HPV testing has a sensitivity of 95 percent and specificity of 80 percent. Assume the sensitivity and specificity of the Pap smear is 50 percent and 95 percent, respectively. Assume that the prevalence of cervical precancer is approximately 2 percent (200 for every 10,000 women screened). In a population of 100,000 women, how many positives and negatives will the Pap smear indicate? Assuming that all true positives are appropriately managed, and all negatives do not get follow-up screening, how many individuals will have cancer with each screening test? Repeat this for HPV testing. Assume the HPV test has a sensitivity and specificity of 95 percent and 80 percent, respectively.
15. Assume the cost for follow-up is $5. How much will be spent in the case of the Pap and HPV test? Based on the response above, what is the cost of each type of test? Which one is more expensive? How many lives are saved (assume that all positives were treated and none of the negatives were treated)?

Cervical Cancer Is a Disease of Health Disparities

16. Seventy percent of cervical cancer deaths occur in LMICs. Does this refer to health disparity or health equity?
17. Assume the exact same care services provided in the US are provided in the countries with the highest burden of disease. What word would best describe this – equity or equality? Why? Disparities in cervical cancer screening place an undue cancer burden on LMIC health systems. Which of the four areas of social determinants of health does this relate to?
18. What will be the projected reduction in deaths in 2040 for a program that has no vaccination or screening program; vaccination only; and vaccination, twice-lifetime HPV screening, and cancer treatment? Why is vaccination alone not as effective as vaccination combined with screening and treatment?
19. Ablative therapies are emerging as possible alternatives to traditional forms of therapy in LMICs. Thermocoagulation was provided as an example for treating cervical precancers in this chapter. What is one advantage of ablative therapies over surgery? What is one disadvantage? What makes a patient ineligible for ablation?

20. Assume the following about Kenya:
    - Average age at diagnosis for cervical cancer is 50.
    - Average age at death from cervical cancer is 59.
    - Number of people diagnosed with cervical cancer per year is 4,000.
    - Number of people who die from cervical cancer each year is 2,000.

    (a) Calculate the DALYs if the discount rate is 5 percent.
    (b) If a new screening and treatment strategy is implemented that reduces the number of women diagnosed with cervical cancer by 80 percent, what is the new DALYs?

REFERENCES

Arbyn, M., Weiderpass, E., Bruni, L., et al. 2020. Estimates of incidence and mortality of cervical cancer in 2018: a worldwide analysis. *The Lancet Global Health*, 8, e191–e203.

Arie, S. 2019. HPV: WHO calls for countries to suspend vaccination of boys. *BMJ*, 367, l6765.

Bednarczyk, R. A., Ellingson, M. K., & Omer, S. B. 2019. Human papillomavirus vaccination before 13 and 15 years of age: analysis of national immunization survey teen data. *Journal of Infectious Diseases*, 220, 730–734.

Blumberg, B. S. 1997. Hepatitis B virus, the vaccine, and the control of primary cancer of the liver. *Proceedings of the National Academy of Sciences*, 94, 7121–7125.

Bruni, L., Diaz, M., Barrionuevo-Rosas, L., et al. 2016. Global estimates of human papillomavirus vaccination coverage by region and income level: a pooled analysis. *The Lancet Global Health*, 4, e453–e463.

Centers for Disease Control and Prevention. 1999. Achievements in public health, 1900–1999: tobacco use – United States, 1900–1999. *MMWR*, 48, 986–993.

Crowley D, L. G. 2012. Emotional aspects of gynecology: depression, anxiety, PTSD, eating disorders, substance abuse, "difficult" patients, sexual function, rape, intimate partner violence, and grief. In Lentz, G., Lobo, R., Gershenson, D., & Katz, V. (eds), *Comprehensive Gynecology*, 6th ed., Elsevier, New York.

Dürst, M., Gissmann, L., Ikenberg, H., & zur Hausen, H. 1983. A papillomavirus DNA from a cervical carcinoma and its prevalence in cancer biopsy samples from different geographic regions. *Proceedings of the National Academy of Sciences*, 80, 3812–3815.

Fusco, E., Padula, F., Mancini, E., Cavaliere, A., & Grubisic, G. 2008. History of colposcopy: a brief biography of Hinselmann. *Journal of Prenatal Medicine*, 2, 19.

Garcia-Moreno, C., Jansen, H. A., Ellsberg, M., et al. 2006. Prevalence of intimate partner violence: findings from the WHO multi-country study on women's health and domestic violence. *The Lancet*, 368, 1260–1269.

Gupta, S., Palmer, C., Bik, E. M., et al. 2018. Self-sampling for human papillomavirus testing: increased cervical cancer screening participation and incorporation in international screening programs. *Frontiers in Public Health*, 6, 77.

IARC. 2012. GLOBOCAN Cervix Uteri ASR (W) per 100,000, all ages [Online]. Available: http://globocan.iarc.fr/old/bar_sex_site.asp?selection=4162&title=Cervix+uteri&statistic=2&populations=6&window=1&grid=1&color1=5&color1e=&color2=4&color2e=&submit=%C2%A0Execute (accessed June 27, 2016).

Joshi, S., Muwonge, R., Kulkarni, V., Deodhar, K., Mandolkar, M., Lucas, E., & Sankaranarayanan, R. 2019. Incidence of cervical intraepithelial neoplasia in women infected with human immunodeficiency virus (HIV) with no evidence of disease at baseline: Results of a prospective cohort study with up to 6.4 years of follow-up from India. *International Journal of Cancer*, 144, 1082–1091. https://doi.org/10.1002/ijc.31826.

Kenny, S. C., Ward, J. L., & Bryan, C. S. 1999. James Marion Sims and the rise of gynaecological surgery. *Journal of Medical Biography*, 7, 217–223.

Kobara, H., Uchita, K., Uedo, N., et al. 2021. Flexible magnifying endoscopy with narrow band imaging for diagnosing uterine cervical neoplasms: a multicenter prospective study. *Journal of Clinical Medicine*, 10(20), 4753. https://doi.org/10.3390/jcm10204753.

Kripke, C. 2008. Pap smear vs. HPV screening tests for cervical cancer. *American Family Physician*, 77, 1740.

Lees, B. F., Erickson, B. K., & Huh, W. K. 2016. Cervical cancer screening: evidence behind the guidelines. *American Journal of Obstetrics and Gynecology*, 214, 438–443.

Lyimo, F. S., & Beran, T. N. 2012. Demographic, knowledge, attitudinal, and accessibility factors associated with uptake of cervical cancer screening among women in a rural district of Tanzania: three public policy implications. *BMC Public Health*, 12, 22.

Maclean, J. S. 1979. The life of Hans Hinselmann. *Obstetrical & Gynecological Survey*, 34, 788–789.

Murray, C. J., & Lopez, A. D. 1996. Evidence-based health policy: lessons from the Global Burden of Disease Study. *Science*, 274(5288), 740–743.

National Vaccine Advisory Committee. 2016. Overcoming barriers to low HPV vaccine uptake in the United States: recommendations from the National Vaccine Advisory Committee: approved by the National Vaccine Advisory Committee on June 9, 2015. *Public Health Reports*, 131, 17–25.

Randall, T. C., & Ghebre, R. 2016. Challenges in prevention and care delivery for women with cervical cancer in Sub-Saharan Africa. *Frontiers in Oncology*, 6, 160.

Safaeian, M., Solomon, D., & Castle, P. E. 2007. Cervical cancer prevention: cervical screening – science in evolution. *Obstetrics and Gynecology Clinics of North America*, 34, 739–760.

Santesso, N., Schunemann, H., Blumenthal, P., et al. 2012. World Health Organization guidelines: use of cryotherapy for cervical intraepithelial neoplasia. *International Journal of Gynaecology and Obstetrics*, 118, 97–102.

Siegel, R. L., Miller, K. D., & Jemal, A. 2020. Cancer statistics, 2020. *CA: A Cancer Journal for Clinicians*, 70, 7–30.

Skloot, R. 2010. *The Immortal Life of Henrietta Lacks*, Broadway Books, Portland, OR.

Wentzensen, N., & Schiffman, M. 2018. Accelerating cervical cancer control and prevention. *The Lancet Public Health*, 3, E6–E7.

Williams, C. M., McCloskey, L. A., & Larsen, U. 2008. Sexual violence at first intercourse against women in Moshi, northern Tanzania: prevalence, risk factors, and consequences. *Population Studies*, 62, 335–348.

Wright Jr, T. C., Gagnon, S., Richart, R. M., & Ferenczy, A. 1992. Treatment of cervical intraepithelial neoplasia using the loop electrosurgical excision procedure. *Obstetrics and Gynecology*, 79, 173–178.

Yang, D. X., Soulos, P. R., Davis, B., Gross, C. P., & Yu, J. B. 2018. Impact of widespread cervical cancer screening: number of cancers prevented and changes in race-specific incidence. *American Journal of Clinical Oncology*, 41, 89–294. doi: 10.1097/COC.0000000000000264. PMID: 26808257; PMCID: PMC4958036.

Yu, L., Sabatino, S. A., & White, M. C. 2019. Rural–urban and racial/ethnic disparities in invasive cervical cancer incidence in the United States, 2010–2014. *Preventing Chronic Disease*, 16, E70.

4 Point-of-Care Assays for Examining Body Fluids and Cells

There is an enormous economic incentive at present to create **point-of-care technologies (POCTs)** for early detection of disease. A recent example of a POCT is the rapid antigen test that uses the concept of a lateral flow assay (LFA), which will be discussed later in this chapter. Figure 4.1 shows some of the advantages of point-of-care diagnostics. Over the last 5–10 years the market size for POCTs has steadily increased. Infectious diseases lead the way for POCT, with the largest market size; however, oncology represents a close second. POCTs have the potential to detect disease at its earliest stages and inform multiple treatment options that can prevent the disease from becoming untreatable. In addition, these POCTs can increase our understanding of molecular mechanisms that underpin cancer, as well as other rare disorders.

An early example of the impact of POCTs is the home pregnancy test. In 1967, Margaret Crane was working at a pharmaceuticals lab when she observed the information flow of pregnancy tests: the patient gives a sample to a physician; the physician ships the sample to a lab; the lab analyzes the sample and sends the results to the physician; and, finally, the physician delivers the results to the patient. She realized this process was quite cumbersome and results were not returned until days or even weeks after the test. Margaret considered what it would be like to relocate this test from the physician's office and the lab to a woman's home. "It was a way for a woman to peer into her own body and find out about her status, without anyone else – husband, boyfriend, boss, doctor – getting in the way" (Kennedy, 2016). But, as is the case with many radical ideas, Ms. Crane's ideas were blocked by higher-ups in the company. The physicians felt threatened: If the women did the tests themselves, it would take away the need for their services. The managers were afraid that if women found out they were pregnant they would become distraught and kill themselves. Despite having her ideas criticized, Ms. Crane persisted; her developed at-home pregnancy tests became available in 1977. "Today, eight out of 10 women learn they are pregnant from a drugstore device" (Kennedy, 2016).

The at-home pregnancy test is one example of a technology that can be implemented in a decentralized location. Chapter 2 discussed a number of

Assays for Examining Body Fluids and Cells

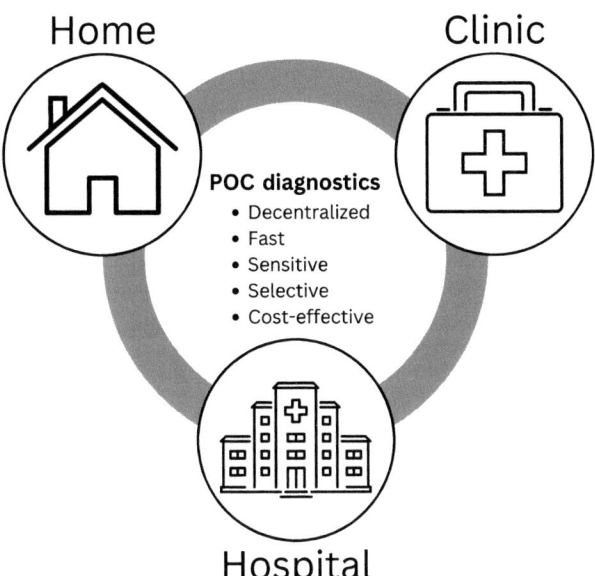

Figure 4.1 Advantages of point-of-care diagnostics. Over the last 5–10 years the market size for POCTs has steadily increased. Infectious diseases lead the way for POCT, with the largest market size; however, oncology represents a close second. The market size for these POCTs is projected to continue to increase through the 2020s.

different advancements in technology that have improved cancer control in the US, but many of them are only accessible in centralized locations, owing to many of the changes in the healthcare system, as described in Chapter 1. Chapter 3 used cervical cancer as an example to show how technological advancements that improve cancer control in the US frequently do not benefit resource-limited settings in low- and middle-income countries (LMICs). Chapter 3 also introduced a POCT for the HPV virus that is likely one of the most effective ways to achieve widespread screening of cervical cancer. This chapter introduces the concept of POCTs as a means to improve access to quality healthcare. Specifically, this chapter will focus on POCT counterparts to laboratory-based tests for examining bodily fluids and cells, like those discussed in Chapter 2. Many of these tests can be performed in a primary care setting or by the individual at home, in the same way that the blood test for pregnancy was performed in the clinic and can now be performed at home.

LEARNING OBJECTIVES

The Origins of Point-of-Care Testing
- The time course of an immune response to a viral infection and how it can be leveraged for molecular testing;
- different types of ELISAs and the specific indication for which each of them might be used;
- different types of samples that can be used for molecular testing and the pros and cons of each.

Point-of-Care Molecular Testing
- The design of a POCT as a surrogate for a gold standard laboratory test;
- the principles behind the LFA, microfluidics, and paper assays;
- the different methods for detecting outputs from POCTs.

Point-of-Care Testing and Cancer: Collecting Appropriate Samples
- The different types of POCTs being used for applications in cancer screening;
- different sample collection methods and what biomarkers they contain;
- circulating tumor cells and circulating tumor DNA for the detection of cancer and for cancer research.

The Origins of Point-of-Care Testing

The modern-day pregnancy test inspired by Margaret Crane is just one example of an improved workflow made possible using a POCT. Another example of at-home testing is the blood glucose test. In 1965, the first blood glucose test strip was created, containing an enzyme called glucose oxidase. A drop of blood was placed on the strip and then washed after 60 seconds. The glucose oxidase enzyme reacts with glucose, water, and oxygen to form gluconic acid and hydrogen peroxide. The hydrogen peroxide oxidizes a colorless organic compound to a stable-colored product, which is then used to estimate the amount of glucose present in the blood. The first glucose meter was used in the 1970s in physicians' offices. By 1980, the first at-home glucose meter was launched. Self-monitoring of blood glucose became the standard of care, especially for patients with type 1 diabetes. The evolution of at-home glucose monitoring was further revolutionized with the introduction of continuous glucose monitoring. Today, continuous glucose monitoring has drastically improved the way diabetes is managed (Clarke and Foster, 2012).

The largest market share for POCTs is infectious disease. The viral DNA or RNA, proteins on the surface of the virus, or proteins such as antibodies that the body produces can all be used as **biomarkers** of viral infection. A **biomarker** is a target that reports on some aspect of disease. For example, a biomarker could report on whether someone is actively infected with a particular virus. The gold standard for the detection of viral infections is the detection of nucleic acids in the virus (i.e., DNA or RNA). This is performed using a method called polymerase chain reaction (PCR), the details of which are described in Chapter 2. PCR requires a centralized facility, sophisticated equipment, and trained technicians. The antibodies or viral proteins are detected using an enzyme-linked immunosorbent assay, or ELISA (also described in Chapter 2). POCTs at present cannot be used to directly test for nucleic acids; however, samples can be self-collected and sent to a laboratory for PCR. On

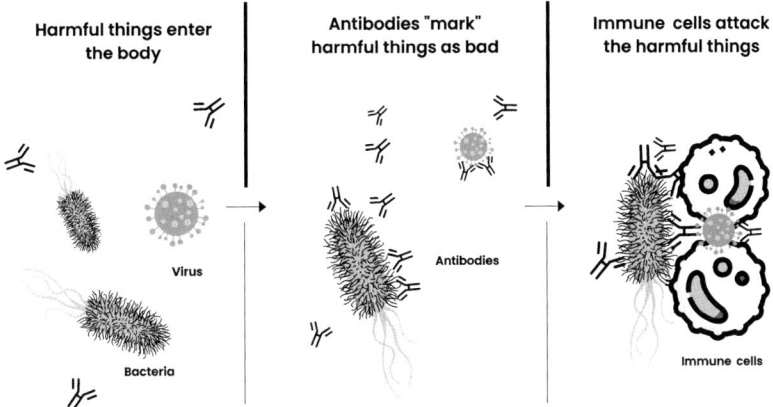

Figure 4.2 Foreign invaders lead to the development of antibodies. The immune system attempts to recognize and label foreign objects within the body for destruction. When a bacteria or virus enters the body, specialized cells in the immune system, called B cells, produce antibodies that can specifically bind to proteins on the surface of the bacteria or virus. These antibodies can then signal to other cells within the immune system that the bacteria, virus, or virus-infected cell needs to be destroyed. Antibodies can persist in circulation for weeks, months, or even years following viral infection.

the other hand, POCTs can be developed to detect antibodies generated in response to the viruses, and serve as a portable, albeit simpler, version of the ELISA test. Though antibody testing is less sensitive than a PCR test, it does offer the advantage of decentralizing the test and providing a rapid turnaround time. POCTs are versatile; they can detect antibodies in blood, saliva, or urine.

Figure 4.2 shows how foreign invaders lead to the development of antibodies. The immune system attempts to recognize and label foreign objects within the body for destruction. When a bacteria or virus enters the body, specialized cells in the immune system, called B cells, produce antibodies that can specifically bind to proteins on the surface of the bacteria or virus. These antibodies can then signal to other cells within the immune system that the bacteria, virus, or virus-infected cell needs to be destroyed. Antibodies can persist in circulation for weeks, months, or even years following viral infection.

There are five different classes of antibodies that can be produced by the immune system: IgG, IgM, IgA, IgD, and IgE. Three of these – IgG, IgM, and IgA – are important with respect to viral infections (Klimpcl, 1996). **IgM** is the first antibody produced during an antiviral immune response and has limited specificity for the virus. **IgG** and **IgA** are the second antibodies produced and have a higher specificity for the virus. Antibody levels can be used to determine when a viral infection has occurred, since their levels are dependent on the time since infection.

An antibody test is not as effective as the PCR test as it can miss the presence of the virus altogether. For instance, if the immune system successfully clears the infection prior to the development of measurable antibody levels, as is the case for viral infections such as influenza (common flu), an antibody test cannot report on an active infection. Viruses that are not rapidly cleared, such as human papillomavirus (HPV), human immunodeficiency virus (HIV), and hepatitis B, can be reliably detected via antibody testing owing to the fact that there is a longer window in which to perform the test. At the same time, because it takes time for antibodies to develop following an infection, a negative antibody test for HPV, HIV, or hepatitis B does not guarantee that a person is not currently infected.

HIV has long dominated the global burden of infectious disease since it was discovered in the 1980s. Just as HPV testing will be central to the elimination of cervical cancer, HIV testing is an integral part of ending the autoimmune deficiency syndrome (AIDS) epidemic, the disease caused by persistent HIV infection. There are three prominent types of HIV tests available: RNA tests, antibody/antigen combined tests, and antibody-only tests. Each test looks for a different target or biomarker. PCR tests, also referred to as nucleic acid amplification tests (NAATs), look for the presence of viral RNA in a collected sample. Antibody/antigen combined tests and antibody tests look for the presence of HIV-specific antigens (p24) and antibodies (anti-gp41 IgM, anti-p24 IgG, and anti-gp120 IgG). Each of these tests is useful at different points during HIV infection (Delaney et al., 2017).

Figure 4.3 shows the target detection levels following HIV transmission. The three main types of HIV testing each look at different biomarkers to determine the presence or absence of HIV. Biomarker expression levels change during the different stages of HIV infection. Viral RNA levels rise the quickest, and are detectable within about a week of HIV infection. Antigen levels (i.e., p24 levels) rise second quickest, around two weeks post-infection. The antibody levels are the slowest to rise, as they require the immune system to respond to HIV infection and then produce antibodies. While RNA and antigen levels are highest initially, persistent HIV infection leads to continual production of antibodies, allowing for HIV diagnoses months or even years after infection. Figure 4.3 also shows the different levels of RNA, antigen, and antibody present within the body following HIV infection and how either NAATs or ELISA can be used to detect HIV. It is important to consider the time since potential infection when deciding which type of test will be most appropriate to use: NAATs are the most sensitive, followed by antigen, and then antibody testing. The least sensitive method, a **Western blot**, uses gel electrophoresis to separate the proteins in a sample. The separated proteins are transferred out of the gel to the surface of a membrane.

How do HIV tests work? We will focus here on antibody and antigen HIV tests, since those are the tests most commonly used for POCT development. Both antigen and antibody HIV tests are performed using an ELISA, which was briefly discussed in Chapter 2. Figure 4.4 shows the different types of ELISAs. The four main types of ELISAs are direct ELISA, indirect ELISA,

The Origins of Point-of-Care Testing

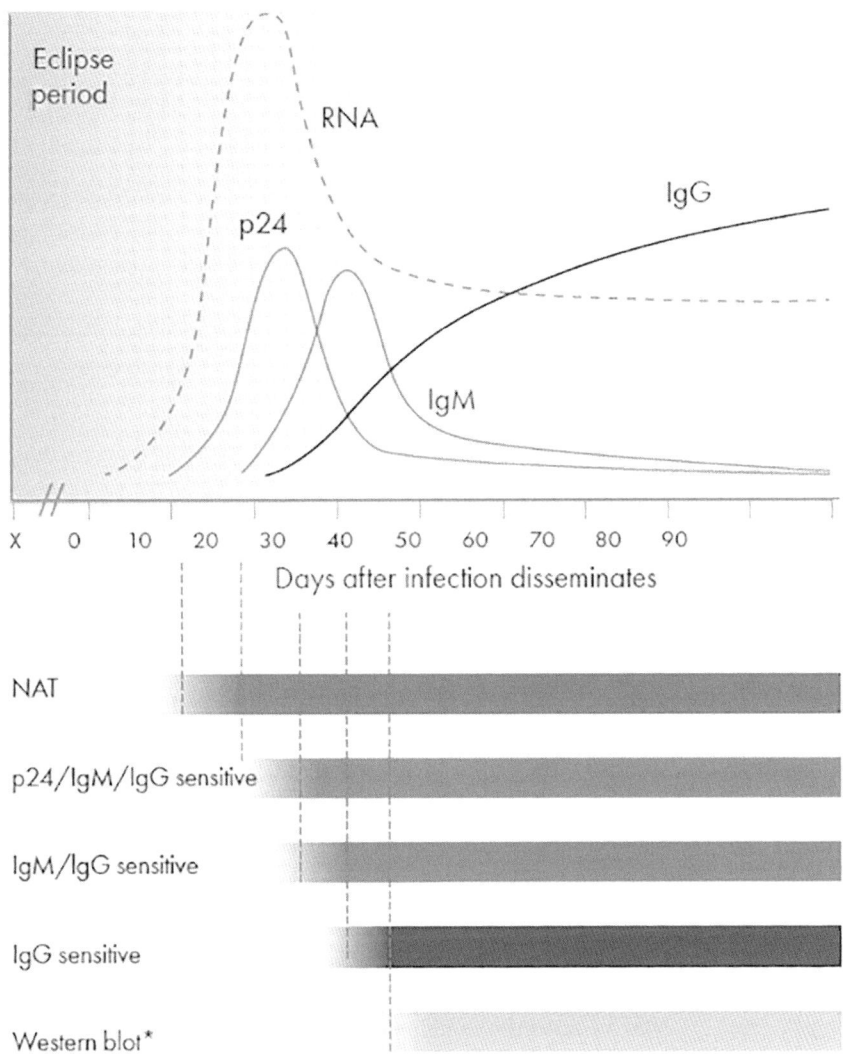

* Western blot is no longer used for HIV.

Figure 4.3 Target detection levels following HIV transmission. The three main types of HIV testing each look at different biomarkers to determine the presence or absence of HIV. Biomarker expression levels change during the different stages of HIV infection. Viral RNA levels rise the quickest, being present at detectable levels within about a week of HIV infection. Antigen levels (i.e., p24 levels) rise second quickest, around two weeks post-infection. The antibody levels are the slowest to rise, as they require the immune system to respond to HIV infection and then produce antibodies. While RNA and antigen levels are highest initially, persistent HIV infection leads to continual production of antibodies, allowing for HIV diagnoses months or even years after infection.
Source: Centers for Disease Control and Prevention.

sandwich ELISA, and competitive ELISA. Direct, indirect, and sandwich ELISAs measure the amount of target (Ag) present in the sample by optically measuring the amount of antibody bound to the target from the sample. As a

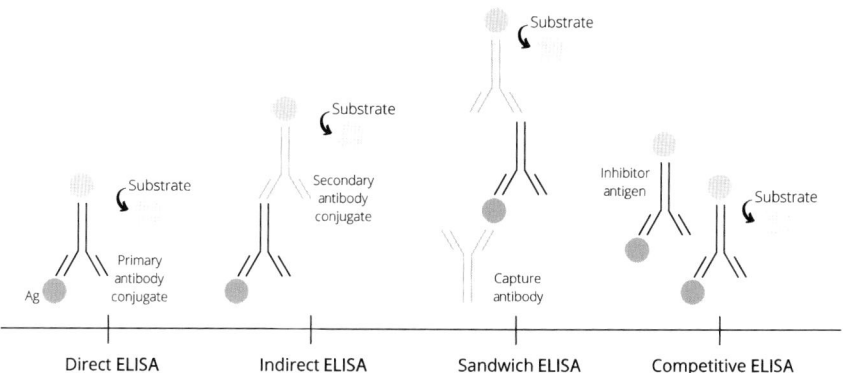

Figure 4.4 Different types of ELISAs. The four main types of ELISAs are direct, indirect, sandwich, and competitive ELISAs. Direct, indirect, and sandwich ELISAs measure the amount of target (Ag) present in the sample by optically measuring the amount of antibody bound to the target from the sample. As a result, the amount of signal present is directly proportional to the amount of target in the sample. Competitive ELISAs measure the amount of unbound antibody present following incubation of the sample. Unlike the other three ELISAs, the signal from a competitive ELISA is inversely proportional to the amount of target present in the sample.

result, the amount of signal present is directly proportional to the amount of target in the sample. Competitive ELISAs measure the amount of unbound antibody present following incubation of the sample. Unlike the other three ELISAs, the signal from a competitive ELISA is inversely proportional to the amount of target present in the sample.

Direct ELISAs look for the presence of a particular antigen or antibody by immobilizing the sample on a plate, adding a target-specific **conjugated antibody** that can be measured optically (either a molecule that has a high absorption or fluorescence to the plate) to determine the amount of primary antibody present. A **conjugated antibody** is a polyclonal or monoclonal antibody that has a molecule attached, which can be used to create a detectable signal. Though a direct ELISA is fairly easy to perform, most antibodies have some level of nonspecific binding, which can lead to a high background signal.

Indirect ELISAs work similarly to the direct ELISA with one small, but important, difference. In an indirect ELISA, the sample is immobilized on the plate, a primary antibody specific to the target is added to the plate, and a secondary detection antibody that specifically binds to the primary antibody is also added to the plate. The addition of the secondary detection antibody improves signal amplification in cases where there is only a small amount of the target present, as multiple secondary antibodies can bind to a single primary antibody to increase the amount of signal present.

The indirect ELISA targets the sample, which is immobilized on the surface of the plate. As a result, indirect ELISAs can have a high background signal caused by nonspecific binding of the primary or secondary antibodies to the plate, which is designed to "stick" to proteins. The sandwich ELISA was developed to help mitigate high background signal. Rather than fixing the sample to the plate, a capture antibody that is specific to the target is immobilized to the plate. The sample is then added and the antibodies in the sample are expected to bind to the capture antibody. Any sample that is not bound to a capture antibody is then washed away. Next, the antibody conjugate is added to the sample for detection. A secondary conjugate antibody is added to amplify the signal from the first.

The final type of ELISA is the competitive ELISA, which is distinct relative to the other three types. Competitive ELISAs are performed by immobilizing the target antigen on a plate. The collected sample is incubated with a detection antibody. In this incubated solution there will be antibody bound to antigen as well as unbound antibody. The solution is added to the plate. Any antibody that is already bound to the target in the sample will not be able to bind with the target on the plate. In other words, only unbound antibody will bind to the plate. The plate is then washed, removing any antibody not bound to the plate. As a result, if more target is present in the sample, less free antibody will be available to bind to the plate. Conversely, if less target is present in the sample, more free antibodies will be available to bind to the plate. As a result, the amount of signal present in the plate is inversely proportional to the amount of target in the sample, unlike direct, indirect, and sandwich ELISAs, where the amount of signal is directly proportional to the amount of target in the sample.

Example: Which ELISA Test Is Better?

Question: A biomedical engineer is tasked with developing an ELISA that could be used to detect a marker in blood that indicates the levels of a breast cancer antigen. The antigen has very low levels in the blood. The engineer is trying to decide between using a direct vs indirect ELISA. Which would be the better choice and why?

Answer: Direct ELISAs use a single antibody to detect the presence of an antigen, whereas indirect antibodies use two antibodies, a primary and a secondary. The addition of a secondary antibody allows for signal amplification when there are low levels of the antigen present; therefore, an indirect ELISA would be more appropriate than a direct ELISA.

Now we will take a closer look at the evolution of ELISA-based HIV tests over time. The earliest generations of HIV testing were based on indirect ELISA and developed in the mid to late 1980s. The tests looked for the presence of HIV IgG antibodies from a blood sample. Both generations had excellent sensitivity and specificity for detecting the two major subtypes of HIV: HIV-1 (generation 1 and 2) and HIV-2 (generation 2 only). The third generation HIV test, which was introduced in the early 1990s, used a sandwich ELISA to test for HIV IgM antibodies, which are produced earlier than HIV IgG antibodies. In the late 1990s, the fourth-generation sandwich ELISA HIV test became available, which added p24 antigen testing. Antigens are detectable in the blood earlier than antibodies and, as a result, indicate an earlier stage of infection. One shortcoming of the fourth-generation test was the inability to differentiate between an antigen-positive result and an antibody-positive result. The fifth generation of HIV testing overcame this obstacle, allowing for both antibody and antigen results to be differentiated through **fluorescence multiplexing**. **Fluorescence multiplexing** refers to the ability to detect the levels of fluorophores with different emission wavelengths. Table 4.1 summarizes the evolution of HIV diagnostic testing (Alexander, 2016). Diagnostic HIV testing is just one example of ELISA-based testing. We will review later in the chapter the use of ELISA-based tests for applications in cancer.

Table 4.1 Evolution of HIV diagnostic tests over time.

Year	1985	1987	1991	1997	2015
Generation	First	Second	Third	Fourth	Fifth
Antigen (ag) source	Virus-infected cell lysate	Recombinant and synthetic peptides	Recombinant and synthetic peptides	Recombinant and synthetic peptides	Recombinant and synthetic peptides
Specificity	95–98%	>99%	>99.5%	99.5%	99.5%
Sensitivity	99%	>99.5%	>99.5%	>99.8%	100%
Negative window	8–10 weeks	4–6 weeks	2–3 weeks	2 weeks	2 weeks
Detects antibody (Ab) and Ag	IgG Anti HIV-1	IgG Anti HIV-1 and HIV-2	IgG and IgM Anti HIV-1, HIV-2, and Group o	IgG Anti HIV-1, HIV-2, and Group o. Also detects HIV-1 p24 Ag	IgG Anti HIV-1, HIV-2, and Group o. Also detects HIV-1 p24 Ag
Results	Single result	Single result	Single result	Single result; does not differentiate Ab from Ag positivity	Separate HIV-1 and HIV-2 and Ag results
Confirming tests	HIV-1 Western blot or immunofluorescence	HIV-1 WB or IFA, HIV-2 ELISA and WB if HIV-1 confirm is negative	HIV-1 WB or IFA, HIV-2 ELISA and WB if HIV-1 confirm is negative	HIV-1/-2 differentiation assay followed by qualitative HIV-1 RNA PCR if differentiation assay is negative	Not determined at the time of this writing

Deeper Look: HIV Testing in Sub-Saharan Africa

Two-thirds of all people infected with HIV live in Sub-Saharan Africa. One of the key metrics for eliminating the spread of HIV is testing so that infected individuals know their status. Unfortunately, HIV infection has minimal symptoms, and many people do not even realize they are currently infected and are potentially spreading the virus to others. Startlingly, in 2000 only around 5.7 percent of infected individuals in Sub-Saharan Africa were aware of their status. Lack of awareness and barriers to HIV testing represented major reasons for this abysmal testing rate. Fortunately, the development of POCTs and integration of HIV testing with other common healthcare visits has drastically improved the testing rates. The improved access to diagnostic testing over the last two decades has resulted in approximately 84 percent of HIV-infected individuals in Sub-Saharan Africa being aware of their status (Giguère et al., 2021). HIV testing is an essential gateway to HIV prevention, treatment with antiretroviral therapy (ART), care, and support services. Figure 4.5 shows the number of deaths per 100,000 between 1990 and 2017 in Sub-Saharan Africa. There has been a steep decline in the number of deaths from AIDS-related illness in Sub-Saharan Africa, which is home to 53 percent of the world's people living with HIV. In short, AIDS-related mortality has declined owing to HIV testing and ART.

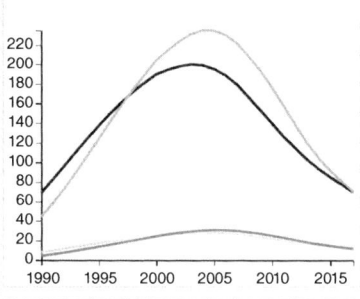
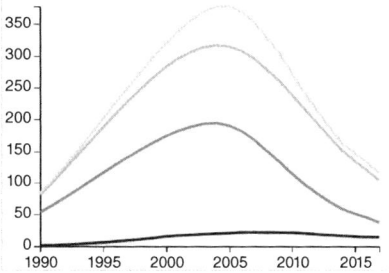

Figure 4.5 Number of deaths per 100,000 between 1990 and 2017 in Sub-Saharan Africa. There has been a steep decline in the number of deaths from AIDS-related illness in Sub-Saharan Africa, which is home to 53 percent of the world's people living with HIV. In short, AIDS-related mortality has declined owing to HIV testing and ART.
Source: Burden and changes in HIV/AIDS morbidity and mortality in Southern Africa Development Community Countries, 1990–2017. BMC Public Health. Licensed under CC BY-SA 4.0.

How can the basic principles that underly ELISA tests be leveraged to develop POCTs? To answer that question, we will first discuss biomarkers. Biomarkers are at the heart of POCT development. Unlike the complex "omics" tests discussed in Chapter 2, which required huge amounts of laboratory resources and

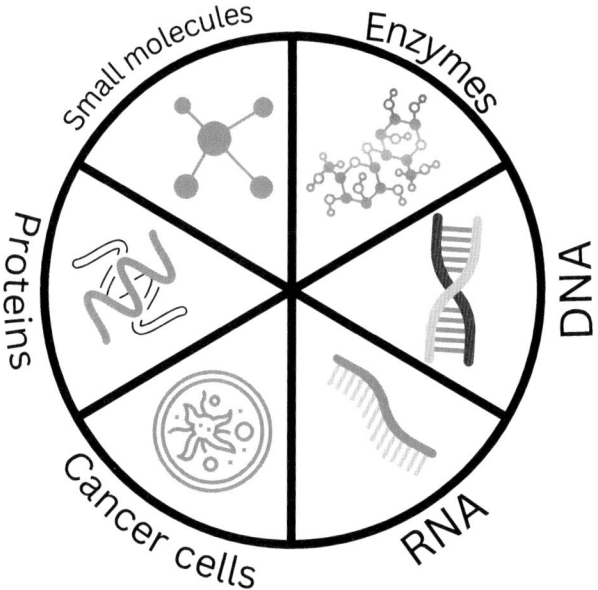

Figure 4.6 Different biomarkers that can be targets for POCTs. Each POCT is designed to test for a specific biomarker that serves as a surrogate to report on the presence/absence of disease or provide additional information about the disease. Examples of different biomarkers that are compatible with POCTs include small molecules such as metabolites, enzymes that catalyze chemical reactions, DNA, RNA, cancer cells, or proteins such as HER2.

computational power to study large amounts of data, POCTs tend to focus on a singular endpoint or biomarker. It is this focus on a single biomarker that makes POCT testing possible. Without the ability to perform "omics" studies to identify specific targets and biomarkers, POCTs for diseases such as cancer would be nearly impossible to develop. Figure 4.6 shows different biomarkers that can be targets for POCTs. Each POCT is designed to test for a specific biomarker that serves as a surrogate to report on the presence/absence of disease or provide additional information about the disease. Examples of different biomarkers that are compatible with POCTs include small molecules like metabolites, enzymes that catalyze chemical reactions, DNA, RNA, cancer cells, or proteins such as HER2. The next section will take a closer look at the different types of POCTs that can be used to detect these biomarkers.

Point-of-Care Molecular Testing

Molecular tests have become more accessible to patients through the evolution of innovative testing procedures, from ones that were expensive and centralized to portable technologies that can be used in decentralized facilities or even an individual's home. In this section we will look at different types

Point-of-Care Molecular Testing

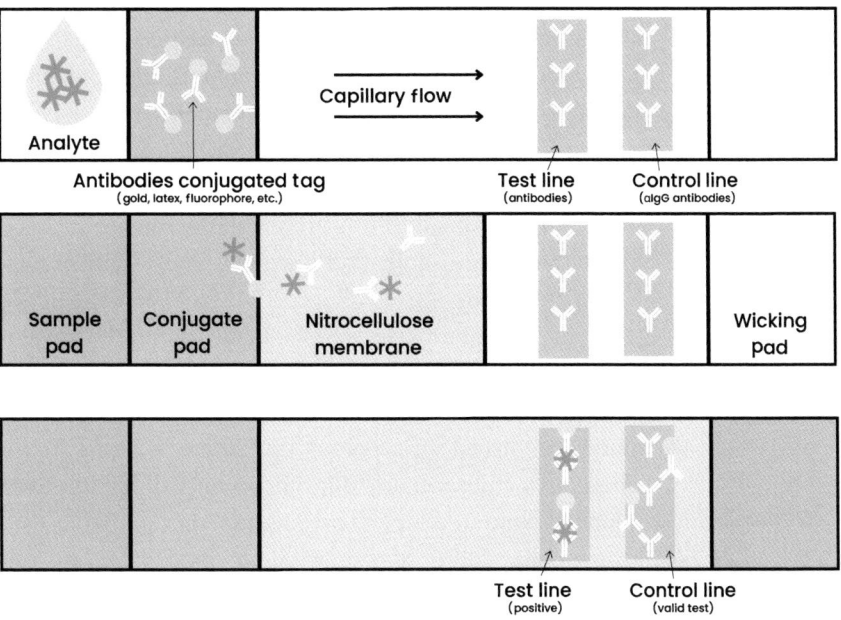

Figure 4.7 Lateral flow assay schematic. The sample, or analyte, is deposited onto a porous membrane that will cause the sample to travel across the membrane through capillary action. As the sample traverses the membrane, it comes into contact with antibodies. As is the case with the ELISA test, if the target biomarker is present in the sample, it will bind to the antibodies. Importantly, the number of antibodies in the LFA will be greater than the number of target antigens present in the sample, such that there are both antigen-bound and -unbound antibodies.

of molecular POCTs and example applications. Specifically, this section will describe LFAs, plasmonic technologies, microfluidics, and paper assays.

The most common portable method for detection of a target specimen is the LFA, which is the key feature of the home pregnancy test. Lateral flow assays are typically quick to perform, with results available on the order of minutes, and made of relatively inexpensive and stable materials. As a result, LFAs are an excellent example of a POCT that can be widely deployed as they are cheap to manufacture, can be stored for long periods of time, and deliver quick results that are easy to interpret (Sajid et al., 2015). The pregnancy test is an example of an LFA.

How do LFAs work? Figure 4.7 shows an LFA schematic. The sample, or analyte, is deposited onto a porous membrane that will cause the sample to travel across the membrane through capillary action. As the sample traverses the membrane, it comes into contact with antibodies. As is the case with the ELISA test, if the target biomarker is present in the sample, it will bind to the antibodies. Importantly, the number of antibodies in the LFA will be greater than the number of target antigens present in the sample, such that there are both antigen-bound and -unbound antibodies.

How are the antibodies detected? The antibodies will flow across the pad and encounter two lines, a test line and a control line. The test line contains another set of antibodies that will bind only to the antigen-bound antibodies (targets of interest); conversely, the control line contains another set of antibodies that will bind only to the unbound antibodies. The control line is used to confirm that the antibodies successfully traveled across the porous membrane and should be visible for every test that is run, regardless of whether or not the target biomarker was present in the sample. The test line will only be visible if the target biomarker is present in the sample.

The pregnancy test developed by Margaret Crane is one example of an LFA that uses urine as the sample. In the case of the pregnancy test, the target biomarker is called **β-chorionic gonadotropin** or β-hCG. β-hCG is a hormone produced during pregnancy and excreted through urine. A urine sample can be placed on a porous membrane in an LFA. As the urine travels across the membrane, any β-hCG present will bind to antibodies, which will ultimately bind to a second set of antibodies on the test line. If no β-hCG is present, there will only be unbound antibodies present, and only the control line will be visible. In addition to at-home pregnancy tests, LFAs are widely used for the qualitative detection of several specimens in fertility and ovulation tests (luteinizing hormone and follicle stimulating hormone), infectious diseases, cardiac testing, drug abuse markers (amphetamines, cocaine, and benzodiazepines), cancer diagnostics, and, of course, most recently in the COVID Rapid Antigen Test that can be used at home.

Deeper Look: COVID-19 Testing

With the onset of the global COVID-19 pandemic in March 2020, contact tracing methods proved highly effective means to reduce virus transmission in previous pandemics; however, reliable contact tracing depends on the ability to accurately test people for infection with SARS-CoV-2, the virus that causes COVID-19. Early in 2020, as COVID-19 rapidly became a pandemic, molecular testing for SARS-CoV-2 emerged as a method for testing potential COVID-19 patients for active viral infection.

The SARS-CoV-2 genome consists of ribonucleic acid (RNA) rather than DNA. Just as DNA samples can be amplified for molecular testing using PCR (discussed in Chapter 2), RNA samples can be converted into DNA samples and amplified using a modified version of PCR called reverse transcription PCR (RT-PCR). RT-PCR adds an initial step prior to DNA amplification, in which the RNA sample undergoes reverse transcription to produce a strand of DNA (the opposite of transcription, which creates a strand of RNA from DNA, hence the name "reverse transcription"). Once a strand of DNA has been derived via reverse transcription, PCR is used to amplify the DNA for testing. RT-PCR became the primary and most reliable method for detecting active SARS-CoV-2 infection.

> A major limitation of widespread testing for COVID-19 was the reliance on expensive technology, such as the thermocycler, required for performing RT-PCR. As a result, researchers seized the opportunity to develop low-cost POCT for diagnosis of COVID-19. Due to their simplicity, an LFA was an obvious choice based on the ASSURED criteria: LFAs are affordable, sensitive, specific, user-friendly, rapid, equipment-free, and deliverable to end users.
>
> As was described above for HIV testing, when a person is infected with a virus there are virus-specific antigens present within the body. In the case of SARS-CoV-2, these antigens can be sampled using a swab of the nasal cavity. After sample collection, the sample is placed on the sample collection pad. Any antigen present within the sample will migrate through the porous membrane and encounter conjugated antibodies specific to SARS-CoV-2 antigens. The antibody–antigen complex will continue to the test line, where it will bind to another antibody specific to the SARS-CoV-2 antigen, much like the sandwich ELISA shown in Figure 4.5.

One important point to note is that the cheaper, faster tests are not as effective as their laboratory counterparts. ELISA has true positive and false positive rates of 84 and 16 percent, respectively, whereas the LFA has true positive and false positive rates of 66 and 34 percent, respectively. However, both tests are equally effective in patients without COVID-19, with a true positive rate of almost 100 percent and a false positive rate of less than 5 percent. Therefore, a negative result with LFA has to be confirmed with additional tests or repeated several times to improve the likelihood of detecting the virus. Table 4.2 shows the different tests for COVID-19. The differences in the properties are compared, specifying the time window of their effectiveness to produce an accurate diagnosis. The assessment of all these characteristics allows for the correct choice of detection method.

Now that we have discussed the principles of LFAs, we will take a closer look at some of the differences between ELISAs and POCTs, such as the LFA. Figure 4.8 shows ELISAs and LFAs. ELISAs and LFAs use the same basic method of leveraging antibodies for sample detection. Unlike LFAs, which are relatively inexpensive and do not require trained personnel, ELISAs depend on expensive equipment and trained operators to perform and interpret results. The major benefits of an ELISA over an LFA are their quantitative nature and improved sensitivity. The main difference between a bench-top ELISA and an LFA is the method of detection. For an LFA, the human eye is the primary method for detecting a positive result. For an ELISA, a bench-top piece of equipment called a plate reader is the primary method for detection. The main reason a plate reader is used for detection during an ELISA is the benefit

Table 4.2 Different tests for COVID-19

The differences in the properties are compared, specifying the time window of their effectiveness to produce an accurate diagnosis. The assessment of all these characteristics allows for the correct choice of detection method.

Sample	Nasopharyngeal/oropharyngeal swabs	Serum/plasma	Serum/plasma/whole blood
Detection	Viral RNA SARS-CoV-2	IgG/IgM/IgA antibodies and antigen	IgG/IgM antibodies
Characteristics	Gold standard test for direct detection of the viral genome performed in a laboratory	Assay for the detection of viral antigen or antibodies in response to viral infection by antigen–antibody interaction performed in a laboratory	Low-cost point-of-care device, portable, free laboratory equipment with results in maximum 15 minutes
Window of use for accurate results	0–14 days after onset	5–30 days after onset	5–30 days after onset
Drawbacks	Expensive, requires specialized equipment, reagents, and personnel, not accessible to the whole population	Laborious assay procedure, requires laboratory environment, unspecific binding can occur	Low sensitivity, results depend on the individual's immune response, may have cross-reactivity

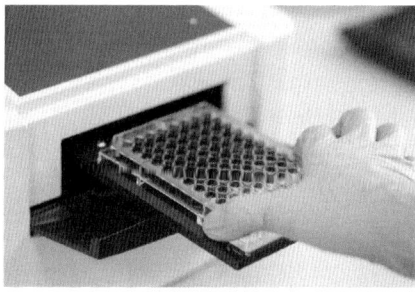 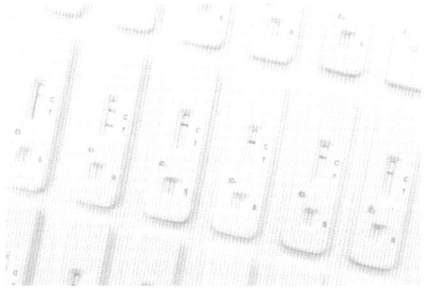

Figure 4.8 ELISAs and LFAs. ELISAs and LFAs use the same basic method of leveraging antibodies for sample detection. Unlike LFAs, which are relatively inexpensive and do not require trained personnel, ELISAs depend on expensive equipment and trained operators to perform and interpret results. The major benefits of an ELISA over an LFA are their quantitative nature and improved sensitivity.
Source: (a) ©TON_AQUATIC, CHOKSAWATDIKORN/SCIENCE PHOTO LIBRARY/Science Photo Library/Getty Images; (b) ©Justin Paget/DigitalVision/Getty Images/Getty Images.

of quantification and higher sensitivity. LFAs are dichotomous tests, having only two possible results: positive or negative. ELISAs can be dichotomous, providing a positive or negative result, but can also quantify the amount of the target biomarker in the sample.

Example: Comparing Different Assays

Question: A biomedical engineer is comparing an ELISA and an LFA to determine the effectiveness of implementing the LFA for detecting a cervical cancer protein that can be sampled with a simple vaginal swab. The sensitivity/specificity of the ELISA and LFA are 90/95 percent and 75/90 percent, respectively. Assuming 100,000 people with cervices are screened with each test and the prevalence of disease is 2 percent, calculate the number of true positives, true negatives, false positives, and false negatives.

Answer: The sensitivity of a test is the true positive rate, which is defined as the ratio of true positives to TP plus false negatives (FN). Based on the prevalence of disease of 2 percent, the total number of people with cervices with the cervical cancer protein is expected to be 2,000. A sensitivity of 90 percent would mean that 90 percent of the people with cervices who have the cervical cancer protein test positive, which would mean 1,800 people with cervixes are TP for ELISA. The remaining 200 people with cervices would test negative and would be considered a FN. Using the same method for LFA with a sensitivity of 75 percent, we get that 1,500 people with cervices are TP and 500 people with cervices are FN. So far we have:

$$TP_{ELISA} = 1{,}800, TP_{LFA} = 1{,}500, FN_{ELISA} = 200, FN_{LFA} = 500.$$

The specificity of a test is the true negative rate, which is defined as the ratio of the true negatives (TN) to TN plus false positives (FP). The number of people with cervices expected to not have the cervical cancer protein is 98,000 (i.e., 100,000 – 2,000). A specificity of 95 percent would mean that 95 percent of the people with cervices who do not have the cervical cancer protein test negative, which would mean 93,100 people with cervices are TN for ELISA. The remaining 4,900 people with cervices would test positive and would be considered FP. Using the same method for LFA with a specificity of 90 percent, we get that 88,200 people with cervices are TN and 9,800 people with cervices are FP, giving:

$$TN_{ELISA} = 93{,}100, TN_{LFA} = 4{,}900, \ FP_{ELISA} = 88{,}200, FP_{LFA} = 9{,}800.$$

The optical biosensor is one of the most commonly used methods for reading signals from POCTs. Fluorescence measurements are perhaps one of the most common optical sensing methods. Most point-of-care LFAs use a colorimetric marker attached to the antibodies that can be viewed with the naked eye. To increase sensitivity, however, the signal can be enhanced by using different labeling agents, such as fluorophores, that can be detected using a microscope or camera (Sajid et al., 2015). To quantify the amount of the biomarker present, ELISAs use an optical biosensor that indirectly detects fluorescence from optically labeled antibodies on the target sample. As a result, the fluorescence measurement can be used to precisely determine the amount of detection antibody present and, by extension, the amount of biomarker present.

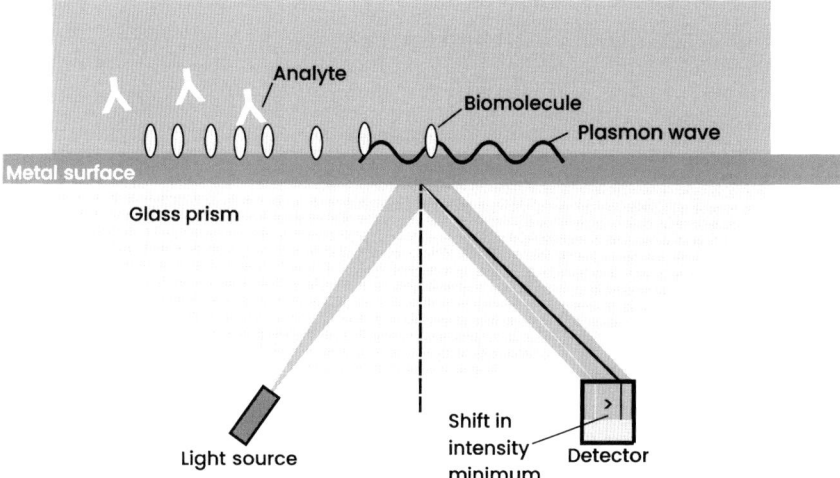

Figure 4.9 Principles of plasmonic sensing. Plasmonic sensing depends on the interactions between molecules and a boundary surface, typically made of a metal such as gold. Light is reflected off the metal surface using a glass prism and detected with an optical detector. When light is incident on the metal surface at a specific angle, the electrons within the metal surface absorb the light, resulting in a minimum intensity at the detector. When the nature of the metal surface changes, the angle for maximum absorption also changes, causing a shift in the minimum intensity on the detector. Changes in the metal surface are caused by the binding of an analyte (typically the biomarker being studied) and a capture molecule (biomolecule).

Another class of optical biosensors, referred to as plasmonic technologies, represents a rapidly developing biosensing technology that is far more sensitive than fluorescence detection. Figure 4.9 shows the principles of plasmonic sensing. Plasmonic sensing depends on the interactions between molecules and a boundary surface, typically made of a metal such as gold. Light is then reflected off the metal surface using a glass prism and detected with an optical detector. When light is incident on the metal surface at a specific angle, the electrons within the metal surface absorb the light, resulting in a minimum intensity at the detector. When the nature of the metal surface changes, the angle for maximum absorption also changes, causing a shift in the minimum intensity on the detector. Changes in the metal surface are caused by the binding of an analyte (typically the biomarker being studied) and a capture molecule (biomolecule).

Different types of plasmonic biosensors include **surface-enhanced Raman scattering** (SERS), and **surface plasmon resonance** (SPR). **Raman scattering** is a method of analyzing chemicals nondestructively by measuring the way light interacts with the chemical bonds in a sample. **Surface-enhanced Raman scattering** uses a surface modified with molecules or nanostructures to enhance the amount of Raman scattering. **Surface plasmon resonance** is electron oscillation on a surface that is induced by the exposure of the surface to light. These sensors are extremely sensitive compared to other optical sensing techniques and are label-free. However, detectors for SERS and SPR tend to be extremely expensive, driving up the cost of the POCT. As a result, resource-stretched settings may not have access to these types of POCTs.

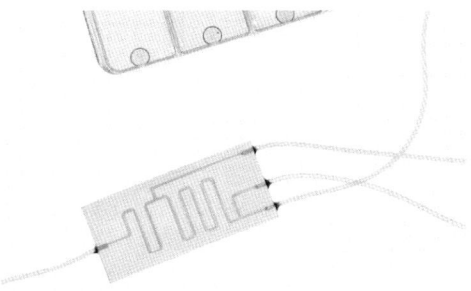

Figure 4.10 Illustration of a microfluidics chip. Chambers are designed and etched into the chip to promote mixing of different solutions. For example, the chip shown here has three inputs on the right and one output on the left. The bottom two inputs are mixed first through a series of U-bends in the chamber prior to the addition of the top input, which is mixed by additional U-bends before being output from the chip.
Source: ©WLADIMIR BULGAR/SCIENCE PHOTO LIBRARY/Science Photo Library.

Lateral flow assays provide a readout of a single assay or interaction. Unlike simple LFAs, microfluidic devices can essentially put an entire laboratory procedure into a simple microsystem, often referred to as a "lab on a chip." The chips on which microfluidic assays are typically performed are analogous to a computer chip in terms of size. Microfluidics systems work by using a pump and a chip. Different types of pumps precisely move liquid inside the chip at a rate of 1 µL / min to 10,000 µL / min. Figure 4.10 shows an illustration of a microfluidics chip. Chambers are designed and etched into the chip to promote mixing of different solutions. For example, the chip has three inputs on the right and one output on the left. The bottom two inputs are mixed first through a series of U-bends in the chamber, prior to the addition of the top input, which is mixed by additional U-bends before being output from the chip.

Microfluidic chips contain a series of chambers and tubes that can mix samples with specific reagents in a desired sequence, allowing for the processing of the liquids via mixing, chemical, or physical reactions (Whitesides, 2006). The liquid may carry tiny particles such as cells or nanoparticles. The microchannels range from submicron to a few millimeters, thereby allowing precise and controlled experiments to be conducted at a lower cost and faster pace compared to laboratory devices. Microfluidic assays are highly repeatable, which is important for POCTs when many microfluidic chips may be needed for screening patients for a variety of conditions. Figure 4.11 shows the different methods through which the output from a microfluidic chip can be measured. These measurements most commonly involve some sort of optical method that can use colorimetry, fluorescence sensing, or plasmonics (SERs or SPR). There are many applications for point-of-care microfluidics, including detection of cancer cells and pathogens (Nasseri et al., 2018).

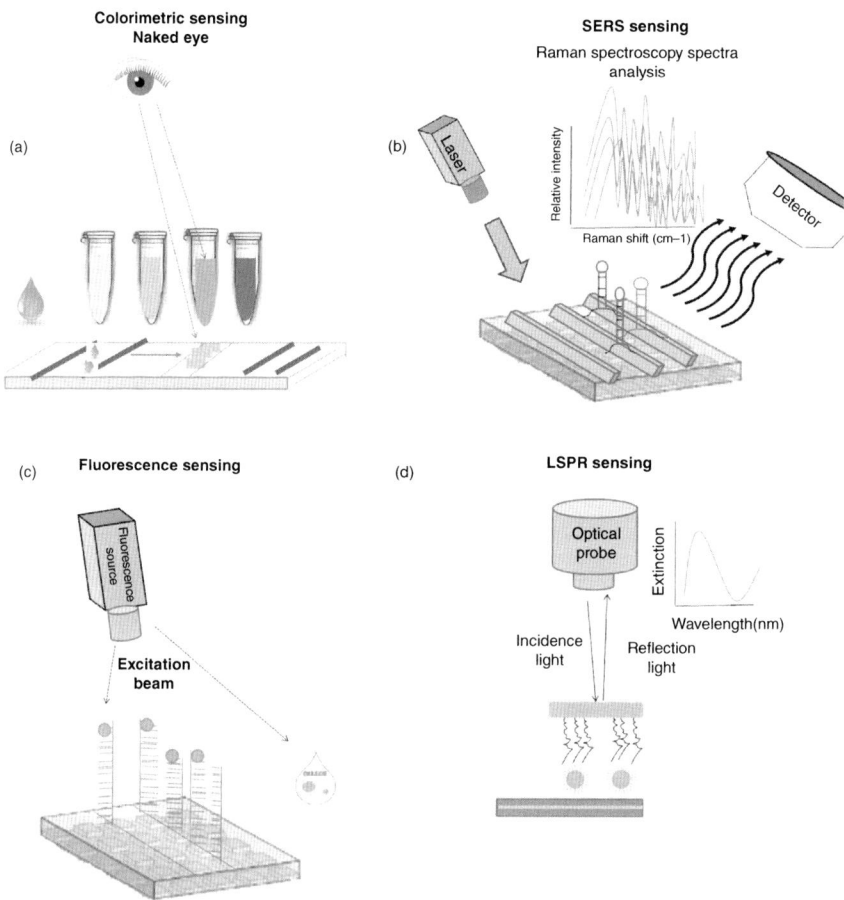

Figure 4.11

Different methods through which the output from a microfluidic chip can be measured (Nasseri et al., 2018). These measurements most commonly involve some sort of optical method that can use colorimetry, fluorescence sensing, or plasmonics (SERs or SPR). There are many applications for point-of-care microfluidics, including detection of cancer cells and pathogens (Nasseri et al., 2018). Source: Nasseri et al. (2018). © Elsevier.

The final point-of-care assay we will discuss are paper assays. Similar to LFAs, the devices are made from cellulose or modified cellulose using inexpensive manufacturing methods, and use capillary action for transport of the analyte. Like microfluidic chips, paper assays can be used to facilitate mixing of different chemicals and compounds with a sample to investigate the presence of a target. The target could be an antigen, antibody, or other protein. Patterning networks that can direct flow to different regions of the device without the need for external pumps makes them an attractive alternative to standard microfluidic devices (Carrell et al., 2019). Figure 4.12 shows an example of a colorimetric paper assay. Capillary action can be used to mix fluids together. For example, if three different fluids are added, one to each of the three channels, they will arrive at the square pad at different times based on capillary flow. The amount of fluid and time that the fluids take to arrive can be dictated by the distance from the initial reservoir to the final square pad. In this manner, fluids can be designed to interact at specific times and in specific orders (Byrnes et al., 2013).

Point-of-Care Testing and Cancer

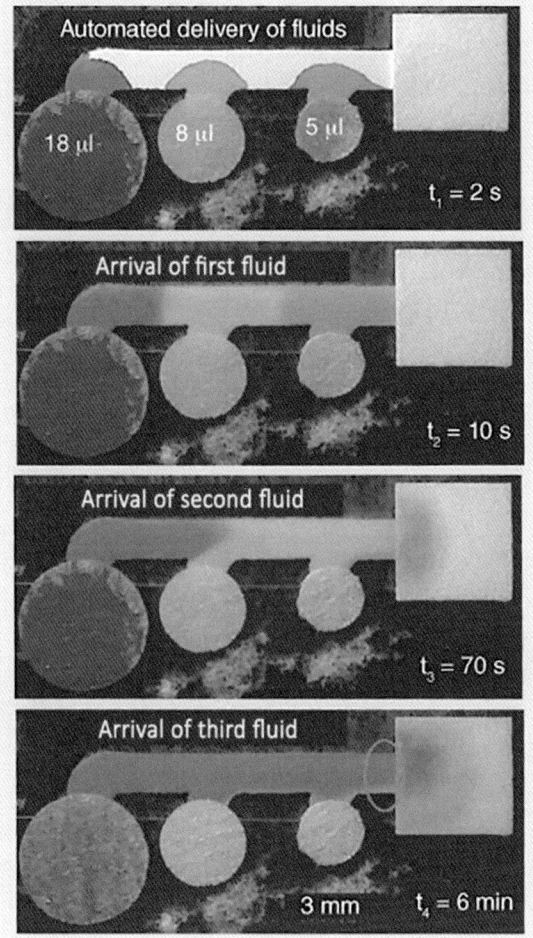

Figure 4.12 Colorimetric paper assay. Capillary action can be used to mix fluids together. For example, if three different fluids are added, one to each of the three channels, they will arrive at the square pad at different times based on capillary flow. The amount of fluid and time that the fluids take to arrive can be dictated by the distance from the initial reservoir to the final square pad. In this manner, fluids can be designed to interact at specific times and in specific orders (Byrnes et al., 2013).
Source: Byrnes, S., Thiessen, G. & Fu, E. 2013. Progress in the development of paper-based diagnostics for low-resource point-of-care settings. Bioanalysis, 5, 2821–2836.

Point-of-Care Testing and Cancer

As described above, the general development process for a POCT starts with biomarker identification. Once a specific biomarker has been identified, the next step is to determine how to obtain a sample from the body that would contain that biomarker. In the example of the at-home pregnancy test, the biomarker for pregnancy is β-hCG and the method for obtaining a sample is urine

Table 4.3 A number of POCTs that have been developed for applications in cancer diagnostics, along with the biomarkers they target

Many of the POCTs listed in the table have a very high sensitivity and specificity for detecting the biomarker of interest, making them excellent candidates for effective screening and diagnostic tools, particularly in settings where routine pathology is not available.

Associated cancer	Cancer biomarker	POC device	Clinical capabilities	Test duration	Sample	Company
Prostate	PSA	PSA semi-quantitative rapid test	4 ng/ml	15 min	WB, S or P	CTK Biotech
Bladder	Nuclear matrix protein 22 (NMP 22)	Alere NMP22® BLADDERCHEK®	99% sensitivity when combined with cystoscopy	30 min	Urine	Abbott (formerly Alere)
Colorectal	Fecal occult blood	FOB Rapid Test CE	hHB > 50 ng/ml >98% specificity for hHB	5–10 min	Stool	CTK Biotech
Cervical	OncoE6	OncoE6™ Cervical Test	Sensitivity 84.6% Specificity 98.5%	2.5 h	Cervical swab	Arbor Vita
HPV causing head and neck cancer	OncoE6	OncoE6™ Oral Test	Still at testing stage	–	Oral swab	Arbor Vita
Liver	AFP	Medical IVD rapid diagnostic test kits AFP test kit	Sensitivity 25 ng/ml Specificity 99%	10 min	WB, S or P	INVBIO (Innovation Biotech)
Colorectal, breast, lung	CEA	CEA Serum Rapid Test	5 ng/ml Sensitivity 97% Specificity 100%	10 min	S or P	Cortez Diagnostics Inc.

AFP, alphafeto protein; CEA, carcinoembryonic antigen; hHB, human hemoglobin; P, plasma; S, serum; WB, whole blood.

collection. One of the key attributes to the successful adoption of the at-home pregnancy test was its ease of use in terms of sample collection. If the test had required blood collection beyond a finger prick, for example, it may not have been so widely adopted. As this anecdote illustrates, the sample collection method is critical for successful development and adoption of a POCT. In this section, we will look at the different biomarkers used in POCTs for cancer applications, as well as how samples can be collected in a noninvasive manner.

Table 4.3 summarizes a number of POCTs that have been developed for applications in cancer diagnostics along with the biomarkers they target. Many

Point-of-Care Testing and Cancer

Deeper Look: Regular Colon Cancer Screening Can Save Lives – Why Is It Not Popular?

About one in three adults aged 50–75 years have not been tested for colon cancer according to a new *Vital Signs* report from the CDC. Colorectal cancer is the second leading cause of cancer deaths, after lung cancer. Figure 4.13 shows the different stages of colon cancer. Screening is essential as colon cancer may not present with symptoms until it has progressed to advanced stages.

Part of the lack of adherence to colon cancer screening is the prep, experience, and recovery. Prior to screening, patients must avoid solid foods the day before the exam and limit themselves to clear liquids. Additionally, a laxative is required to empty the bowels, necessitating multiple visits to the bathroom. This is only a prelude to the actual exam, which

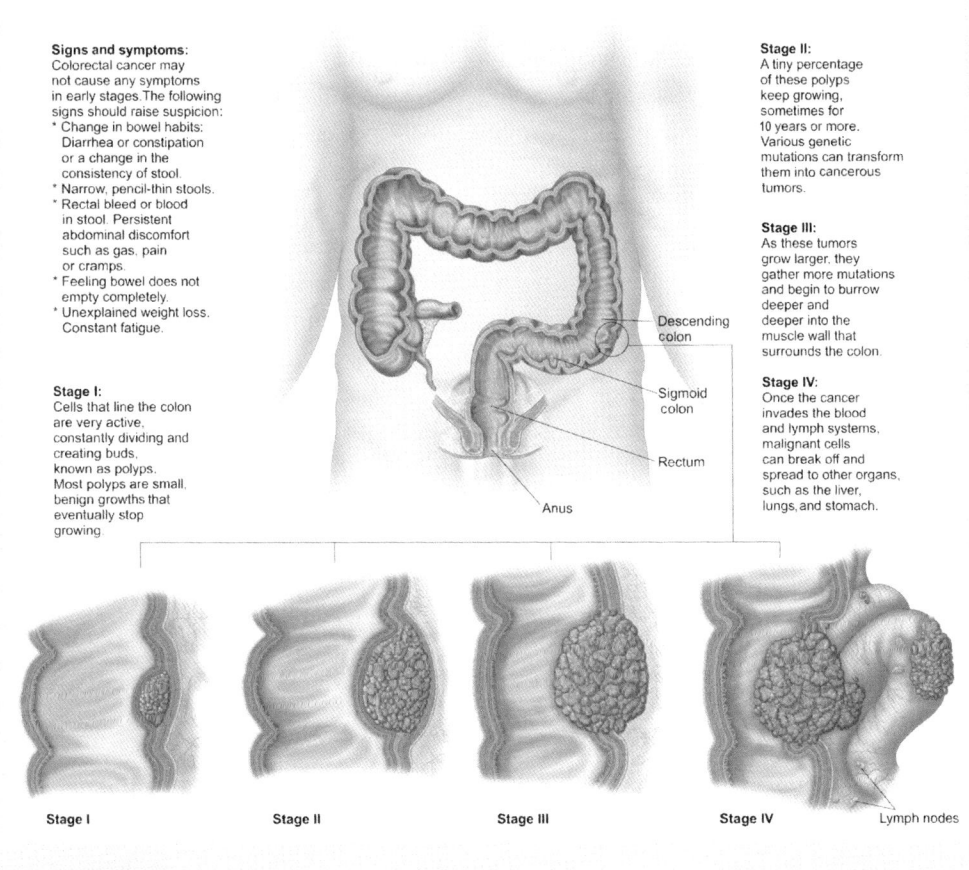

Figure 4.13 Different stages of colon cancer. Screening is essential as colon cancer may not present with symptoms until it has progressed to advanced stages.
Source: ©Stocktrek Images/Stocktrek Images/Getty Images.

involves the insertion of a long, flexible endoscope into the colon to look for abnormalities, as well as the additional discomfort after the exam.

POCTs can be life savers. There are two types of POCTs for colon cancer screening – the fecal occult blood test (FOBT) and the fecal immunochemical test (FIT). Both tests look for occult blood in the stool, which can be an early indicator for precancer or cancer. In FOBT, a chemical substance called guaiac is infused into a small paper card that is part of the FOBT at-home kit. After samples are collected and smeared onto the card, they are sent to a lab for testing. The FIT is an LFA test that is considered more sensitive than FOBT. The FIT LFA kit has a membrane precoated with an anti-hemoglobin. A liquid sample in which the stool is mixed is added to the LFA, following which it migrates upward by capillary action to react with the anti-hemoglobin antibody. The results can be seen shortly after the test. The FIT is similar to an at-home COVID-19 test kit.

of the POCTs listed in the table have a very high sensitivity and specificity for detecting the biomarker of interest, making them excellent candidates for effective screening and diagnostic tools, particularly in settings where more advanced laboratory tests are not readily available. Chapter 3 covered cervical cancer screening and that effective and widely available testing for cervical precancer and cancer are central to meeting the WHO metrics to eradicate cervical cancer in the next century. As you can see in Table 4.3, a variety of tests have been developed to detect proteins expressed by precancerous and cancerous cells.

What are the different methods for biomarker sample collection? Prostate cancer will be used as an example to illustrate the different sample collection methods and their relative pros and cons. Prostate cancer has been extensively studied and is very well characterized. Many prostate cancers are slow-growing, with a minimal risk for metastases to vital organs; however, there are a subset of prostate cancers that can be very aggressive, with a high risk of metastases (Bubendorf et al., 2000). Table 4.4 shows several different options for prostate cancer detection. A comparison of advantages and limitations and the sample required is presented. In general, collected samples are in the form of either tissue or a liquid.

Solid tissue samples can often provide the most information about a tumor's biology. How are tissue samples collected? Generally, tissue samples have to be excised from the body using either a biopsy or surgical procedure. The location of the tissue dictates how invasive the procedure required is. Sampling a lesion on the skin with a scrape biopsy, for example, can be performed in a doctor's office under a local anesthetic, whereas collecting a tissue sample within the colon would require the use of a colonoscope while a patient is under some form of general anesthesia. In some instances the invasive nature of a biopsy may even require full surgery. Brain tumors are a good example of a surgical biopsy, as a surgeon will need to perform a craniotomy

Table 4.4 Several different options for prostate cancer detection

A comparison of advantages and limitations and the sample required is presented. In general, collected samples are in the form of either tissue or a liquid.

	Markers	Advantages	Limitations
Tissue	Histopathological features Cellular proliferation Molecular factors Genetic aberrations or patterns	Direct evaluation of protein or gene expression Potential insights into prostate cancer biology	Invasive method of collection Snap-frozen or formalin-fixed paraffin-embedded samples Highly complex
Whole blood, serum, or plasma	PSA Circulating tumor cells Circulating tumor DNA microRNA Soluble proteins	Noninvasive method of collection Large quantities possible	Large dynamic range Dilution of markers Complex Distal from site of tumor
Urine or urinary EPS	microRNA RNA (e.g., *PCA3*) Soluble proteins Exosomes	Noninvasive method of collection Large quantities possible Proximal to site of tumor	Dilution of markers Nonstandardized method of collection Intrapatient variability
EPS of seminal fluid	Soluble proteins Exosomes	Proximal to site of tumor Presumably more concentrated in prostatic proteins	Invasive procedure Routine collection not possible

to remove a portion of the skull to access the tissue. Tissue collection can often only be performed in more centralized healthcare settings such as specialized clinics or hospitals. Results from tissue testing are also frequently not available for days or even weeks.

Once solid tissue has been collected, how can it be used for biomarker analysis? Collected tissue can be stained for different biomarkers using immunohistochemical staining (IHC, discussed in Chapter 2) and analyzed by a highly trained pathologist. Additionally, tissue can also be used for many of the "omics" studies covered in Chapter 2. Both IHC and "omics" analysis have the potential to provide significant information about a particular tumor, making collected tissue an excellent option for analysis. Tissue also has the advantage of remaining stable when stored properly for long periods of time, with minimal degradation. As a result, if a new test needs to be performed, even a tissue sample collected years prior could be used for that test without the need to collect new tissue.

Now that we have discussed how solid tissue samples are collected and analyzed, what are some of the drawbacks for tissue sampling? The major downsides for tissue analysis are: (1) the requirement for experienced personnel to perform IHC and "omics" analysis and to interpret the results; and (2) the invasive nature of collecting tissue either via a biopsy or surgery. Tissue samples are also not compatible with many of the POCT molecular tests described in the previous section without some form of preprocessing. For example, to use tissue as a sample for an LFA, the tissue would need to undergo some form of digestion and suspension steps to convert the sample from a solid to a liquid.

Liquid samples encompass a broader range of sample types compared to solid tissue samples. Common liquid samples include blood, urine, and saliva, though there are many other samples for specialized indications, such as cerebral spinal fluid (CSF) or genital secretions. Many liquid samples are less invasive to collect than solid tissue samples; for example, urine and saliva can be collected noninvasively and small blood samples can be collected with a simple finger prick, depending on the volume required for testing. If a large amount of blood is required, a venous puncture may be required, which is more invasive than a finger prick, though still less invasive than a biopsy or excisional procedure. Some types of liquid samples still require highly invasive procedures; for example, CSF collection typically requires a lumbar puncture to collect liquid from the spinal column.

Tissue sampling provides a very direct means to probe a tumor. Liquid sampling, on the other hand, provides a more indirect means of sampling the tumor. The biomarkers in liquid samples are frequently byproducts of processes occurring within the tumor that are absorbed by or shed into the blood. These are downstream effects from altered processes within the body that are a direct or indirect result of the tumor. Liquid sampling that is closest to tissue sampling is one that detects **circulating tumor cells** (CTCs) and/or **circulating tumor DNA** (ctDNA). Circulating tumor cells are cells from the primary tumor that are found within the bloodstream, whereas circulating tumor DNA (ctDNA) is DNA from the primary tumor that is found within the bloodstream. Collecting these types of liquid samples to screen for, diagnose, or otherwise investigate tumors is referred to as a **liquid biopsy**, where a sample of liquid collected from the body is used to screen for, diagnose, or otherwise study a tumor. Liquid biopsies also include circulating microRNAs, circulating proteins, and extracellular vesicles.

Figure 4.14 shows how both CTCs and ctDNA can provide insights into the biology of the primary tumor and how advanced the disease is. Circulating tumor cells and ctDNA can, therefore, play an important role in cancer, including cancer diagnostics, measuring treatment response, and detecting early metastases. More specifically, CTCs and ctDNA can be used to study the genetic makeup of the tumor, while CTCs can also be used to study alterations to RNA and gene transcription, as well as protein expression. Additionally,

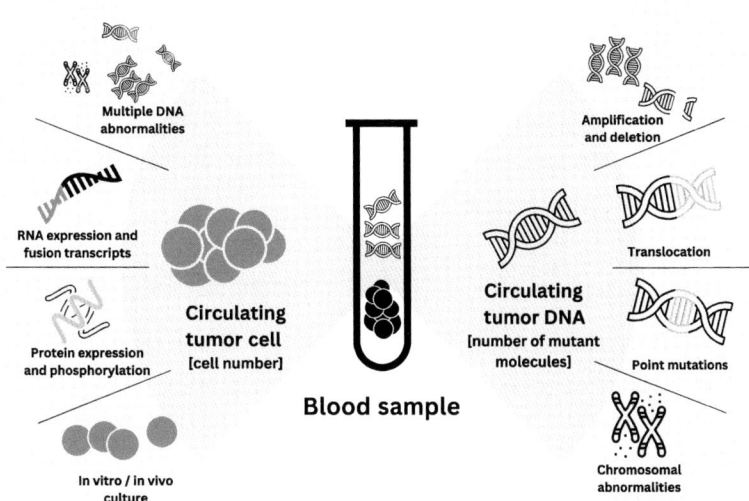

Figure 4.14

CTCs and ctDNA can provide insights into the biology of the primary tumor and how advanced the disease is. CTCs and ctDNA can therefore play an important role in cancer, including cancer diagnostics, measuring treatment response, and detecting early metastases.

CTCs could be collected and grown in a laboratory setting to test possible therapies to predict if the tumor will respond, or to perform laboratory experiments to help future patients with a similar condition. Taken together, the information provided to both physicians and researchers by CTCs and ctDNA can help inform patient care and improve outcomes (Haber and Velculescu, 2014).

In addition to providing information about the identity of a tumor, CTCs can be used to detect metastases. One of the early steps in metastatic tumor spread is shedding of tumor cells into the bloodstream. The shed CTCs can then travel to a distant site from the primary tumor and form a new tumor (metastasis). The majority of cancer deaths occur because of metastases to a vital organ such as the lungs, liver, or brain. Catching disease before metastases form can greatly increase the chances of survival. The number of CTCs in circulation correlates with the presence of metastases, making CTCs an important surrogate marker for metastatic spread, particularly in settings where advanced imaging techniques such as PET, CT, and MRI are not available.

As you can see, liquid samples can offer great insights into tumor biology, albeit in a less direct manner than solid tissue sampling. One of the major benefits of collecting liquid samples is that the procedure is typically much less invasive than solid tissue sampling (generally blood collection vs. a biopsy or surgical excision). Additionally, liquid samples can be used more easily with many of the POCTs described in the previous section, with fewer complicated preprocessing steps than are required for solid tissue. The major drawbacks for liquid sampling are that: (1) liquid sampling involves biomarkers that are indirectly related to the tumor (with the exception of CTCs and ctDNA); (2) CTCs and ctDNA that are directly related to the tumor are often found at extremely low levels in patients, potentially requiring large volumes of blood to adequately sample them; and (3) in some cases there may not be any CTCs or ctDNA in the blood at all, leaving nothing to test.

Example: Developing a Point-of-Care Molecular Test for Breast Cancer

Question: Describe how you would develop a POCT or series of POCTs to test whether a woman with breast cancer has a tumor that overexpresses HER2, making her eligible for treatment with trastuzumab. Include the type of sample you would need and the type of assay you would use.

Answer: When present, HER2 is expressed on the surface of breast tumor cells. As a result, either a sample of tissue or a sample of CTCs would be required to test for HER2 expression. To make the test minimally invasive, we will use CTCs as the sample since they can be collected via a blood draw. Blood is filled with other types of cells and CTCs are found in limited numbers within the blood. As a result, it will be important first to concentrate the CTCs as much as possible. A microfluidic chip can be developed to sort CTCs out of the blood using size exclusion to remove smaller objects such as red and white blood cells. Once the CTCs have been concentrated, an LFA could be developed that uses antibodies that target HER2 for detection. The CTCs will move through the porous membrane, binding to the detection antibodies only if HER2 is present on the cell surface. Capture antibodies on the test line will be used to establish whether or not HER2 was present on the CTCs. This combinatorial approach with the microfluidic chip as the first step is critical for two reasons: First, the microfluidic chip will concentrate the CTCs for testing on the LFA, which is important because CTCs are rare in blood. Second, the microfluidic chip will determine whether or not CTCs were present in the blood sample, which will improve the overall testing sensitivity (true positive rate), because a lack of CTCs would cause a negative result by LFA testing regardless of whether or not the patient actually has a HER2-positive tumor.

Looking Ahead

Point-of-care technologies can greatly increase access to molecular testing in settings where traditional methods like PCR and ELISA are difficult to access due to a lack of equipment, personnel, or both. Some types of POCTs – such as LFAs, basic microfluidic chips, and paper assays – can be interpreted by the naked eye. If greater sensitivity is warranted, these tests can be greatly enhanced using optical techniques. This can potentially be done inexpensively using smartphone cameras, which are becoming ubiquitous globally. This demonstrates the synergy between molecular assays and optical sensors. Further, with low-cost treatment technologies (for example, ablation therapy), patients are not left without an option for treatment following a positive screening and/or diagnostic test.

There is always a trade-off between accuracy, accessibility, and affordability, and each should be considered depending on which level of the healthcare system the test will be used in. Tests prioritizing accuracy typically require complex instrumentation and infrastructure, so these are not accessible or affordable to individuals seeking care in primary health clinics. These lower-level settings require tests that are user-friendly and which provide results quickly, even if they are not as accurate as their hospital-based counterparts. POCTs can fill this important gap as they are well-suited to widespread screening, testing, and – in the case of cervical precancer – treatment.

The molecular POCTs described in this chapter all require some type of sampling of either solid tissue or liquid from the body. Developing optical imaging POCTs has the potential to not only augment the capabilities of these molecular tests, they can be directly used to image different parts of the body. Optical POCTs can range from microscopes (to image cells) to endoscopes (to image body cavities). POCTs based on optical imaging will be the focus of Chapter 5. The next chapter also includes POCTs based on ultrasound imaging, which have distinct attributes compared to optical imaging.

SUMMARY

One of the ways in which molecular tests can be used is to look at the response of the immune system to foreign invaders – for example, the COVID-19 virus. When a bacteria or virus enters the body, specialized cells in the immune system, called B cells, produce antibodies that can specifically bind to proteins called antigens on the surface of the bacteria or virus, and signal to other cells within the immune system to orchestrate an attack. Both antigens and antibodies can be used as biomarkers. The gold standard method for detecting biomarkers such as antibodies is an ELISA. The four main types of ELISAs are direct, indirect, sandwich, and competitive ELISAs. The initial HIV tests for the detection of antigens and antibodies were based on ELISAs. Other biomarkers that are amenable to molecular testing include small molecules such as metabolites, enzymes that catalyze chemical reactions, DNA, RNA, cancer cells, or proteins such as HER2.

The most common POCT for detection of a target specimen is the LFA. These are quick to perform, with results available on the order of minutes, and made of relatively inexpensive and stable materials. Unlike simple LFAs, microfluidic devices can essentially put an entire laboratory procedure into a simple microsystem, often referred to as a "lab on a chip." Similar to LFAs, paper assays are testing platforms made from cellulose or modified cellulose using inexpensive manufacturing methods, and they use capillary action for transport of the analyte. Like microfluidic chips, paper assays can be used to facilitate mixing of different chemicals and compounds with a sample to investigate the presence of a target. Optical biosensors are used to read the results of the POCT, particularly to increase sensitivity. Fluorescence detection is the most common method – and perhaps the least expensive, second to colorimetry. An alternate approach is to use plasmonic sensing, which is extremely sensitive and label-free, but relatively more expensive.

Chapter 3 covered cervical cancer screening – in particular, the HPV test for detecting different HPV strains, some of which indicate a high risk for developing cervical cancer. It should be noted that HPV testing, which can be performed as a self-test or as a clinic test, does require the samples to be processed by a PCR machine. However, there are molecular cancer screening tests that are self-contained – that is, the samples do not have to be sent somewhere for processing and instead operate as a rapid diagnostic test. There are now molecular tests for a variety of cancers, including prostate, lung, and colon. Another important point to note is that molecular testing can be performed on different types of samples, both solid and liquid. Solid tissue samples can often provide the most information about a tumor's biology; however, the removal of biopsies is an invasive procedure. Liquid samples encompass a broader range of sample types, including blood, urine, and saliva. However, the samples provide systemic rather than local information, as would be the case with biopsies. Liquid sampling that is closest to tissue sampling is one that detects CTCs and/or ctDNA. Collecting these types of liquid samples to screen for, diagnose, or otherwise investigate tumors is referred to as a liquid biopsy.

PROBLEMS

The Origins of Point-of-Care Testing

1. What type of ELISA test can be used to detect an antibody in an immobilized sample?
2. What type of ELISA test improves sensitivity to the presence of an antibody?
3. What role do B cells play in mounting an attack on the COVID-19 virus?
4. Why is antigen testing used for active infection and antibody testing used for previous COVID-19 infection?

5. A COVID-19 test is performed and antibodies are detected. Does that mean you are immune to the virus? Why or why not?
6. Pregnancy tests detect the hCG hormone, which is important in the early stages of pregnancy and continues to increase after fertilization. A pregnancy test comes back negative. What could be two reasons why it might be negative?
7. Figure 4.3 shows different levels of detectable targets following HIV infection. Based on this graph, which target(s) are best during the first 23 days following HIV infection? Which are best from 38 days and beyond?

Point-of-Care Molecular Testing

8. What are three sources of user error that can cause an LFA colorimetry test to report a false negative?
9. What would you expect to see in an LFA if not all of the conjugated antibodies were bound to an antigen?
10. What are three different ways in which the sensitivity of the readout of a POCT can be improved over standard colorimetry? What are the pros and cons?
11. An individual has all of the symptoms of COVID-19 and wants to perform a test to confirm that indeed she has COVID-19. She uses an at-home test for COVID-19 that provides a result in 20 minutes. The result is negative. The individual gets a second test during which she collects the sample at home and then sends it to the clinic for PCR. The second test indicates that the individual is positive. Which test is more reliable and why?
12. An individual performs an at-home HPV test and mails the sample to a central lab to be analyzed. She repeats the test in the clinic, where a provider performs the test and sends it to the lab. The home test indicates that she is negative, but the clinic test indicates that she is positive. The clinical lab assumes that the discordance between the tests is due to quality control issues of the home test. What are three potential sources of quality control that could have affected the integrity of the home test?
13. Of the types of POCTs described in this chapter, which is the easiest to manufacture? Why?

Point-of-Care Testing and Cancer

14. A patient's biopsy is sent to pathology and the presence of a tumor is confirmed. However, on a prior blood test, no CTCs were detected. What are two reasons for the discordance between the biopsy test and the blood test?
15. What type of biomarker would be tested for cervical cancer screening vs. colon cancer screening? What type of test would be needed?

Use the following excerpt for questions 16–20:

Pathological assessment of a biopsy is generally considered the gold standard diagnostic for many types of cancer, including breast cancer. Assume: (1) pathological assessment has a sensitivity of 98 percent and specificity of 95 percent for diagnosing breast cancer; (2) the prevalence of disease is 20 percent for women who screen positive on mammography; and (3) 100,000 women undergo mammographic screening.

16. Pathological assessment of a biopsy is largely unavailable in LMICs due to a dearth of trained pathologists. Suppose you innovate a POCT that uses microfluidics to assess the biopsy sample for the presence of cancer with a sensitivity of 75 percent and a specificity of 90 percent. Calculate the number of true positives, true negatives, false positives, and false negatives for each test.
17. Calculate the cost per positive test for diagnostic biopsy and for your POCT using your answers from the previous question. Assume pathological assessment of a biopsy costs $100 and the POCT costs $8.
18. Now assume that the pathology test is only performed on patients who test positive with the POCT. Calculate the number of true positives, true negatives, false positives, and false negatives.
19. What is the cost per positive test based on the response to the previous question? Again, assume that the cost of pathological assessment of a biopsy costs $100 and the POCT costs $8.
20. In the previous two scenarios, what are the implications for the individual if the test is positive, but the individual does not actually have the disease? What if the test is negative and the individual has the disease? What is the terminology used to characterize the inaccuracy of the first scenario and that of the second scenario?

REFERENCES

Alexander, T. S. 2016. Human immunodeficiency virus diagnostic testing: 30 years of evolution. *Clinical and Vaccine Immunology*, 23, 249–253.

Bubendorf, L., Schöpfer, A., Wagner, U., et al. 2000. Metastatic patterns of prostate cancer: an autopsy study of 1,589 patients. *Human Pathology*, 31, 578–583.

Byrnes, S., Thiessen, G., & Fu, E. 2013. Progress in the development of paper-based diagnostics for low-resource point-of-care settings. *Bioanalysis*, 5, 2821–2836.

Carrell, C., Kava, A., Nguyen, M., et al. 2019. Beyond the lateral flow assay: a review of paper-based microfluidics. *Microelectronic Engineering*, 206, 45–54.

Clarke, S., & Foster, J. 2012. A history of blood glucose meters and their role in self-monitoring of diabetes mellitus. *British Journal of Biomedical Science*, 69, 83–93.

Delaney, K. P., Wesolowski, L. G., & Owen, S. M. 2017. *The Evolution of HIV Testing Continues*. Lippincott Williams & Wilkins, Philadelphia, PA.

Giguère, K., Eaton, J. W., Marsh, K., et al. 2021. Trends in knowledge of HIV status and efficiency of HIV testing services in sub-Saharan Africa, 2000–20: a modelling study using survey and HIV testing programme data. *The Lancet HIV*, 8, e284–e293.

Haber, D. A., & Velculescu, V. E. 2014. Blood-based analyses of cancer: circulating tumor cells and circulating tumor DNA. *Cancer Discovery*, 4, 650–661.

Kennedy, P. 2016. Could women be trusted with their own pregnancy tests. *New York Times*.

Klimpel, G. R. 1996. Immune defenses. In Baron, S. (ed.), *Medical Microbiology*, 4th ed., University of Texas, Galveston, TX.

Nasseri, B., Soleimani, N., Rabiee, N., et al. 2018. Point-of-care microfluidic devices for pathogen detection. *Biosensors and Bioelectronics*, 117, 112–128. https://doi.org/10.1016/j.bios.2018.05.050.

Sajid, M., Kawde, A.-N., & Daud, M. 2015. Designs, formats and applications of lateral flow assay: a literature review. *Journal of Saudi Chemical Society*, 19, 689–705.

Whitesides, G. M. 2006. The origins and the future of microfluidics. *Nature*, 442, 368–373.

5 Point-of-Care Technologies for Imaging Applications

The previous chapter provided a comprehensive summary of molecular tests that can provide rapid diagnostics at a local clinic or even at home. Rapid diagnostics can serve as frontline screening to triage patients who need additional evaluation. Often this is done through some sort of visualization technology, whether it be anatomical or molecular, to learn more about the source of the problem. This was discussed in detail in Chapter 2 and included a variety of systems such as computed tomography (CT), magnetic resonance imaging (MRI), and positron emission tomography (PET). This, along with in vitro testing, provides an important framework for treatment. An excellent example is the case where screening for colon cancer is performed as a home test, and for those who need a confirmatory diagnosis, colonoscopy can be used to visualize disease. Similarly, following a positive prostate cancer screening test, transrectal ultrasound and/or MRI can be used for the same purpose.

Optical and ultrasound imaging are low-cost counterparts to systems such as MRI or CT. They can be used at the bedside to visualize anatomical features such as cancer of the colon or the prostate. These technologies do not replicate the capabilities of systems that can perform whole-body imaging, but they can be life-saving tools in a wide variety of scenarios. In fact, light and sound have been integral to the diagnosis and management of COVID-19 symptoms. Portable ultrasound can be used as a screening tool to identify fluid in the lungs. The pulse oximeter allows for quick evaluation of individuals with potential respiratory distress. Figure 5.1 shows a comparison of different imaging technologies. Clearly, there is a trade-off between spatial resolution and cost, underscoring the point that no single technology will have all of the desirable features. Also important to note is that optical and ultrasound imaging are safer to use. CT imaging requires high-frequency radiation, rendering it more dangerous to use.

As mentioned in previous chapters, high-resource settings can be notoriously cost-inefficient. In countries like the US, those living in rural areas, lacking healthcare coverage, or of low socioeconomic status (SES) are often left with limited access to healthcare resources. As an alternative, portable

Point-of-Care Technologies for Imaging Applications

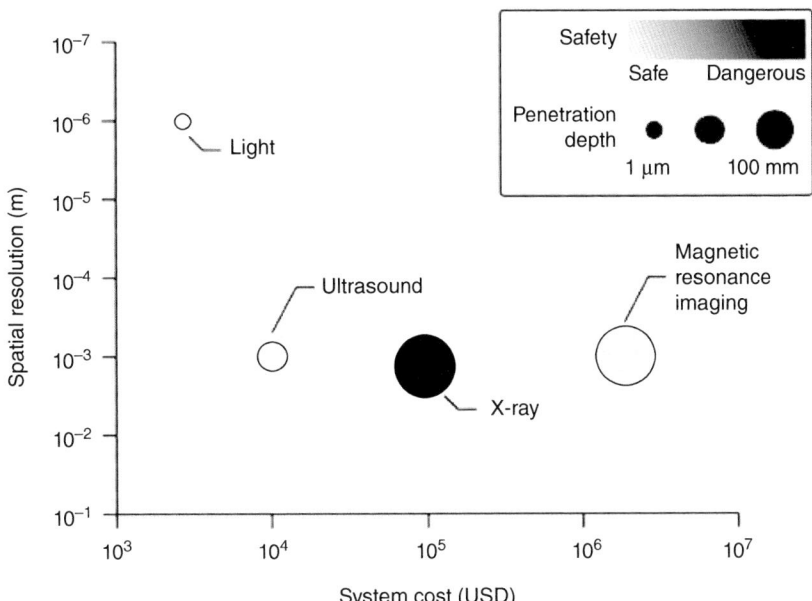

Figure 5.1
A comparison of different imaging technologies. Clearly, there is a trade-off between spatial resolution and cost, underscoring the point that no single technology will have all of the desirable features. Also important to note is that optical and ultrasound imaging are safer to use. CT imaging requires high-frequency radiation, rendering it more dangerous to use.

imaging systems can enable a hub-and-spoke model. In this model, hospitals serve a similar function as air traffic control; providers using portable technologies would act as metaphorical planes to reach different destinations (patients) within a guided framework. This chapter will focus on the development of imaging-based POCTs, as well as some of the underlying physical principles that each technology is based on. The three technologies covered will be microscopy, endoscopy, and ultrasound.

LEARNING OBJECTIVES

POCT for Microscopy of Cells and Tissue
- The principles of single and multiple lens systems to create magnified images;
- the differences between brightfield and darkfield fluorescence microscopy;
- the innovations behind low-cost, portable microscopes.

POCT for Imaging Internal Body Cavities
- The basic components of an endoscope;
- different types of endoscopes and the differences between them;
- novel POCTs for operator-free imaging, speculum-free imaging, and in vivo pathology.

Ultrasound Imaging and POCTs
- The piezoelectric effect and its use in operation of an ultrasound machine;
- the interaction of ultrasound with different types of tissue to create anatomical images;
- the principles of portable ultrasound systems.

POCT for Microscopy of Cells and Tissues

The most common use of light is in microscopes. Microscopes are widely used in healthcare, most notably in pathology labs where they are used to read histology slides. Microscopes can use three different types of contrast to visualize samples: absorption, scattering, or fluorescence. Photon absorption is the process that occurs when a photon of light interacts with a compound or molecule and transfers its energy into the molecule. The energy is generally emitted as heat when relaxation back to the original energy level occurs. Photon scattering is the process that occurs when a photon of light interacts with a compound or molecule and is directed either in the same or different direction than it was originally traveling. Fluorescence is the process that occurs when a photon of light is absorbed by a compound or molecule, moving electrons into a higher energy level. When the electrons relax to their original energy level, a new photon of light at a longer wavelength is emitted. The amount of light absorbed or scattered varies with the wavelength of light and the component that the light is interacting with.

Lenses play a critical role in magnifying microscopic objects that are not resolvable to the unaided eye. Let's consider a system with an object and a single lens. One of the properties of a lens is its **focal length**. The focal length of a lens is a measure of how effectively it converges or diverges light. A lens with a short focal length will converge light at a shorter distance than a lens with a long focal length. Depending on where an object is placed relative to the lens' focal length, the resulting image can be larger, smaller, or the same size, or no image may be formed at all. The actual process of identifying where an image of an object is within a lens system is determined using ray-tracing.

Figure 5.2 shows a ray-tracing diagram for a single-lens system. The focal lengths are labeled. The object can be placed within the system. Three rays are drawn to determine where the resulting image will be and how large it will be. The first ray is drawn from the top of the object, parallel to the **optical axis** toward the lens. The optical axis is the line that runs perpendicularly through the center of a lens system. From the lens, the ray then goes through the focal length (F) on the other side. The second ray is drawn from the top of the object directly through the center of the lens. The final ray is drawn from the top of the object through the focal length until it hits the lens and follows a parallel path to the optical axis. The point where the three rays intersect on the opposite side of the lens will correspond to the top of the object's image. When an object is placed at two times the focal length (also called the second focal length, or 2F), the resulting image will be real, inverted, and the same size as the original object. When an object is placed between the focal length and two times the focal length, the resulting image will be real,

POCT for Microscopy of Cells and Tissues

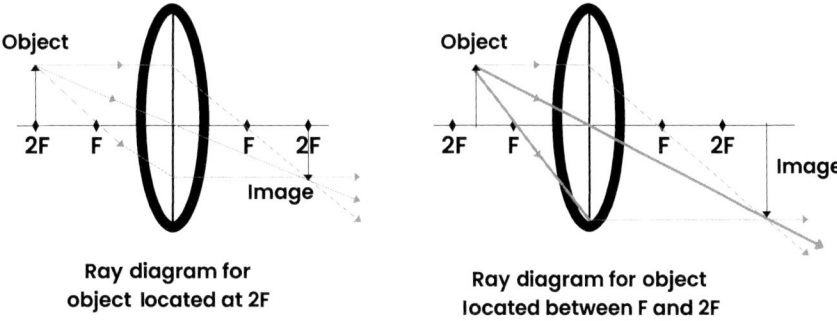

Figure 5.2 Ray-tracing diagram for a single-lens system. The focal lengths are labeled. The object can be placed within the system. Three rays are drawn to determine where the resulting image will be and how large it will be. The first ray is drawn from the top of the object, parallel to the **optical axis** toward the lens. The optical axis is the line that runs perpendicularly through the center of a lens system. From the lens, the ray then goes through the focal length (F) on the other side. The second ray is drawn from the top of the object directly through the center of the lens. The final ray is drawn from the top of the object through the focal length until it hits the lens and follows a parallel path to the optical axis. The point where the three rays intersect on the opposite side of the lens will correspond to the top of the object's image. When an object is placed at two times the focal length (also called the second focal length, or 2F), the resulting image will be real, inverted, and the same size as the original object. When an object is placed between the focal length and two times the focal length, the resulting image will be real, inverted, and larger than the original object.

inverted, and larger than the original object. Both of the resulting images in Figure 5.2 are referred to as **real images**. Real images are created when rays from an object pass through a lens and converge on the opposite side of the lens from the object. In a single-lens system, real images will be inverted relative to the original object. Real image creation results when the object is placed beyond the focal length of the lens (for example, at 2F or between 2F and F) (Sanderson, 2019).

What happens if the object is placed between the first focal length and the lens? Figure 5.3 shows ray-tracing for an object between the lens and the focal length. The first two rays are drawn exactly in the same way as shown in Figure 5.2: One ray runs parallel from the top of the object to the lens and then through the focal length; the second ray runs from the top of the object directly through the center of the lens. The third ray must be drawn differently, however, as it is not possible to draw a ray from the top of the object through the focal length since the object is between the lens and the focal length. In this case, ray 3 originates at the focal length and runs through the top of the object until it reaches either the lens or the plane through the center of the lens. The ray then runs parallel to the optical axis. As shown in Figure 5.3, the rays on the opposite side of the lens from the object appear to diverge; therefore, there is no image created on the opposite side of the lens. Instead, the rays can be projected backward behind the object to a point where they all intersect. The image that results from this set up is referred to as a **virtual image**. A virtual image is an image created at the point where light rays

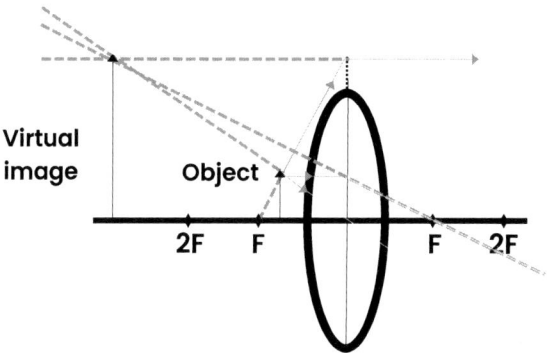

Ray diagram for object located in front of F

Figure 5.3 Ray-tracing for an object between the lens and the focal length. The first two rays are drawn exactly in the same way as shown in Figure 5.2: one ray runs parallel from the top of the object to the lens and then through the focal length; the second ray runs from the top of the object directly through the center of the lens. The third ray must be drawn differently, however, as it is not possible to draw a ray from the top of the object through the focal length since the object is between the lens and the focal length. In this case, ray 3 originates at the focal length and runs through the top of the object until it reaches either the lens or the plane through the center of the lens. The ray then runs parallel to the optical axis. the rays on the opposite side of the lens from the object appear to diverge; therefore, there is no image created on the opposite side of the lens. Instead, the rays can be projected backward behind the object to a point where they all intersect. The image that results from this set up is referred to as a virtual image.

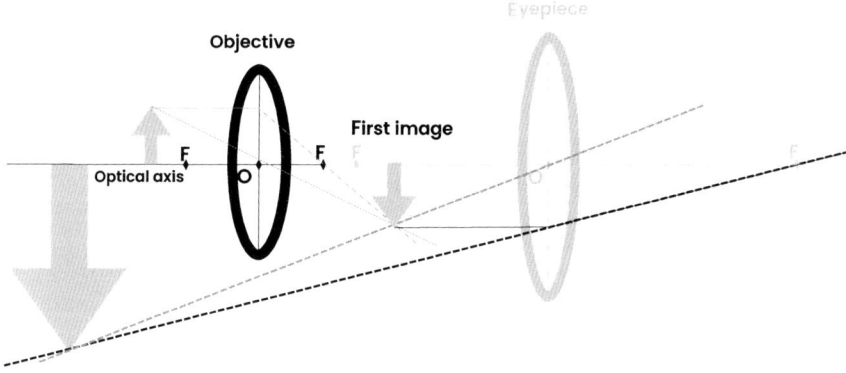

Figure 5.4 Example of image formation in a two-lens system. The two-lens system is a simple way to magnify an image of an object. The first lens, also called the objective, is used to create a real, inverted, magnified image by placing the sample between the focal length and two times the focal length. The second lens, called the eyepiece, is placed such that the resulting real image is between the lens and the focal length, creating a magnified virtual image that can be seen by the user.

converge in the direction opposite to which they are traveling. Importantly, no light rays are actually present at the point where the image is formed (Northrup Grumman, 1963).

How are lenses used to create a microscopy system to magnify an object? A compound microscope uses two lenses or lens systems to create both real and virtual images. Figure 5.4 shows an example of image formation in a two-lens system. The two-lens system is a simple way to magnify an image of an object. The first lens, also called the objective, is used to create a real, inverted, magnified image by placing the sample between the focal length and two times the focal length. The second lens, called the eyepiece, is placed such that the resulting real image is between the lens and the focal length, creating a magnified virtual image that can be seen by the user.

Example: Performing Ray-Tracing for a Two-Lens System

Question: Two converging lenses with focal lengths $f_1 = 10$ cm and $f_2 = 15$ cm are placed 40 cm apart. An object is placed 60 cm in front of the first lens. Draw the lens system and perform ray-tracing to show where the final image will be located. Determine whether the image is real or virtual and upright or inverted.

Answer: Figure 5.5(a) shows the lens system before any ray-tracing has been performed, with each distance labeled. First, we will perform ray-tracing on the first lens to establish where the first image will be formed, as shown in Figure 5.5(b). As you can see, the first

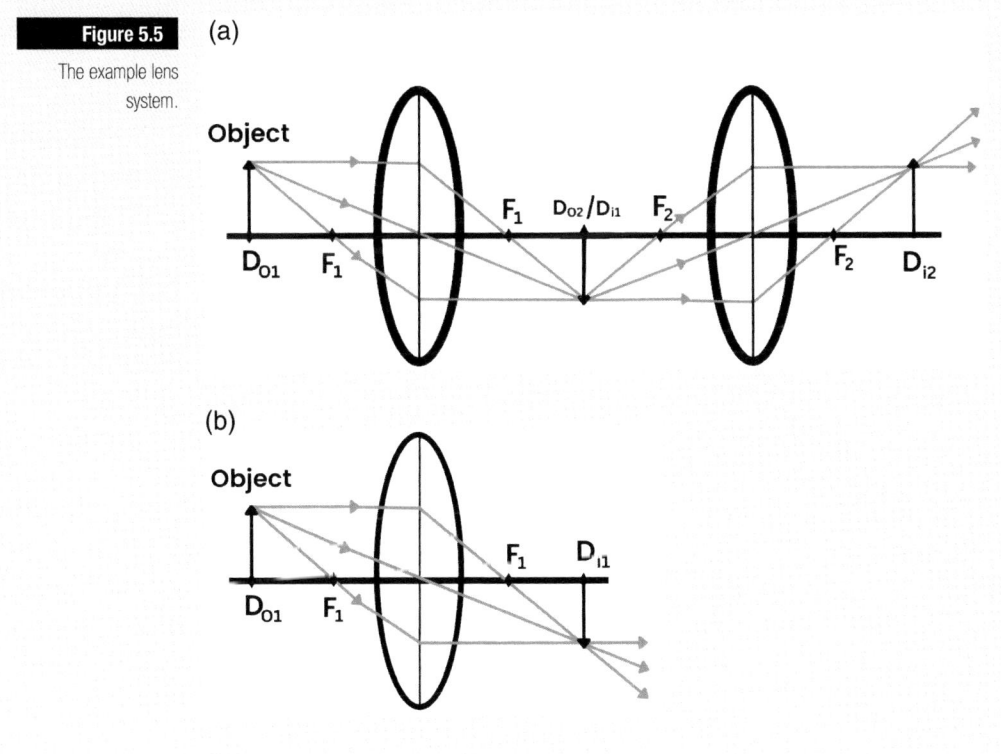

Figure 5.5 The example lens system.

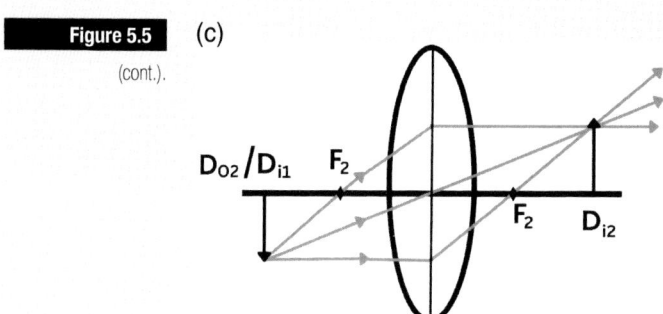

Figure 5.5 (cont.).

image formed is real because the image is formed at the point where the rays converge, and inverted because the image is formed on the opposite side of the optical access from the original object. Next, we will perform ray-tracing on the second lens using the formed image as the object (Figure 5.5(c))

As you can see, the final image formed is real because the image is formed at the point where the rays converge and upright because the image is formed on the same side of the optical access as the original object.

Figure 5.6 shows how a multi-lens system can be used to make a light microscope. The main components in a basic light microscope are the condenser to focus light onto the sample, an objective lens or lens system, and an ocular lens or lens system (also called an eyepiece). The objective and the eyepiece can be made up of a single lens or a system of lenses. The magnified virtual image is what is seen by an observer looking through the eyepiece at the sample.

How do you calculate the magnification of a two-lens system, given lens 1 (L_1), lens 2 (L_2), and the corresponding distance and height of the final image?

The image distances can be calculated from the lens equation (Equation 5.1), which relates the focal length (f), object distance (d_o), and image distance (d_i):

$$\frac{1}{f} = \frac{1}{d_o} + \frac{1}{d_i}. \quad (5.1)$$

Lens magnification can be found using the relationship between the magnification and distance, shown in Equation 5.2, where m is the magnification, d_i is the image distance from the lens, and d_o is the object distance from the lens:

$$m = \frac{d_i}{d_o}. \quad (5.2)$$

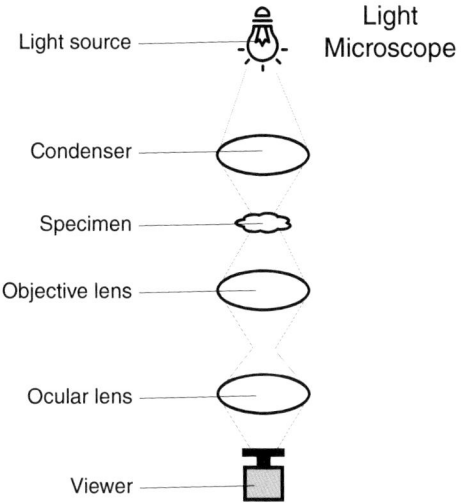

Figure 5.6 A multi-lens system can be used to make a light microscope. The main components in a basic light microscope are the condenser to focus light onto the sample, an objective lens or lens system, and an ocular lens or lens system (also called an eyepiece). The objective and the eyepiece can be made up of a single lens or a system of lenses. The magnified virtual image is what is seen by an observer looking through the eyepiece at the sample.

The height of the image can also be determined from the magnification, as shown in Equation 5.3, where m is the magnification, h_i is the image height from the optical axis, and h_o is the object height from the optical axis:

$$m = \frac{h_i}{h_o}. \tag{5.3}$$

These same equations can be applied to the case where an image is the input to the lens. In this case, the object distance in Equation 5.2 or object height in Equation 5.3 would be replaced with the input image.

Now that we have demonstrated how optical systems can be used to magnify objects, let's take a closer look at how a microscopy system could be set up and the differences between a brightfield microscope and a darkfield microscope. Figure 5.7 shows the differences between darkfield and brightfield microscopy configuration and images. The main components in a basic **brightfield light microscope** are the condenser to focus light onto the sample, an objective, and an eyepiece. The magnified virtual image is what is seen by an observer looking through the eyepiece at the sample. In a **darkfield microscope**, a central aperture is placed between the light source and the sample, and the objective only captures the indirect scattered light, and therefore the sample looks bright on a dark background. Brightfield microscopy works on the principle of absorption and, as such, light focused on the specimen is absorbed and the image appears dark against a bright background. Unlike brightfield microscopes, darkfield microscopes are dark in regions where there is no sample present and bright when light scatters from a sample. Light microscopes are routinely used for pathology slides. Since many organic specimens are transparent or opaque, staining is required to cause the contrast that allows them to be visible under the microscope.

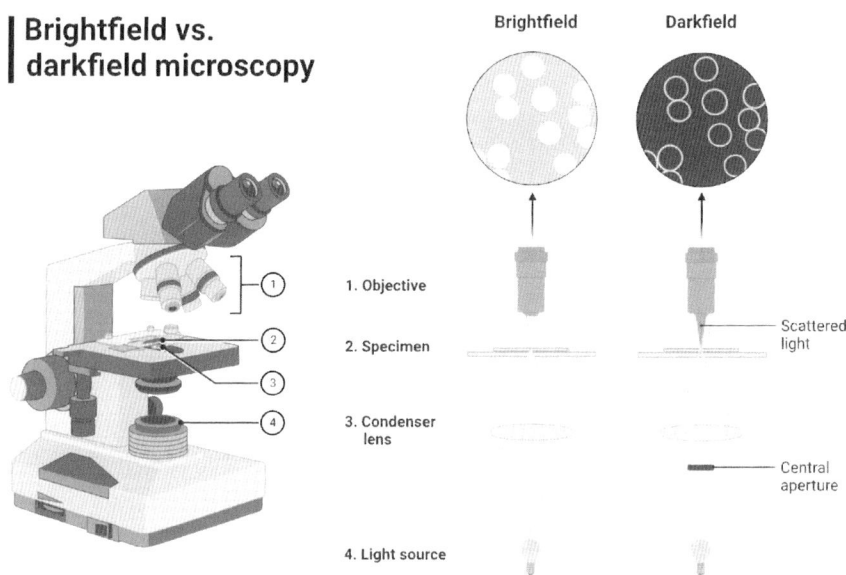

Figure 5.7 Differences between darkfield and brightfield microscopy configuration and images. Brightfield microscopy works on the principle of absorption and, as such, light focused on the specimen is absorbed and the image appears dark against a bright background. With **darkfield microscopy**, a central aperture is placed between the light source and the sample, and the objective only captures the indirect scattered light, and therefore the sample looks bright on a dark background.
Source: Created with BioRender.com.

Example: Darkfield or Brightfield?

Question: A biomedical engineer is trying to decide whether to use a brightfield or darkfield microscope to image two different samples: (1) blood smeared on a slide and (2) adipocytes smeared on a slide. Which type of microscope setup would provide better contrast in each case?

Answer: Brightfield microscopes use absorption as the primary source of contrast, and therefore would be more suitable to image a blood smear, which will absorb light. Darkfield microscopes use scattering as the primary source of contrast, and therefore would be more suitable to image adipocytes, which tend to scatter light.

POCT for Microscopy of Cells and Tissues

A fluorescence microscope is similar to a conventional brightfield microscope but with more features to enhance its capabilities. Illumination light, also referred to as the excitation light, at one or multiple wavelengths excites electrons within the sample to a higher energy level. As the electrons relax back to their original state, they release fluorescence at a longer wavelength. The conventional microscope uses a lamp or a laser to illuminate and produce a magnified image of a sample. **Oblique and epi-illumination** configurations are used to position the light source and the detector. With an oblique illumination setup, the illumination light and detected light pass through different objectives and/or lens systems. Conversely, with an epi-illumination setup, the illumination and detected light pass through the same objective and/or lens system (i.e., the illuminated and detected light travel parallel to each other). In a properly configured microscope only the emission light should reach the eye or detector. This is limited by the sensitivity of the detector and the excitation light, which is typically several hundred thousand to one million times brighter than the emitted fluorescence. Fluorescence microscopy

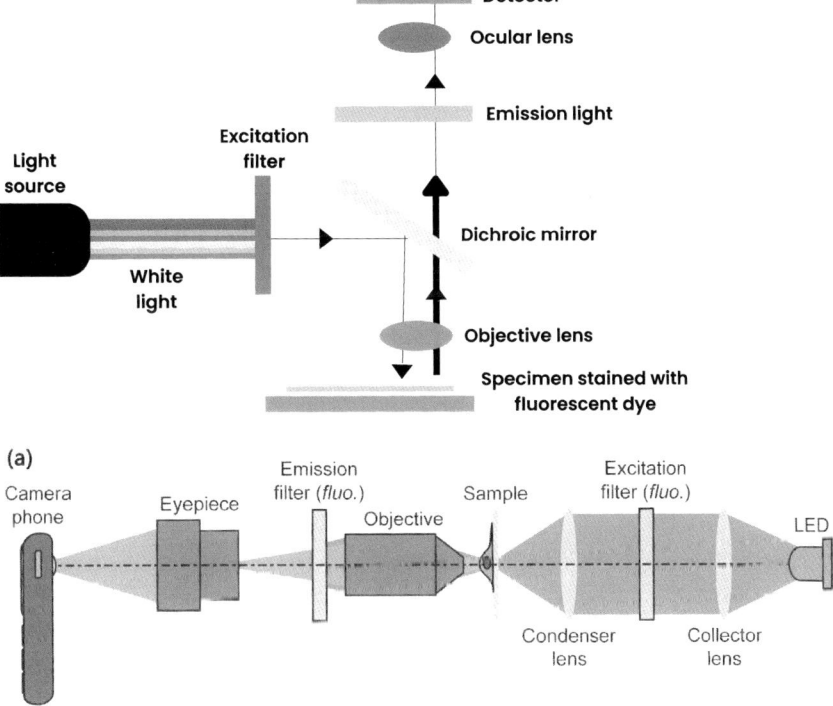

Figure 5.8 A schematic of (a) a standard fluorescence microscope and (b) a portable cell phone-based counterpart. The layouts are very similar, with three exceptions: different light sources, detectors, and the optical path – specifically, the excitation and emitted light share the same optical path in the former whereas they are separate in the latter owing to the fact that transmission is used.
Source: (b) Breslauer et al. (2009). © 2009 Breslauer et al. Licensed under the Creative Commons Attribution License.

is often applied to imaging cell structures or structural features, checking the viability of cells, imaging genetic material (both DNA and RNA), and imaging particular cells in a larger population.

Now that the basic principles of microscopes and the different types of contrast have been discussed, the question is how these principles can be applied to the development of portable imaging technologies, microscopes, and endoscopes. Cell phones are gaining wider use globally, and they serve as an excellent scaffold for microscopes. Further, the majority of cell phones are now equipped with high-quality cameras that can be leveraged as detectors within a microscopy system. **Light-emitting diodes** (LEDs) are great alternatives to lasers or lamps as a means for fluorescence excitation in POCTs, as they are relatively inexpensive and can often be run on battery power. LEDs can be easily swapped out to provide different excitation wavelengths for fluorescence excitation or broad-spectrum coverage for brightfield imaging. Figure 5.8 shows a schematic of (a) a standard fluorescence microscope and (b) a portable cell phone-based counterpart. The layouts are very similar, with three exceptions: different light sources, detectors, and the optical path – specifically, the excitation and emitted light share the same optical path in the former whereas they are separate in the latter owing to the fact that transmission is used.

Deeper Look: Democratizing Microscopy with the Foldscope

Health providers in some of the poorest parts of the world lack access to high-quality diagnostic instruments – most notably the microscope. Cell phone microscopes provide an alternative solution to traditional microscopy and are more accessible within these communities. However, even cell phones are bulky and expensive compared to the miniature Foldscope, an invention that could a put a versatile microscope in anyone's hand. Figure 5.9 shows different configurations of the Foldscope, which was developed at Stanford University. This foldable microscope captures brightfield, darkfield, and fluorescence images ((a)–(d)). The system consists of an LED at the base (the square box shown at the bottom), a sample port above the LED, and a ball lens at the top to focus the light either onto a camera or the eye ((e)–(h)). The system uses mechanical tabs that can be pushed or pulled to change the orientation of the LED, sample, and ball lens to change between imaging configurations and to focus the sample.

The Foldscope has already had far-reaching impacts. The tiny microscope has been distributed to over 135 countries. Not only is it enhancing research and healthcare initiatives, it has become a powerful educational tool. The Foldscope gives students, particularly those in LMICs, the opportunity to go beyond verbal learning to visual learning. Students from around the world have created an online community to share their explorations and experiments.

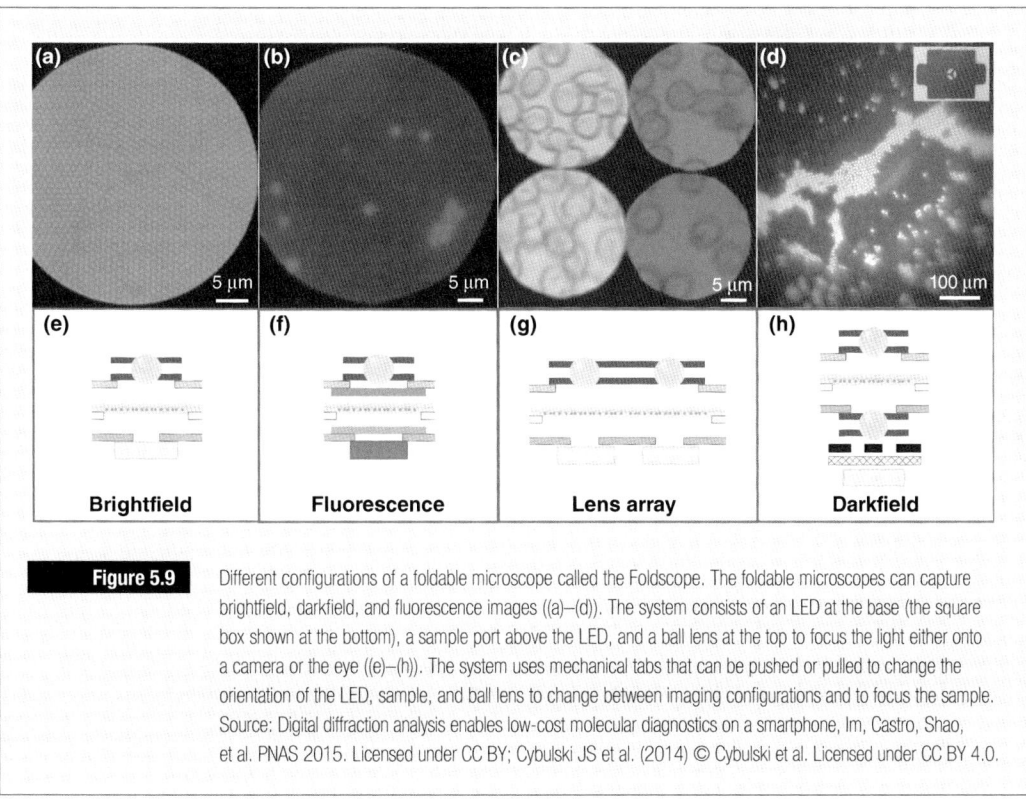

Figure 5.9 Different configurations of a foldable microscope called the Foldscope. The foldable microscopes can capture brightfield, darkfield, and fluorescence images ((a)–(d)). The system consists of an LED at the base (the square box shown at the bottom), a sample port above the LED, and a ball lens at the top to focus the light either onto a camera or the eye ((e)–(h)). The system uses mechanical tabs that can be pushed or pulled to change the orientation of the LED, sample, and ball lens to change between imaging configurations and to focus the sample. Source: Digital diffraction analysis enables low-cost molecular diagnostics on a smartphone, Im, Castro, Shao, et al. PNAS 2015. Licensed under CC BY; Cybulski JS et al. (2014) © Cybulski et al. Licensed under CC BY 4.0.

Cell phone microscopy systems, like those shown in Figure 5.8, can be used for a wide variety of applications in cancer diagnosis and prognosis. There are numerous colorimetric and fluorescence antibodies available on the market today that are in use with some of the POCTs described in Chapter 4. Taking breast cancer as an example, microscopic imaging of immunohistochemical staining (IHC) slides stained for HER2 could be used to rapidly assess whether a patient is a good candidate for therapy with a HER2-targeted inhibitor, like trastuzumab. Another test discussed in earlier chapters is the Pap smear, which requires imaging of a sample of cells taken from the cervix. Cell phone microscopy systems could be used to image Pap smear samples and either to send them to a provider via a mobile phone application or to analyze them directly using artificial intelligence algorithms to provide a diagnosis.

POCTs for Imaging Internal Body Cavities

The microscopy technologies described in the previous section are primarily for use on samples taken out of the body, much like the POCTs described in Chapter 4. A subset of microscopy systems, referred to as **endoscopes**,

162 Point-of-Care Technologies for Imaging Applications

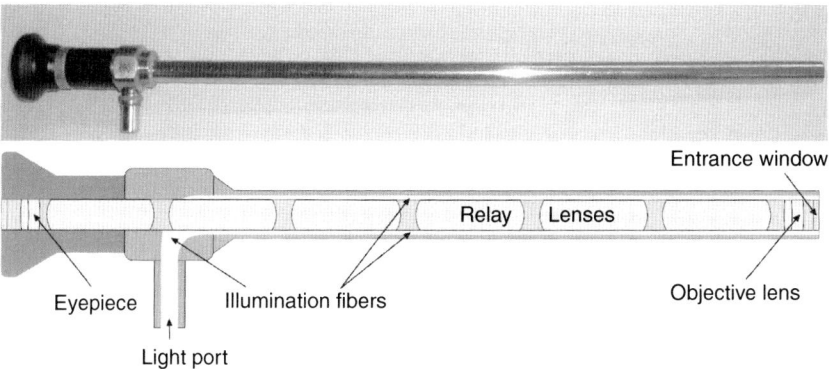

Figure 5.10 Example of a rigid endoscope. Rigid endoscopes have a tube that contains the optical components required to relay light from the source to the end of the tube, as well as light from the entrance window back to the detector. The eyepiece can be used by a healthcare provider to directly visualize objects through the rigid endoscope or attached to a camera to acquire images.
Source: Tobias C. Wood and Daniel S. Elson (2010). Shared by Optica Publishing Group under a CC BY license.

are designed to image within the body. Optical technologies that are used to explore different anatomical sites on or in the human body are referred to as endoscopes. Examples of endoscopes include arthroscopes, bronchoscopes, laryngoscopes, laparoscopes, gastroscopes, hysteroscopes, and colposcopes. As a general rule, an **endoscope** contains a light source to illuminate the desired structure, an optical mechanism to capture an image, and an opening for the use of tools. The specifics of each system vary; however, images may be captured and relayed back using a series of lenses or a flexible bundle of wires. There are two major classes of endoscopes: rigid and flexible.

Figure 5.10 shows an example of a rigid endoscope. Rigid endoscopes have a tube that contains the optical components required to relay light from the source to the end of the tube, as well as light from the entrance window back to the detector. The eyepiece can be used by a healthcare provider to directly visualize objects through the rigid endoscope or attached to a camera to acquire images. Rigid endoscopes, the first type of endoscope developed, are still routinely used during surgery to visualize internal organs without the need for making large incisions.

Figure 5.11 shows an example of a flexible endoscope. Flexible endoscopes have the same functions and basic components as rigid endoscopes (a). The main difference is the light delivery and collection method (b). Rather than using a series of lenses to relay light back and forth, flexible endoscopes use a fiber optic bundle to transport light to and from the sample. Fiber optic delivery of light is achieved by encasing a large number of small fiber light guides together, a **fiber optic bundle** that consists of multiple individual fibers. Light is coupled into the fiber optic bundle and transferred to the sample. Similarly,

Figure 5.11

Example of a flexible endoscope. Flexible endoscopes have the same functions and basic components as rigid endoscopes (a). The main difference is the light delivery and collection method (b). Rather than using a series of lenses to relay light back and forth, flexible endoscopes use a fiber optic bundle to transport light to and from the sample.

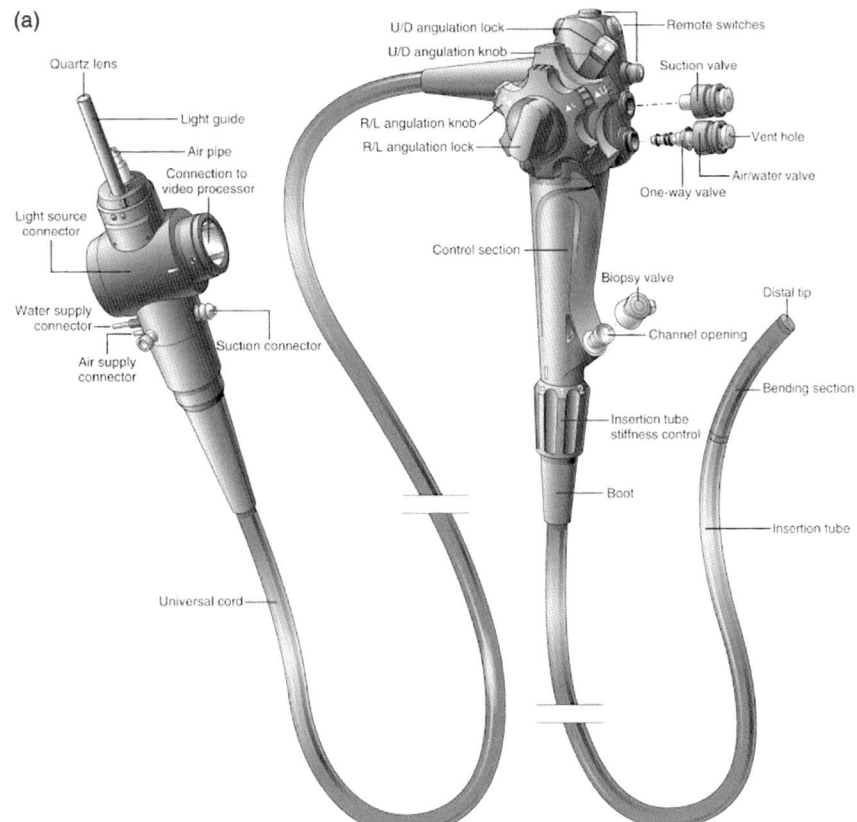

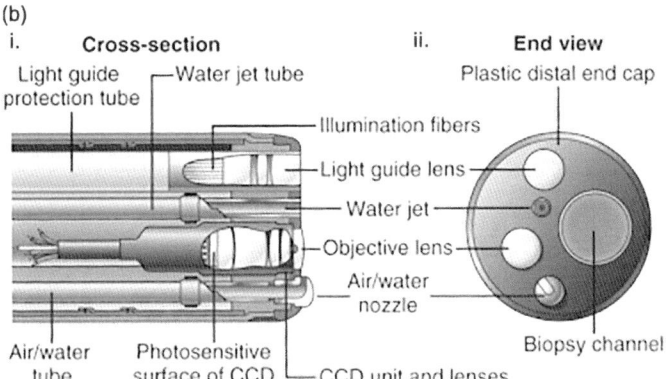

collected light from the sample is transferred back either to a camera or an eyepiece for visualization.

Another type of endoscope that fits in a pocket is a capsule endoscope. Figure 5.12 shows a capsule endoscope and representative images of the colon. The system consists of a camera, LED, lenses, and a transmitter to send data to the provider (a). Representative images are shown for adenocarcinoma of the small bowel (b), neuroendocrine tumor of the small bowel (c),

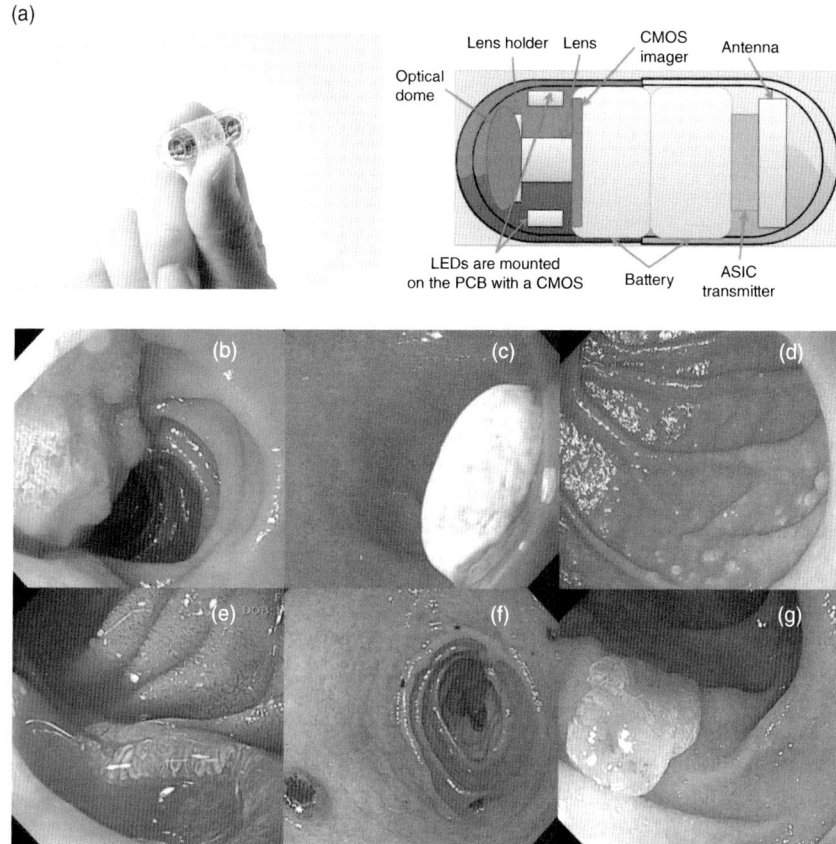

Figure 5.12 A capsule endoscope and representative images of the colon. The system consists of a camera, LED, lenses, and a transmitter to send data to the provider (a). Representative images are shown for adenocarcinoma of the small bowel (b), neuroendocrine tumor of the small bowel (c), follicular lymphoma of the small bowel (d), gastrointestinal stromal tumor of the small bowel with active bleeding (e), secondary small bowel malignancy originating from malignant melanoma (f), and adenoma of the small bowel (g).
Sources: (a) ©Yuuji/E+/Getty Images; (b) Umay et al. (2017); (c) Kim and Kim (2022). Shared under an open access license.

follicular lymphoma of the small bowel (d), gastrointestinal stromal tumor of the small bowel with active bleeding (e), secondary small bowel malignancy originating from malignant melanoma (f), and adenoma of the small bowel (g) (Kim and Kim, 2021). The capsule is swallowed just like any other pill and allowed to pass through the entire gastrointestinal system, capturing images as it travels. It should be noted that unlike the rigid or flexible endoscopes, the capsule has less control over where images are obtained. A variation of the capsule endoscope, a tethered capsule endomicroscope involves swallowing a small, tethered pill that provides relatively more control to the operator than the untethered version. This device uses an optical technique called optical coherence tomography (OCT) to capture high-resolution images of the whole esophagus. The OCT images show structural features of the tissue microanatomy, thus providing histopathology-like images rather than just the surface anatomy (Gora et al., 2013).

The colposcope originally developed by Hinselmann was described in Chapter 3. The modern colposcope is used to examine the internal female reproductive anatomy. The optical components of the colposcope are encased in a head attached to a rigid stand. The colposcope head comprises an objective lens, two eyepieces, a light source, and, in more recent versions, a camera. Either halogen bulbs or LEDs are used as the light source. Most colposcopes have white light and green light illumination. The former provides anatomical information and the latter delineation of blood vessels. The colposcope has a working distance of 30 cm and three or four different magnifications between 4× and 15×. The factor that makes the colposcope large and expensive (high-end colposcopes can cost more than $10,000) is the distance between the colposcope head and the cervix, which necessitates high optical powers, a high-resolution camera, and optics with long working distances.

A variety of portable colposcopes have been developed. These colposcopes have a smaller form factor compared to a standard colposcope, but operate using the same principles as their original counterpart. Many of these colposcopes leverage the light source and camera on a smartphone and some use additional lens attachments to the cell phone for magnification. Both standard-of-care colposcopes and portable colposcopes operate similarly – outside of the speculum. Often, the low-cost versions have inferior image quality to that of a high-end traditional colposcope owing to the fact that the device is outfitted with lower-cost components. While portable colposcopes can be hand-held when used during an examination, they are prone to instability.

A portable colposcope called the Pocket Colposcope has been developed by Duke University (Lam et al., 2015). The Pocket Colposcope is shaped like a tampon and can be inserted through and stabilized on the speculum, such that it is 30–40 mm away from the cervix, removing the need for powerful light sources, high-resolution cameras, and long working distances. Additionally, USB-enabled data transfer allows for images to be transferred to a cell phone. Figure 5.13 shows photos of an upright colposcope, the Pocket Colposcope, the positioning of the devices to capture an image of the cervix, and representative images from both devices. The Pocket Colposcope is portable and a fraction of the size of the upright colposcope. The colposcope has a microscope mounted on an upright stand, whereas the Pocket Colposcope can be directly inserted into the vaginal canal. The images of a precancerous cervix captured with both colposcopes have comparable image contrast and fields of view.

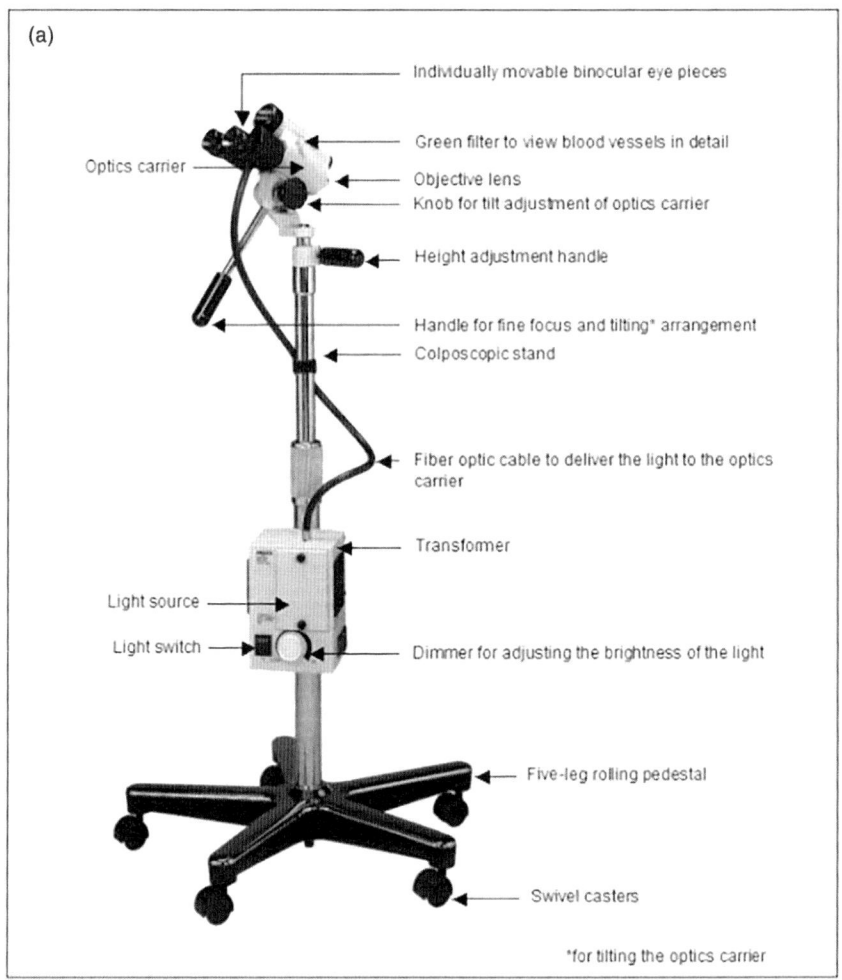

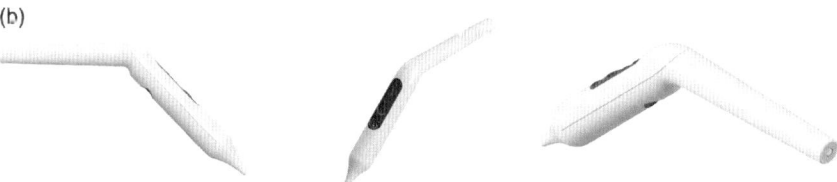

Figure 5.13 Photos of an upright colposcope (a), the Pocket Colposcope (b), the positioning of the Pocket Colposcope to capture an image of the cervix (c), and representative images from both devices (d). The Pocket Colposcope is portable and a fraction of the size of the upright colposcope. The colposcope has a microscope mounted on an upright stand, whereas the Pocket Colposcope can be directly inserted into the vaginal canal. The images of a precancerous cervix captured with both colposcopes have comparable image contrast and fields of view.
Source: (a) Colposcopy and treatment of cervical intraepithelial neoplasia: a beginners' manual, Edited by J.W. Sellors and R. Sankaranarayanan, Chapter 4 © IARC.

(c)

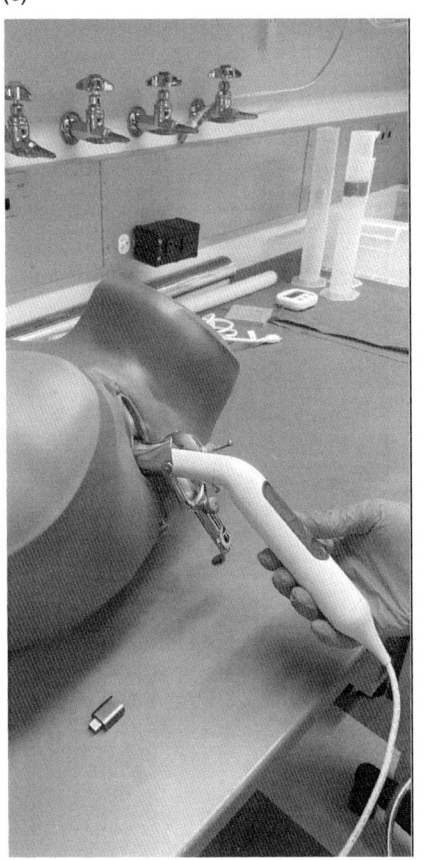

(d)

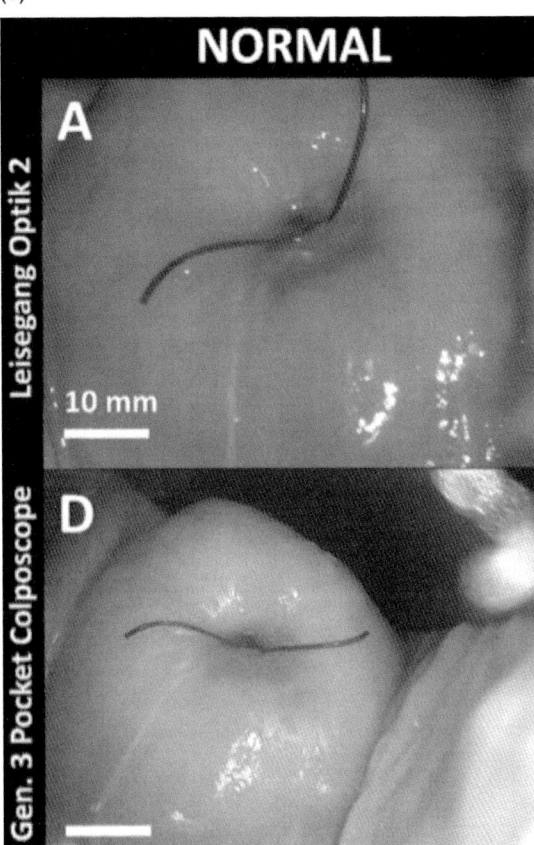

Figure 5.13 (cont.)

Deeper Look: The Speculum as a Barrier to Screening

A speculum is essential to a colposcopy procedure. The speculum parts the vaginal walls such that the colposcope has a clear line of sight to the cervix. Figure 5.14 illustrates the modern duck bill speculum, which can be made of metal or plastic. Despite rapid technological advances over the last century, the mechanism by which the speculum operates has been largely unchanged since its invention over 150 years ago (see Chapter 3).

The speculum-based exam has been reported to create anxiety, fear, discomfort, pain, embarrassment, and vulnerability during the procedure. In the US, middle-aged African American women have the second highest rate of cervical cancer incidence and the highest cervical cancer mortality rate, nearly double that of their white counterparts. The perceived pain of the screening procedure among African American women and the cost of office visits are associated with a six-fold increase in nonadherence to screening relative to the general population. These barriers to screening in the US are echoed globally. In Ghana, cervical cancer is the most common cancer in women. The high prevalence has been attributed to issues including inadequate awareness of the disease, limited access to care, fear, and cultural taboos surrounding the exam and reproductive health. A study of women in Moshi, Tanzania showed that key barriers to obtaining gynecological exams were concerns about embarrassment and pain due to the speculum and physician gender. In Australia, a study of women's attitudes toward physician-insertion versus self-insertion of a speculum found that 91 percent of women preferred self-insertion, and that having another person insert the device caused discomfort, embarrassment, and vulnerability (Asiedu et al., 2020).

A derivative of the Pocket Colposcope, the Callascope, obviates the need for a speculum. This technology has similar components to the Pocket Colposcope, except that it has a thinner form factor, which allows it to be inserted through a Calla Lily (flower)-shaped introducer that obviates the need for a speculum. Figure 5.14 shows a comparison of the design of the Callascope and the conventional speculum and corresponding images. A traditional gynecological exam uses a speculum to part the vaginal walls (a) and orient the cervix into the line of sight of the colposcope (b) to capture an image (c). The Callascope achieves the same goal using a Calla Lily tip (d) that orients the cervix into the line of sight (e) for image capture with the Callascope camera (f).

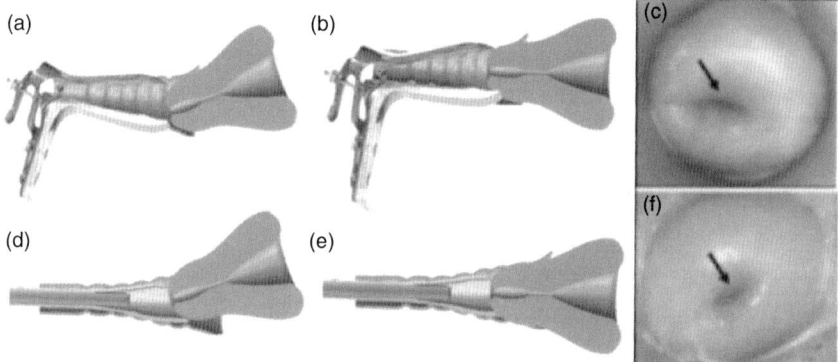

Figure 5.14 Comparison of the design of the Callascope and the conventional speculum and corresponding images. A traditional gynecological exam uses a speculum to part the vaginal walls (a) and orient the cervix into the line of sight of the colposcope (b) to capture an image (c). The Callascope achieves the same goal using a Calla Lily tip (d) that orients the cervix into the line of sight (e) for image capture with the Callascope camera (f).
Source: Calla Health.

Histopathology remains the gold standard for cancer diagnosis. Traditional histopathology requires a multistep process to remove tissue from the body, process and stain the tissue, and then examine the tissue using a high-powered microscope. This ex vivo method for cancer diagnosis is highly restrictive due to the high cost of the equipment involved and the number of highly trained individuals required during each step of the process. In situ tissue examination with microscopy has the advantage of not requiring removal of tissue from the body and can be performed with relatively inexpensive microscopes and labeled contrast agents. A group out of Rice University has developed a portable confocal microscope that can take high-resolution images of labeled contrast agents in situ, demonstrating the ability to differentiate tumor from nontumor tissue, similar to histopathology. Figure 5.15 shows a schematic of

(a)

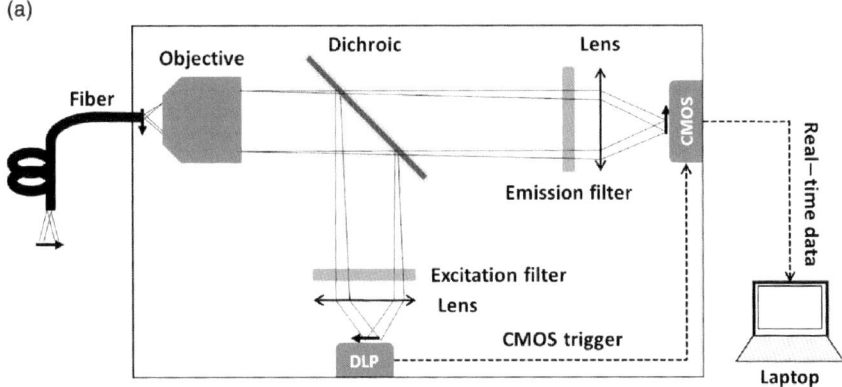

(b)

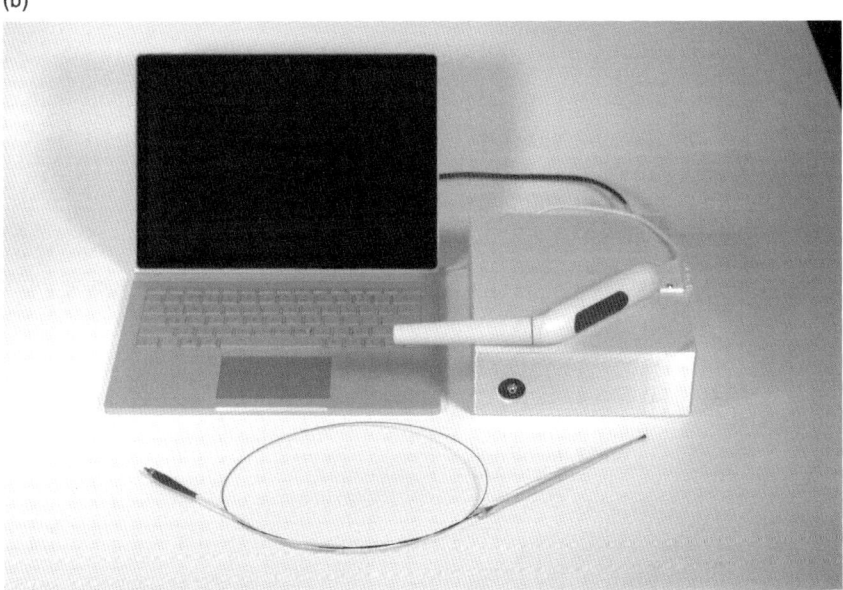

Figure 5.15 Schematic of the high-resolution microendoscope (HRME), photo of the actual HRME with the Pocket Colposcope, and images obtained with both devices. The HRME uses traditional optics in a compact form factor to achieve high-resolution imaging at the point of care (a). The HRME system is battery-powered, connects to a laptop for image capture and display (Tang et al., 2017), and can be coupled with the Pocket Colposcope for widefield, high-resolution imaging (b). The Pocket Colposcope can identify suspicious areas on the cervix and the HRME can image in situ tissue pathology. The HRME images capture the density and size of cell nuclei, which are larger and more crowded in precancerous tissues.
Source: (a) Line-scanning confocal microendoscope for nuclear morphometry imaging, Tang, Carns, Richards-Kortum et al. (2017). Licensed under CC BY-SA 3.0.

(c)

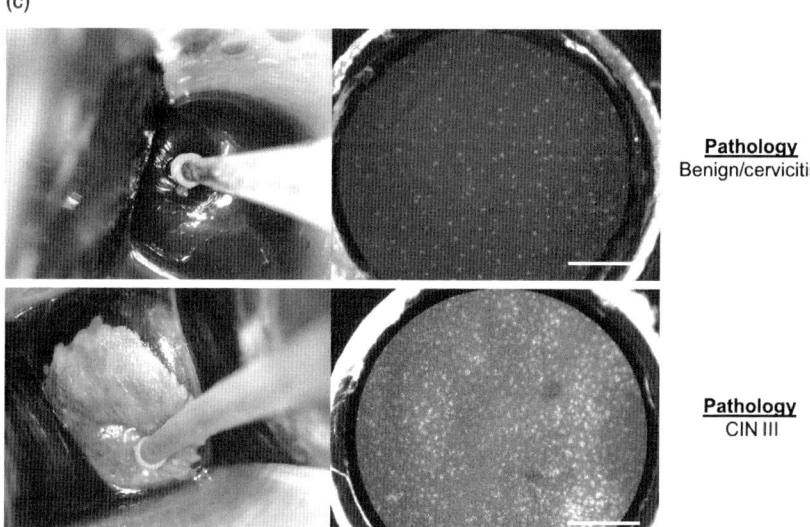

Pathology
Benign/cervicitis

Pathology
CIN III

*Scale bars on HRME images represent 200 μm

Figure 5.15 (cont.)

the high-resolution microendoscope (HRME), a photo of the actual HRME with the Pocket Colposcope, and images obtained with both devices. The HRME uses traditional optics in a compact form factor to achieve high-resolution imaging at the point of care (a). The HRME system is battery-powered, connects to a laptop for image capture and display (Tang et al., 2017), and can be coupled with the Pocket Colposcope for widefield, high-resolution imaging (b). The Pocket Colposcope can identify suspicious areas on the cervix and the HRME can image in situ tissue pathology. The HRME images capture the density and size of cell nuclei, which are larger and more crowded in precancerous tissues. Microscopy systems like the HRME system are attractive POCTs that use imaging as a method to perform rapid diagnosis at the point of care, reducing time between diagnosis and treatment.

Ultrasound Imaging and POCTs

Perhaps the most iconic example of a POCT is the ultrasound. In this section we will explore the fundamental principles behind ultrasound, as well as the transition from large ultrasound to portable ultrasound devices that can be used at the point of care. The underlying physical principle that ultrasound imaging leverages is called the piezoelectric effect. Figure 5.16 shows the piezoelectric effect used in ultrasound and an ultrasound wave moving through tissue. The piezoelectric effect is used in ultrasound probes to emit sound

Ultrasound Imaging and POCTs

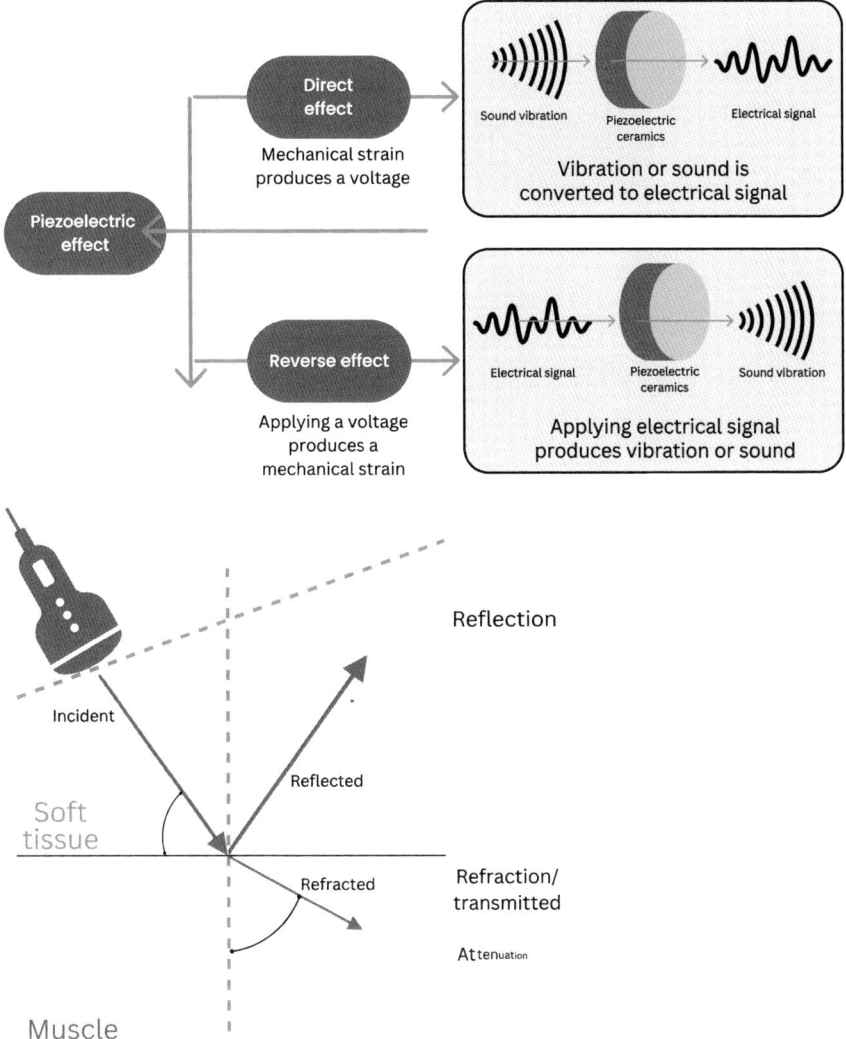

Figure 5.16
The piezoelectric effect used in ultrasound and an ultrasound wave moving through tissue. The piezoelectric effect is used in ultrasound probes to emit sound waves into the body through conversion of an electrical signal into a mechanical vibration (via a **reverse effect**) and to receive sound waves through conversion of a mechanical vibration into an electrical signal (via a **direct effect**) (a). When a sound wave enters the body and encounters a **boundary surface**, part of the wave's energy is reflected back by the surface, while the remaining energy is transmitted through the boundary into the new tissue type (b).

waves into the body through conversion of an electrical signal into a mechanical vibration (via a **reverse effect**) and to receive sound waves through conversion of a mechanical vibration into an electrical signal (via a **direct effect**) (a). When a sound wave enters the body and encounters a **boundary surface**, part of the wave's energy is reflected back by the surface, while the remaining energy is transmitted through the boundary into the new tissue type (b). A **boundary surface** is the place where the physical properties of tissue change, either because the tissue type changes or because the tissue structure changes.

A number of parameters are used to describe sound waves, including frequency, period, wavelength, amplitude, power, and intensity, all of which were covered in Chapter 2. These parameters are briefly described below. The wavelength is the distance traveled by one complete wave (in millimeters, mm),

Table 5.1 Impedance values for different tissue types within the body

The acoustic impedance of a medium is directly proportional to the density and the propagation velocity of the medium.

Tissue	Density (kg/m^3)	US velocity (m/s)	z (106 Rayls)
Air	1.21	330	0.0004
Fat	952	1,450	1.34
Water	1,000	1,480	1.48
Soft tissue av.	1,058	1,540	1.63
Kidney	1,038	1,560	1.63
Blood	1,025	1,570	1.65
Liver	1,065	1,550	1.65
Muscle	1,076	1,580	1.71
Bone	1,912	4,080	7.8

Impedance (Z) = medium density (ρ) × US velocity (v) in medium.

the period is the time required for one complete wave to pass (seconds, s), the frequency is inversely related to period and wavelength and reported in hertz (Hz), and the propagation velocity is the product of the wavelength and frequency (mm/s). **Amplitude** is the height of the wave reported in megapascals (MPa), the **power** of the sound wave is the total amount of energy in the ultrasound beam and proportional to the square of the amplitude in watts (W), and **intensity** is the power per unit area (W/cm^2). The sound waves create a pressure field within the tissue. The higher the voltages converting electric signals to acoustic pressure waves, the higher the amplitude, intensity, and power. Higher-frequency sound waves (5–15 MHz) yield better resolution than lower-frequency waves (2–5 MHz). However, this improved resolution for higher-frequency sound waves is at the expense of lower penetration depth.

The propagation velocity is assumed to be that of air, which is 1,540 m/s (1.54 mm/μs), which means the time for sound to travel 1 cm in the body is approximately 6.5 μs, and the roundtrip is double. In reality, the actual speed of sound varies significantly from the assumed 1,540 m/s, and therefore, this results in an error on the displayed image (higher than assumed values lead to shallower images and vice versa). **Impedance** is a measure of how much resistance an ultrasound wave experiences as it moves through a medium and affects how deep the ultrasound wave will penetrate into tissue (transmission), and how much will be reflected back. Table 5.1 shows impedance for different tissue types within the body. The acoustic impedance of a medium is directly proportional to the density and the propagation velocity of the medium.

173 Ultrasound Imaging and POCTs

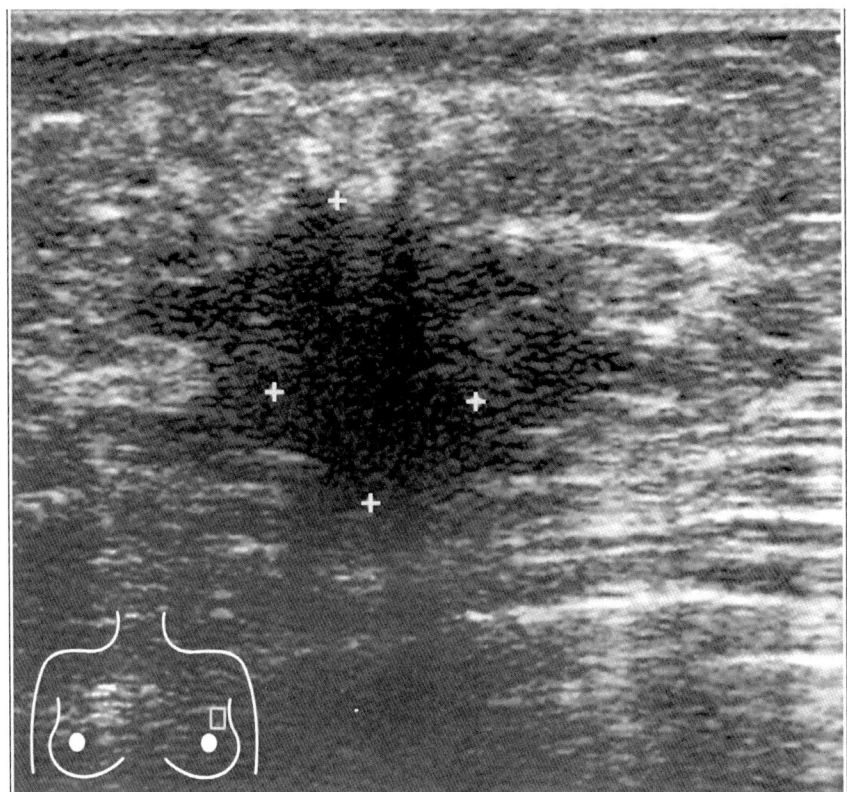

Figure 5.17

A representative ultrasound image of breast cancer. The dark hypoechoic area in the middle is the tumor and the brighter areas are fat. Source: ©BSIP / Contributor/Universal Images Group/Getty Images.

The percent reflection, which is the ratio of reflected intensity and total intensities (reflection + transmission), is related to the impedance mismatch of two different media such as air and tissue, and is represented by Equation 5.4. The larger the impedance mismatch, the larger the reflection. Denser tissues, such as muscle or fibrous tissues, absorb more of the sound wave (hypoechoic and correspond to dark areas on an image) and fatty tissue or fluid-filled cysts are less dense and reflect more of the sound wave (hyperechoic and corresponds to bright areas on the image). Figure 5.17 shows a representative ultrasound image of breast cancer. The dark hypoechoic area in the middle is the tumor and the brighter areas are fat.

Two of the largest changes in acoustic impedance in the body are when ultrasound encounters air or bone (relative to soft tissue). Consequently, if the ultrasound waves encounter air between the transducer and the skin, the vast majority of the ultrasound energy will be reflected back to the transducer owing to the large impedance mismatch between the two. Ultrasound gel, which provides impedance matching, addresses this problem. Ultrasound gel is a thick substance composed of **water and propylene glycol**, a synthetic compound often found in food and cosmetic or hygiene products. It has a sticky consistency, allowing it to be spread over the skin without dripping or running off. For diagnostic ultrasound, the gel has acoustic impedance comparable to soft tissue. The reflection coefficient (R) at a boundary can be related to the impedance of the first and second mediums using Equation 5.4:

$$R = \frac{Z_2 - Z_1}{Z_2 + Z_1}. \tag{5.4}$$

Example: How Impedance Affects Ultrasound Image Interpretation

Question: A biomedical engineer is examining a series of four images she recorded with a low-cost ultrasound system she designed. The first image was taken in a tank of water with a solid bead in the middle with an impedance of 1.53. The second image was taken with the same bead submerged in fat. The third image was taken of a bead with an impedance of 1.43 submerged in water. The fourth image was taken of the same bead submerged in fat. Quantitatively explain whether the bead would appear brighter or darker than the surrounding medium for each image. In which image would there be the most contrast between the bead and the surrounding medium?

Answer: For image 1, the bead has a higher impedance than water, which will reflect more sound waves back to the probe. As a result, the bead will appear brighter. We can see this quantitatively using Equation 5.4:

$$R = \frac{1.53 - 1.48}{1.53 + 1.48} = 0.017.$$

For image 2, the bead has a higher impedance than fat and will, therefore, appear brighter. Using Equation 5.4:

$$R = \frac{1.53 - 1.34}{1.53 + 1.34} = 0.066.$$

For image 3, the bead has a lower impedance than water and will, therefore, appear darker. Using Equation 5.4:

$$R = \frac{1.43 - 1.48}{1.43 + 1.48} = -0.017.$$

For image 4, the bead has a higher impedance than fat and will, therefore, appear brighter. Using Equation 5.4:

$$R = \frac{1.43 - 1.34}{1.43 + 1.34} = 0.032.$$

Because there is the greatest difference in impedance between the bead and medium for image 2, that image would contain the highest contrast.

(a)   (b)

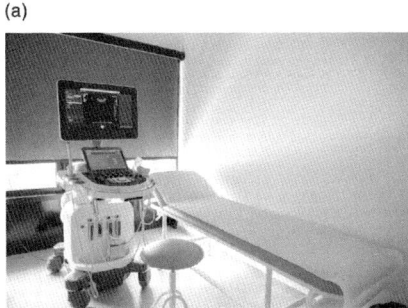 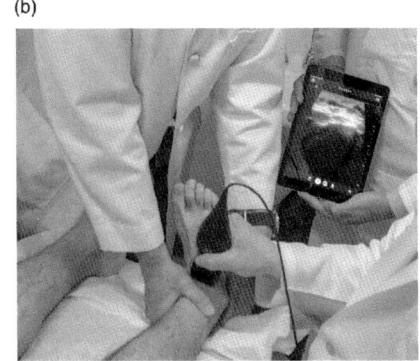

Figure 5.18 Bench-top vs. portable ultrasound. The original ultrasound units and those still found primarily in hospitals and centralized health facilities are large devices situated either on a bench-top or a large rolling cart (a). Recently, more portable ultrasound probes have been developed that can be connected directly to a smartphone or tablet for image reconstruction (b).
Source: (a) ©miodrag ignjatovic/E+/Getty Images; (b) Portable ultrasound devices: A method to improve access to medical imaging, barriers to implementation, and the need for future advancements, Tang, Guss, Tanaka, Lubberts. Clinical Imaging, 2022-01-01, Volume 81, Pages 147–149, Copyright © 2021.

Anatomical ultrasound imaging has become routine in maternity clinics throughout the developed world. The technology has undergone extensive development over the last few decades, from large bench-top systems that require a large and constant power supply to ones that are battery-powered, hand-held, less expensive, and lighter weight. Figure 5.18 shows a bench-top and a portable ultrasound system. The original ultrasound units and those still found primarily in hospitals and centralized health facilities are large devices situated either on a bench-top or a large rolling cart. Recently, more portable ultrasound probes have been developed that can be connected directly to a smartphone or tablet for image reconstruction. The evolution of bench-top ultrasound systems to portable ultrasound devices has expanded applications of the technology beyond specialized facilities to medical school anatomy classes, battlefields, and even patients' homes.

Having discussed the principles of ultrasound, let us examine what makes portable ultrasound systems so mobile. Figure 5.19 shows a photo of a microelectromechanical system (MEMS) for ultrasound. The basic principle of MEMS is similar to the piezoelectric effect. MEMS uses a **capacitor** to generate small vibrations. A **capacitor** is a device that stores electrical energy in an electric field. When a current is applied and removed, the terminals of the capacitor move toward and away from each other, respectively, generating an ultrasonic wave when performed rapidly. The same system can be used to measure a received ultrasonic wave because a current is generated when a wave displaces one terminal toward the other. Many MEMS can be placed in an array to create a low-cost, portable ultrasound transducer.

176 Point-of-Care Technologies for Imaging Applications

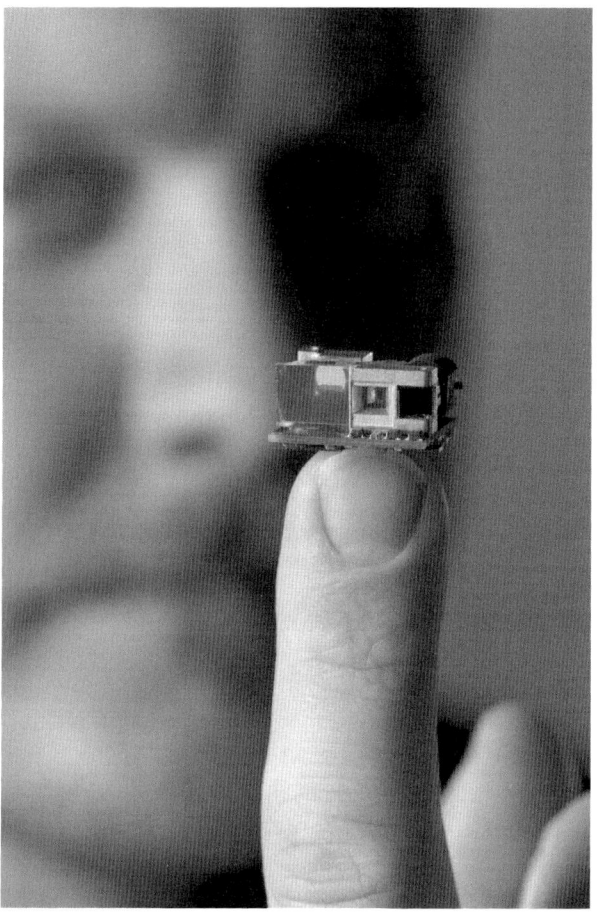

Figure 5.19 A photo of a micro-electromechanical system (MEMS). MEMS uses charge applied to a capacitor to generate small vibrations. When a current is applied and removed, the terminals of the capacitor move toward and away from each other, respectively, generating an ultrasonic wave when performed rapidly. The same system can be used to measure a received ultrasonic wave because a current is generated when a wave displaces one terminal toward the other. The basic principle is similar to the piezoelectric effect. Many of these MEMS can be placed in an array to create a low-cost, portable ultrasound transducer.
Source: ©Business Wire / Handout/Getty Images Publicity/Getty Images.

In its basic form, a capacitor consists of two conductive (metal) plates which are electrically separated either by air or a good insulating material. Figure 5.20 shows a capacitor in a circuit, where the battery serves as the voltage source. The capacitor is fully charged when the voltage of the power supply is equal to that at the capacitor terminals. The capacitor is fully charged when current stops flowing through the electrical circuit. When the power supply is removed from the capacitor, the discharging phase begins. The formula for capacitance C is shown in Equation 5.5:

$$C = Q/V = \varepsilon (A/d) \tag{5.5}$$

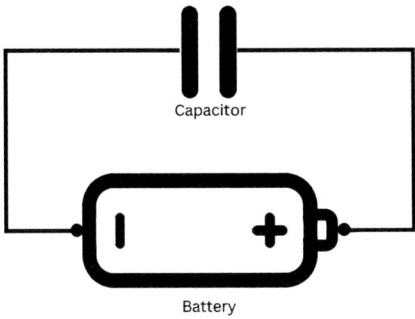

Figure 5.20 A capacitor in a circuit, where the battery serves as the voltage source. The capacitor is fully charged when the voltage of the power supply is equal to that at the capacitor terminals. The capacitor is fully charged when current stops flowing through the electrical circuit. When the power supply is removed from the capacitor, the discharging phase begins.

where Q is the charge, V is the voltage, A is the area of the capacitor, and d is the distance between the plates. ε represents the absolute permittivity of the dielectric material being used. The dielectric constant, ε_o, also known as the "permittivity of free space" has the value 8.854×10^{-12} farads per meter.

The MEMS used in portable ultrasounds employ piezoelectric materials that act similarly to a capacitor. When a charge is applied to the capacitor, it expands or contracts, depending on the type of charge applied. When the charge is removed, the capacitor contracts or expands in the opposite manner. Rapid changes in charge can cause mechanical fluctuations that can generate sound waves. The magnitude and frequency of these sound waves can be changed by selecting different types of capacitors, applying different voltages and currents, and changing the frequency of applying voltages and currents.

Example: Changes in Capacitance Change Distance Between Plates

Question: How would the distance between the two plates within a capacitor change if the capacitance was increased by a factor of five?

Answer: We can answer this question using Equation 5.5. Let's call the initial capacitance and distance C_1 and D_1, and the final capacitance and distance C_2 and D_2. Plugging both into Equation 5.5:

$$C_1 = \varepsilon \frac{A}{D_1},$$

$$C_2 = \varepsilon \frac{A}{D_2}.$$

We know from the question that C_2 is five times higher than C_1, so $C_2/C_1 = 5$; therefore, we can divide the two equations and set that equal to 5:

$$\frac{C_2}{C_1} = \frac{\varepsilon \frac{A}{D_2}}{\varepsilon \frac{A}{D_1}} = 5.$$

Canceling out terms that are in both the numerator and denominator gives:

$$\frac{\frac{1}{D_2}}{\frac{1}{D_1}} = 5.$$

Simplifying:

$$\frac{1}{D_2} = 5 \frac{1}{D_1},$$

$$D_2 = \frac{1}{5} D_1.$$

Therefore, a five times increase in capacitance would reduce the distance between the two plates of the capacitor by a factor of five.

Deeper Look: Ultrasound Imaging During the COVID-19 Pandemic

Chest CT has a high sensitivity for the diagnosis of COVID-19 pneumonia, and it is considered the gold standard imaging method. During the pandemic, CT systems underwent high usage owing to the large influx of patients to hospitals. The ability to rapidly triage, monitor, and manage patients was essential so that patients with the greatest need could be advanced to CT imaging.

Ultrasound has not previously been considered for lung imaging, but since the onset of the pandemic, it has been instrumental to tracking the course of lung disease in patients with COVID-19-related respiratory symptoms. Figure 5.21 shows a hand-held ultrasound scanner being used to image the lung in a pediatric patient. Ultrasound images are correlated with the progression of clinical and radiological deterioration in patients with COVID-19 respiratory problems (Smith et al., 2020), and therefore present a simple way in which to determine the course of action for a provider – for example, whether the patient needs to go to the ER or the ICU.

The availability of hand-held ultrasound scanners has also helped hospitals reduce cross-contamination and risk of infection spread. Because it can be used where the patient is, it minimizes the need to move the patient, and the number of healthcare professionals exposed to the patient (as CT requires more personnel than ultrasound). Further, portable ultrasound scanners are easier to disinfect than traditional cart-based systems. Another significant benefit is the ability to monitor patients at regular intervals without the risk of the ionizing radiation used in CT imaging. Additionally, hand-held systems are a fraction of the cost of a standard ultrasound system, which can cost upward of $100,000.

Hand-held ultrasound can be viewed as a tool to extend hospital-based services. As footprints of current systems get smaller and the cost lower, ultrasound is poised to impact a larger population. Tele-ultrasound facilitated by the US Food and Drug Administration (FDA) emergency use authorization enabled many healthcare providers to expand tele-ultrasound services, where a trained professional can remotely see the scan and talk a nontrained professional through the process. This is a particularly important service for older adults living in nursing homes with suspected COVID-19 pneumonia or for occupational health surveillance of healthcare workers affected by COVID-19 at the home or the workplace.

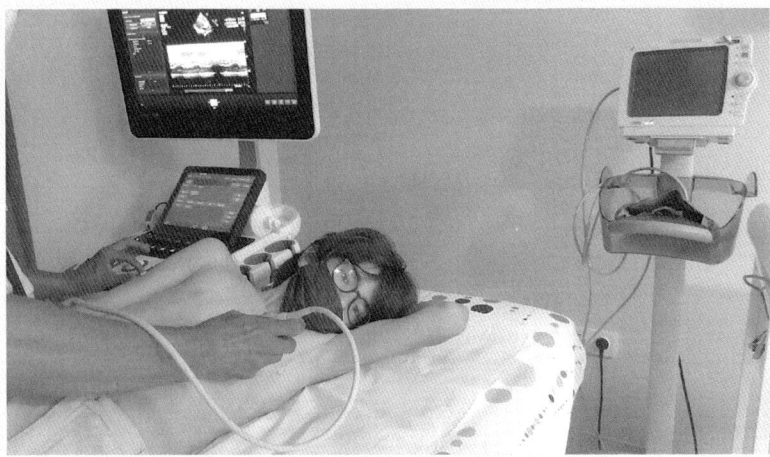

Figure 5.21 Hand-held ultrasound scanner being used to image the lung. Ultrasound images are correlated with the progression of clinical and radiological deterioration in patients with COVID-19 respiratory problems, and therefore present a simple way in which to determine the course of action for a provider – for example whether the patient needs to go to the ER or the ICU.
Source: ©mgstudyo/E+/Getty Images.

Looking Ahead

Earlier, we discussed that to truly democratize access to care, a hub-and-spoke model must be implemented. In this model, a subset of the tasks routinely performed by physicians is shifted to less experienced personnel who can consult with the experts to make decisions. Telemedicine is a powerful way to carry this out. For example, if a nurse or midwife performs imaging with a portable colposcope or ultrasound system in a mobile clinic or a community clinic, the images can be relayed to an expert who can then render a decision. Over time, through mentoring and counseling, the nurse or midwife can learn the patterns that discern diseased from normal tissue and, as a result, might rely less on the expert except for difficult cases or for quality control. Telemedicine will be described in greater detail in Chapter 10.

Ultrasound and optical techniques can be used in diverse healthcare settings. Increased demand, simpler technological requirements, and multiple-use design can drive down overall costs as well as costs per procedure. Cost minimization is important in low-resource settings due to supply chain limitations and the frequent lack of infrastructure (power, water, disinfection protocols, extreme environmental conditions). Caution is still needed with the currently available portable technologies as these devices may provide information that the providers are not able to act on, owing to lack of follow-up care. Another important issue is access to experts to interpret images. Telemedicine is emerging as a promising way in which to connect midwives and nurses who are closest to the patients to remote experts who can comment on the images. However, if there is unreliable access to the internet and/or a lack of availability of experts, this could further limit the utility of these diagnostic procedures.

Increased development of low-cost POCTs for use in LMICs, such as HPV molecular testing, hand-held colposcopes, and portable ultrasound, have enabled early screening and diagnosis of diseases at the point of care. Treatment, however, continues to be a challenge. For example, in high-income countries cervical cancer is effectively prevented through the curative treatment of the disease at its precancerous stage, as described in Chapter 3. The primary method used to treat localized cancer involves surgical removal of the diseased tissue. In fact, the primary frontline treatment for the vast majority of cancers involves some form of surgery. Unfortunately, 9 out of 10 people in LMICs lack access to essential surgery, the primary life-saving treatment for cancer. Chapter 6 will describe alternatives to surgery for treatment of cancer in LMICs, because, without methods to effectively treat cancer, what is the utility of POCTs for cancer diagnosis?

SUMMARY

There is a growing need for POCTs for cancer diagnosis in LMICs. Optical and ultrasound imaging are well suited for development of imaging POCTs, as they are relatively inexpensive, safe, and easy to use. The microscope, a ubiquitous optical instrument, is widely used in healthcare, most notably in pathology labs where they are used to read histology slides. Lenses play a critical role in magnifying microscopic objects that are not resolvable to the unaided eye. The two-lens system is the basic element of a microscope. There are three major types of microscopes: brightfield, darkfield, and fluorescence. Brightfield microscopes use absorption as the source of contrast between the sample and background. Darkfield microscopes, on the other hand, use scattered light as the source of contrast. Fluorescence microscopes use fluorescence as the source of contrast. Optical microscopy can be readily implemented at the point of care by swapping out expensive lasers and lamp sources for cheaper LEDs, and detectors with cell phone cameras.

Optical technologies that are used to explore different anatomical sites on or in the human body are referred to as endoscopes. Examples of endoscopes include arthroscopes, bronchoscopes, laryngoscopes, laparoscopes, gastroscopes, hysteroscopes, and colposcopes. As a general rule, an endoscope contains a light source to illuminate the desired structure, an optical mechanism to capture an image, and an opening for the use of tools. The specifics of each system vary; images may be captured and relayed back using a series of lenses or a flexible bundle of wires. There are two major classes of endoscopes, rigid and flexible. An endoscope called a microendoscope can merge microscopy and endoscopy into one unit. The system referred to as a high-resolution microendoscope (HRME) can visualize pathological features in the body with the use of an inexpensive contrast agent. The capsule, a miniaturized endoscope, can be swallowed and captures images as it passes through the entire gastrointestinal system. The images are then transmitted to the healthcare provider for interpretation. The Pocket and Callascopes use the concept of an endoscope to provide images of the cervix without the need for an expensive clinical microscope, called the colposcope. They both capture equivalent images to their clinical counterparts at a fraction of the cost, and in the case of the Callascope, colposcopy can be performed without a gynecological speculum.

Ultrasound systems complement optical imaging both in terms of the contrast they provide and greater penetration depth. Ultrasound probes emit sound waves into the body through conversion of an electrical signal into a mechanical vibration, and receive sound waves through conversion of a mechanical vibration into an electrical signal. The impedance of each tissue type affects how deep the ultrasound wave will penetrate into tissue, as well as how much of the ultrasound wave will be reflected back toward the probe; this serves as the basis for the visualization of different anatomical structures. The original ultrasound units are large devices situated either on a bench-top or a large rolling cart. Recently, more portable ultrasound probes have been developed that can be connected directly to a smartphone or tablet for image reconstruction. One of the major advancements that allowed for the development of portable ultrasounds has been the creation and use of MEMS.

PROBLEMS

POCT for Microscopy of Cells and Tissue

1. What three key features differentiate ultrasound and optical imaging from larger systems such as MRI and CT?
2. An object is placed along the optical axis of a converging lens at its focal length. Would an image be formed? Use a ray-tracing diagram to determine your answer.
3. The human eye is analogous to a single-lens system. Explain why the human eye is unable to see microscopic objects. Hint: Consider what the focal length for the eye would need to be to visualize microscopic objects.
4. What range of the electromagnetic spectrum does optical imaging use? What characteristics of light change as it travels through tissue and what characteristics of the light do not? Explain your answers.
5. Why are the objects in a brightfield image dark and those in a darkfield image bright? What is the difference in the setup that differentiates darkfield from brightfield microscopes?
6. Explain what needs to be changed in a brightfield microscope to convert it into a fluorescence microscope. Why are additional components required for fluorescence microscopy?
7. Nuclei are highly scattering and red blood cells are highly absorbing. What types of microscopes are best suited to each of these biological samples? What would the images look like if the systems were switched?

POCT for Imaging Internal Body Cavities

8. An engineer is designing a "pill camera" to take magnified images of the digestive tract. The engineer is using a two-lens system to accomplish magnification. Design a two-lens system that fits within a 1 cm space that could accomplish 4× magnification. Assume the distance between the object and the first lens is 0.5 cm.
9. What is the main feature of an endoscope that allows it to relay light to and from body cavities?
10. What is one advantage and one disadvantage of a capsule endoscope versus a traditional endoscope?
11. What advances in lenses were required to go from a traditional endoscopy system to a system like a capsule endoscope? Hint: Consider the changes in focal lengths.

12. How does reducing the distance between an imaging system and the target (e.g., going from a colposcope outside the body to a colposcope that works inside the body) simplify the optics of a colposcopy system?

Ultrasound Imaging and POCTs

13. Why is an ultrasound wave more suitable to monitor a tumor located in the liver than an optical endoscope?
14. Explain quantitatively why it would be difficult to visualize a bone metastasis with ultrasound. Assume the impedance of the metastasis is the same as water.
15. What happens to the transmission and reflection of an ultrasound wave as it encounters a boundary surface where there is a high-impedance mismatch and a low-impedance mismatch, and why are they different?
16. In an ultrasound image of a normal breast, there is a dark region in the middle and a white region around the black region. What is the most likely tissue that gives rise to the black image and the white image? What is the impedance mismatch between the two media?
17. How long would it take for an ultrasound wave to reach the transducer if it travels through 1 cm of fat and 1 cm of muscle before reflecting off a bone and traveling back to the transducer?
18. Explain using impedance mismatch how a tumor (assume impedance of water) surrounded by fat would look different on ultrasound from a tumor surrounded by muscle.
19. A biomedical engineer is designing a portable ultrasound. They would like to have the ability to change the voltage by a factor of four. How much play would there need to be within the capacitor for the distance between the plates to be able to accommodate the change in voltage, assuming the charge on the capacitor does not change?
20. Repeat question 19 for the case where the charge on the capacitor simultaneously increases by a factor of 24 when the voltage increases by a factor of 4.

REFERENCES

Asiedu, M. N., Agudogo, J. S., Dotson, M. E., et al. 2020. A novel speculum-free imaging strategy for visualization of the internal female lower reproductive system. *Scientific Reports*, 10, 1–16.

Breslauer, D. N., Maamari, R. N., Switz, N. A., Lam, W. A., & Fletcher, D. A. 2009. Mobile phone based clinical microscopy for global health applications. *PLoS ONE* 4(7): e6320. https://doi.org/10.1371/journal.pone.0006320.

Cybulski, J. S., Clements, J., & Prakash, M. 2014. Foldscope: origami-based paper microscope. *PLoS ONE* 9(6): e98781. https://doi.org/10.1371/journal.pone.0098781 © Cybulski et al. Licensed under CC BY 4.0.

Gora, M. J., Sauk, J. S., Carruth, R. W., et al. 2013. Tethered capsule endomicroscopy enables less invasive imaging of gastrointestinal tract microstructure. *Nature Medicine*, 19, 238–240.

Kim, S. H., & Kim, J. W. 2021. Small bowel malignancies in patients undergoing capsule endoscopy for iron deficiency anemia. *Diagnostics*, 12, 91.

Lam, C. T., Krieger, M. S., Gallagher, J. E., et al. 2015. Design of a novel low cost point of care tampon (POCkeT) colposcope for use in resource limited settings. *PLoS One*, 10, e0135869.

Northrup Grumman. 1963. Basic optics and optical instruments. Proceedings of SPIE Image Enhancement, 1–160.

Sanderson, J. 2019. *Understanding Light Microscopy*, Wiley, Chichester.

Smith, M., Hayward, S., Innes, S., & Miller, A. 2020. Point-of-care lung ultrasound in patients with COVID-19: a narrative review. *Anaesthesia*, 75, 1096–1104.

Tang, Y., Carns, J., & Richards-Kortum, R. R. 2017. Line-scanning confocal microendoscope for nuclear morphometry imaging. *Journal of Biomedical Optics*, 22, 116005.

Wood, T. C., & Elson, D. S. 2010. Polarization response measurement and simulation of rigid endoscopes. *Biomed. Opt. Express*, 1, 463–470.

Umay, I., Fidan, B., Barshan, B. 2017. Localization and Tracking of Implantable Biomedical Sensors. *Sensors*, 17(3):583. https://doi.org/10.3390/s17030583 MDPI. Shared under a CC BY license.

6 New Approaches to Vaccination and Cancer Treatment

Prevention is an integral component of cancer control and a crucial and cost-effective step toward decreasing the cancer incidence rate. If cancer can be prevented from occurring in the first place, a tremendous amount of money, time, and resources can be saved. Chapter 3 discussed primary and secondary prevention of cervical cancer. Over 30 percent of cancers in low- and middle-income countries (LMICs) have viral origins, as compared to under 5 percent in high-income countries (HICs); cervical cancer is a prime example. Cervical cancer, which is caused by the HPV virus, can be prevented entirely by HPV vaccination. Another cancer that is caused by a virus is liver cancer; the hepatitis B vaccine can prevent liver cancer.

Not all cancers have vaccinations, and therefore secondary prevention is essential. For example, a three-tiered strategy for cervical cancer is: (1) screening women frequently for cervical precancer; (2) performing a diagnostic test for women who screen positive; and (3) treating women diagnosed with cervical precancer. As a result, cervical cancer incidence in the US is at an all-time low. What if the patient has cancer when diagnosed? If surgery, radiation, and drugs are accessible, this provides the patient with a number of treatment options. This is often not the case in LMICs, where 9 out of 10 people do not even have access to surgery. Alternative approaches are needed to fill this gap, and ablation is a promising solution to the problem.

This chapter will explore vaccines (primary prevention) and secondary prevention, as well as local cancer control (ablation), and their underlying mechanisms. With respect to vaccines, we are at a time in society where transformative technologies have made vaccine manufacture faster than it has ever been. The COVID-19 pandemic drew in the resources needed to make this a reality. Ablation is not new to countries like the US. A mainstay in liver cancer treatment, ablation is a particularly useful approach for inoperable cancers and refractory disease. There are trade-offs with ablation with respect to cost and efficacy. This will be discussed in detail in this chapter.

LEARNING OBJECTIVES

Cancer Prevention and Treatment
- The underlying principles of vaccine development;
- vaccine efficacy and herd immunity;
- the mechanisms of cell death.

Thermal Ablation
- Different types of thermal ablation technologies and how they are similar and different from each other;
- principles behind thermal and cryoablation;
- modulation of the ablation zone.

Chemical Ablation
- Different types of chemical ablation;
- comparison of photodynamic therapy and ethanol ablation;
- the effect of ablation on the immune system.

Cancer Prevention and Treatment

The fundamental principle behind vaccination is introduction of an antigen into the body in such a way that the body will recognize the antigen as foreign and mount an immune response against it to learn how to fight it off in the future. **Antigen presenting cells** (APCs) are cells within the immune system that survey the body for foreign objects and show them to the rest of the immune system. The process of alerting the immune system to the presence of an antigen is called antigen presentation, and is performed by **APCs** such as dendritic cells. **Dendritic cells** are the first cell type in the adaptive immune system to come into contact with antigens. The role of the dendritic cell is to survey the body for antigens and, when it finds one, to alert the rest of the immune system to the presence of the foreign entity. Dendritic cells are constantly and randomly sampling the environment for possible antigens to present to the immune system. Any cellular debris, such as extracellular proteins and circulating DNA, can be consumed by a dendritic cell for presentation. As a result, many of the presented "**antigens**" are actually naturally occurring within the body and should not be recognized by the immune system as foreign.

T cells, the second type of immune cell involved in vaccination, assist with identifying foreign antigens. Dendritic cells present possible antigens to the immune system in lymph nodes, where T cells spend a majority of their time. T cells contain a receptor that is expressed on the cell surface that is specific to a particular antigen. During immune system development, any T cell that reacts with something in the body is destroyed, such that the only remaining T cells are reactive to foreign antigens. As a result, a T cell will only recognize an antigen presented by a dendritic cell if it does not naturally occur in the body.

Helper T cells (Th cells) are the first to come into contact with dendritic cells and are responsible for recognizing antigens. When an antigen is found by a dendritic cell, it will present that cell to helper T cells (Th cell) in the lymph nodes on a protein called major histocompatibility complex (MHC) I or II. If the Th cell interacts with a dendritic cell presenting an antigen it recognizes, the Th cell becomes activated to prime the immune system to respond to the antigen. As part of the priming process, the Th cell will replicate to create more Th cells specific to the antigen, activate cytotoxic T lymphocytes (CTLs) that are specific to the antigen, and activate B cells, the third immune cell type, to create antibodies that are specific to the antigen. The antibodies bind to the antigens and flag them for destruction, thus helping to fight future infections.

How does the process described here apply to vaccines? Once an antigen is introduced into the body, picked up by a dendritic cell, and presented to the immune system, the activated immune cells will directly attack and clear the antigen from the body. As the antigen is cleared from the body and the immune response is no longer needed, the activated CTLs and B cells are converted into memory T cells and B cells (also called plasma cells) so that the immune system can mount a more rapid response in the event that the antigen is ever present again. If the antigen is introduced by a vaccine, the memory T cells and B cells will be ready to attack it again if an infection occurs. Figure 6.1 summarizes the immune activation process.

Now that we have covered how an antigen is recognized inside the body, how is the correct antigen selected for vaccination and how does the antigen get introduced to the body? We will use the HPV vaccine, introduced in Chapter 3, as an example. Viruses have two basic components: genetic material, consisting of either DNA or RNA, encoding the necessary machinery for entering a cell and replication; and a capsule encasing the genetic material. The capsule contains spike proteins on the surface that can bind to a receptor on a cell as a means for transmitting genetic material into the cell. Since the spike protein is expressed on the surface of the viral particle, it makes an excellent antigen choice for a vaccine since it will be easily "seen" by the immune system. Figure 6.2 shows the process for creating the HPV vaccine. The L1 gene, which encodes the HPV viral envelope, is introduced into the DNA of a yeast cell via a process called transfection. The yeast cell then transcribes the newly inserted DNA and translates the resulting RNA into the capsid proteins that assemble into an empty viral envelope. The empty viral envelopes with the spike proteins are then injected into the body to elicit an HPV envelope-specific immune response without the risk of HPV infection.

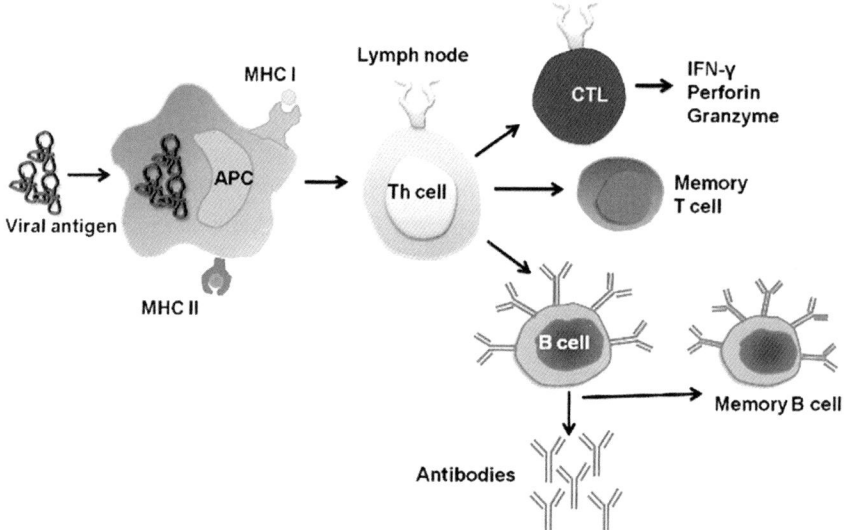

Figure 6.1 The immune activation process. An antigen found by a dendritic cell is presented to helper T cells (Th cell) in the lymph nodes on a protein called major histocompatibility complex (MHC) I or II. If the Th cell recognizes the antigen, it will activate cytotoxic T lymphocytes or CD8+, and B cells to mount an immune response. Eventually, memory T and B cells will be generated to activate future immune responses if the antigen is ever present again.
Image from: The potential of nanoparticles for the immunization against viral infections, Sokolova, Westendorf, Buer, Überla, Epple. *Journal of Materials Chemistry* B 3(24) DOI: 10.1039/C5TB00618J.

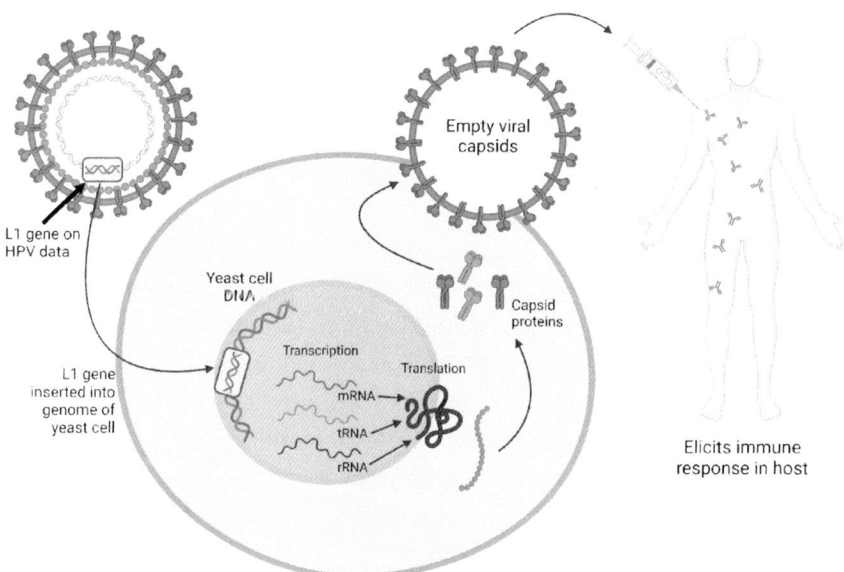

Figure 6.2 The process for creating the HPV vaccine. The L1 gene, which encodes the HPV viral envelope, is introduced into the DNA of a yeast cell via a process called transfection. The yeast cell then transcribes the newly inserted DNA and translates the resulting RNA into the capsid proteins that assemble into an empty viral envelope. The empty viral envelopes are then injected into the body to elicit an HPV envelope-specific immune response without the risk of HPV infection.
Source: Created with BioRender.com.

Cancer Prevention and Treatment

Table 6.1 shows different methods of vaccine production (including that for the HPV vaccine) and their advantages and disadvantages. Vaccines are made using several processes. They may contain live viruses that have been attenuated (weakened or altered to not cause illness); inactivated or killed organisms or viruses; inactivated toxins (for bacterial diseases where toxins generated by the bacteria cause illness, rather than the bacteria themselves); or merely segments of the pathogen. In all cases a spike protein of some

Table 6.1 Different methods of vaccine production and their advantages and disadvantages

In all cases, a spike protein of some kind is introduced to elicit an immune response. Vaccines based on mRNA technology were introduced for the first time as COVID-19 vaccines and therefore are not included in this table.

Vaccine type	Method	Advantages	Disadvantages	Examples
Inactivated virus	Use killed viruses	Vaccine virus cannot cause disease	Immune response not as strong, so several doses usually needed	Polio shot, hepatitis A
Live, weakened virus	Use viruses grown repeatedly in the laboratory in a different cell type than they typically infect so they change and become weaker when given as a vaccine	Strong immune response Typically only one or two doses needed for immunity	May cause side effects due to low-level viral replication	Measles, mumps, rubella, rotavirus, chickenpox
Recombinant	Gene that codes for surface protein is put into a plasmid in yeast or bacterial cells. Purified protein is used for the vaccine	Since no genetic material is used in the vaccine it cannot cause disease	Technically complicated and expensive to produce	Hepatitis B, HPV
Conjugate	Isolate a protein from the pathogen and attach a "helper" protein to cause immune response	Cannot cause disease	Typically requires multiple doses	Pneumococcal *Haemophilus influenzas* type b
Toxoid	Use inactive disease-causing toxins produced by the bacteria (called toxoids)	Cannot cause disease	Typically require multiple doses	Diphtheria, tetanus, pertussis

kind is introduced to elicit an immune response. Vaccines based on mRNA technology are distinct in that they don't involve the introduction of a spike protein. Rather, the vaccines introduce a piece of mRNA that corresponds to a viral protein, found on the virus' outer membrane. Using this mRNA blueprint, cells in the human body produce the viral protein. mRNA vaccines were introduced for the first time as COVID-19 vaccines manufactured by Pfizer-BioNTech and Moderna.

A key goal of immunization programs is to protect as many people as possible. Vaccination among the entire population is difficult, if not impossible. Some people may be unable to be vaccinated due to illness or a compromised immune system, while still others may choose not to vaccinate due to religious beliefs or skepticism of science. However, the principle of herd immunity relies on the fact that populations with higher rates of protected individuals are more protected. If a high enough proportion of the population is immunized, even unvaccinated people will be protected from the disease, simply because there are so few opportunities for the spread of infection.

What proportion of the population must be vaccinated for herd immunity? The **basic reproduction number**, R_0, of the disease helps determine the percentage of the population that needs to be vaccinated in order to have herd immunity. Let us consider three scenarios. For $R_0 > 1$ (e.g., $R_0 = 2$) a single infected person infects two other people and the number doubles with successive infections. This can be generalized to 2^n new infections in the nth round of new infections. When $R_0 < 1$ (e.g., 0.5), the infection rate is 0.5^n new infections in the nth round of infections. When $R_0 = 1$, the disease is considered to be **endemic**. It is always present in the population. R_0 makes the assumption that everyone in the population is susceptible to the disease. Based on this assumption, for $R_0 > 1$, the infection rate will continue to grow until everyone is infected; for $R_0 < 1$, the number of infected individuals will become smaller and smaller as the number of generations becomes larger and therefore, the infection will fizzle out. In reality, not everyone in the population is susceptible. For instance, once a person has recovered from the disease they will gain some immunity. Therefore, the **effective reproduction number**, R, is the product of R_0 and the proportion of the population that is susceptible, S, as shown in Equation 6.1:

$$R = S \times R_0. \tag{6.1}$$

As shown in Equation 6.2, in order for herd immunity to occur,

$$S < 1/R_0. \tag{6.2}$$

The high-end R_0 estimate for COVID-19 is approximately 2.5; therefore, 60 percent of the population must be vaccinated for herd immunity.

Other important terms are vaccine effectiveness and efficacy. **Vaccine effectiveness** is measured by observing how well the vaccines work to protect communities. However, this is difficult to predict. **Vaccine efficacy** applies to specific outcomes in a clinical trial. Equation 6.3 shows the calculation for vaccine efficacy, where c is the cases among unvaccinated people, a is the cases among vaccinated people, N_1 is the number of vaccinated people, and N_2 is the number of unvaccinated people:

$$\text{Efficacy} = 1 - \frac{N_2 a}{N_1 c}. \tag{6.3}$$

Example: How Many People Need to be Vaccinated Against HPV?

Question: The HPV vaccine has the potential to eliminate cervical cancer, as nearly all cervical cancer cases are caused by sustained HPV infection. Assuming R_0 for HPV is 2, the prevalence of HPV among vaccinated people is 5 percent and the prevalence of HPV among unvaccinated people is 70 percent, what percentage of the population must be vaccinated to see a downward trend in HPV cases?

Answer: To see reduction in cervical cancer cases, the effective R must be <1. From Equation 6.1 we know we need to calculate the proportion of the population that is susceptible. The susceptible population is the percentage of the population that is unvaccinated that will get an HPV infection plus the percentage of vaccinated people who will get an HPV infection:

$$S = S_{\text{unvax}} + S_{\text{vax}}.$$

We can calculate S_{unvax} as the percentage of the population that is unvaccinated times 0.7 (since 70 percent of unvaccinated people will get HPV):

$$S_{\text{unvax}} = 0.7 \times P_{\text{unvax}}.$$

We can calculate S_{vax} as the percentage of the population that is vaccinated times 0.05 (since 5 percent of vaccinated people will get HPV):

$$S_{\text{vax}} = 0.05 \times P_{\text{vax}}.$$

We also know that the percentage of the population vaccinated plus the percentage of the population unvaccinated totals to 100 percent:

$$P_{\text{unvax}} + P_{\text{vax}} = 1.$$

Solving for P_{unvax} and plugging into the equation for S gives:

$$P_{\text{unvax}} = 1 - P_{\text{vax}},$$
$$S_{\text{unvax}} = 0.7 \times (1 - P_{\text{vax}}),$$

> $$S = 0.7 \times (1 - P_{vax}) + 0.05 \times P_{vax},$$
> $$S = 0.7 - 0.65 \times P_{vax}.$$
>
> Now we are ready to plug S into Equation 6.1:
>
> $$R = (0.7 - 0.65 \times P_{vax}) \times 2.$$
>
> We know that HPV cases only decrease for $R < 1$, so replacing R with 1 gives the lower limit for P_{vax}:
>
> $$1 = (0.7 - 0.65 \times P_{vax}) \times 2,$$
> $$P_{vax} = 31 \text{ percent}.$$
>
> Therefore, at least 31 percent of the population would need to be vaccinated to see a decrease in HPV cases.

Vaccinations against cancer are only available for the immunization against cervical and liver cancer, both of which are induced by a virus. The majority of cancers cannot be prevented by vaccination. Surgery, radiation therapy, and chemotherapy form the foundation of effective cancer treatment in HICs. Adapting treatment modalities that are commonly used in HICs to LMICs is problematic because of the costly and resource-intensive nature of cancer treatment, especially for cancers that are diagnosed at a more advanced stage. As of 2015, a majority of the world's population – over five billion people – did not have access to surgery (Jain and Puranik, 2022). As a result, there is a dire need for therapies to treat cancer when vaccination and surgery are not options.

Surgery is the cornerstone treatment for the majority of cancers. Unfortunately, 9 out of 10 people in LMICs do not have access to essential surgery. How do we solve this problem? Conventional wisdom would suggest bolstering infrastructure, but this is unsustainable in the short term. The cost of basic surgical care would outstrip the **gross domestic product** (GDP) of many of the countries where these resources are lacking. Fortunately, there are alternatives to surgery for cancer treatment, which will be the focus of this section. **Tumor ablation** is an attractive alternative to surgery because it accomplishes cell death by the destruction of tumor cells through either thermal or chemical means. Some types of tumor ablation can even be performed in the absence of highly trained providers, rendering them excellent tools for use in resource-constrained settings.

Before we cover the specific types of tumor ablation, we will first look at how ablation kills cells. Figure 6.3 shows the three methods by which cells can die: apoptosis, necrosis, and autophagy. **Apoptosis** is the normal process for cell death that occurs in a highly organized fashion as a cell ages.

Cancer Prevention and Treatment

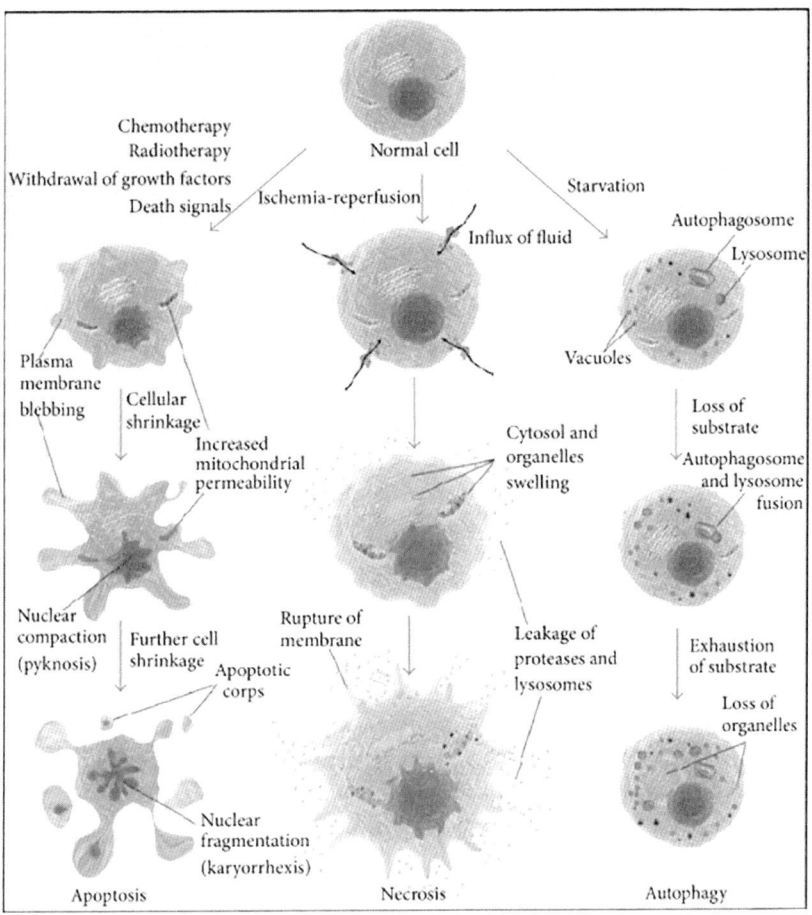

Figure 6.3 The three methods by which cells can die: apoptosis, necrosis, and autophagy. Apoptosis is the normal process for cell death that occurs in a highly organized fashion as a cell ages. Necrosis is a process for cell death that occurs in a disorganized manner that results in cell rupture. Autophagy is a process for cell death that occurs when a cell starves due to a lack of energy resources.
Source: Cell Death and Inflammatory Bowel Diseases: Apoptosis, Necrosis, and Autophagy in the Intestinal Epithelium, Nunes, Bernadazzi, de Souza. Hindawi BioMed Research International. Copyright © 2014 Tiago Nunes et al. Shared under the Creative Commons Attribution License.

Necrosis is a process for cell death that occurs in a disorganized manner that results in cell rupture. **Autophagy** is a process for cell death that occurs when a cell starves due to a lack of energy resources. Apoptosis is the most common form of cell death and is the preferred method by which cells die when they reach senescence. **Apoptotic** death is a highly organized process that begins with cellular blebbing and shrinkage. The nucleus and organelles are sequestered within small cell membrane capsules, which are then consumed by cells within the immune system. Chemotherapies cause apoptosis. **Necrosis** occurs when there is disruption of the cellular membrane, leading

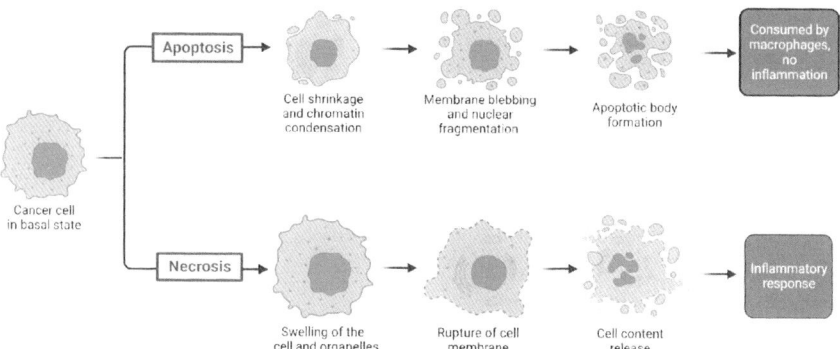

Figure 6.4 The differences between necrosis and apoptosis with respect to immune activation. Necrotic cell death is a disorganized process that results in cell membrane (also called plasma membrane) rupture, spilling cellular contents outside of the cell. The cellular contents, in the case of a tumor, may contain TAAs that the immune system could recognize as foreign to the body. Apoptosis, on the other hand, is a highly organized process that breaks the cell into smaller chunks to be consumed by macrophages, another type of immune cell, without antigen presentation to the immune system.
Source: Created with BioRender.com. Image from Abou-Ghali and Stiban (2015).

to an influx of fluid into the cell. During necrosis, the organelles swell and the cell membrane ruptures. The contents of the cell are then released into the extracellular space. **Autophagy** is a self-destructive process that is important for balancing sources of energy at critical times in development and in response to nutrient stress. Autophagy also plays a housekeeping role in removing misfolded or aggregated proteins, clearing damaged organelles, such as mitochondria, endoplasmic reticulum and peroxisomes, as well as eliminating intracellular pathogens. Thus, autophagy is generally thought of as a survival mechanism.

Ablation kills cells through the mechanism of necrosis. Necrotic cell death is an attractive means for killing tumor cells for two reasons. First, necrosis is a rapid process leading to quick cellular death almost immediately after an ablative treatment is administered. Second, since necrosis is an unregulated process, cellular contents are dumped into the extracellular space. As a result, **tumor associated antigens** (TAAs) can activate the immune system to fight any residual tumor following treatment, or tumor cells that have left the primary tumor and begun to form metastases. Why does cellular necrosis allow the immune system to recognize TAAs, but apoptosis does not? Figure 6.4 illustrates the differences between necrosis and apoptosis with respect to immune activation. Necrotic cell death is a disorganized process that results in cell membrane (also called plasma membrane) rupture, spilling cellular contents outside of the cell. The cellular contents, in the case of a tumor, may contain TAAs that the immune system could recognize as foreign to the body.

Apoptosis, on the other hand, is a highly organized process that breaks the cell into smaller chunks to be consumed by macrophages, another type of immune cell, without antigen presentation to the immune system.

Now that we have established ablative therapies kill cells via necrosis, how do ablative therapies actually induce necrosis within a tumor? There are two main methods that ablative therapies leverage to induce necrosis: physical and chemical cell membrane disruption. Physical damage to the cell membrane can be accomplished thermally, by either heating or cooling the tissue, or electrically, through a process called electroporation, which uses an electromagnetic field to create holes in the cell membrane. Technologies that use temperature to ablate tissue are referred to as **thermal ablation** technologies, and these are by far the most commonly used methods. **Thermal ablation** is the process of destroying tumor cells using either extreme heat or cold as the method of inducing cell death. Technologies that use chemicals to ablate tissue are referred to as **chemical ablation** technologies. **Chemical ablation** is the process of destroying tumor cells using chemicals to disrupt the cell membrane or cellular processes. Thermal ablation and chemical ablation technologies will be discussed in detail in the following sections.

Deeper Look: A New Era of Vaccine Development

It was during the COVID-19 pandemic that mRNA vaccines came to the forefront. These vaccines are potent, can be rapidly developed, and can be manufactured at low cost. Unlike attenuated or inactivated vaccines, mRNA is precise as it will only express a specific antigen and induce a directed immune response. Compared with DNA-based vaccines, mRNA is more effective, since expression does not require nuclear entry (only needs to enter cytoplasm), and safer, since the likelihood of random genome integration is low. Additionally, the antigen is safe as it is quickly degraded by cellular processes, within 2–3 days. Since production is based on cell-free transcription reaction, there is no risk of cell-derived impurities and viral contaminants commonly found in other vaccine production methods. Production can be standardized, and vaccines can be synthesized rapidly as a change in the antigen does not affect the mRNA backbone characteristics (Rosa et al., 2021) [24].

The development of mRNA vaccines began several decades earlier, when the in vivo expression of a protein was observed after injecting the coding mRNA into mouse skeletal muscle. During the following 10 years, several studies demonstrated that mRNA could induce an immune response to the expressed protein in many mammalian cell types, both in vitro and in vivo. The biggest challenge with translation was that mRNA would be quickly degraded before it could reach the cells. The solution to this problem was the development of lipid nanoparticle carriers that transport the mRNA into cells. Once inside the cell, the mRNA message could be translated into spike proteins (Rosa et al., 2021).

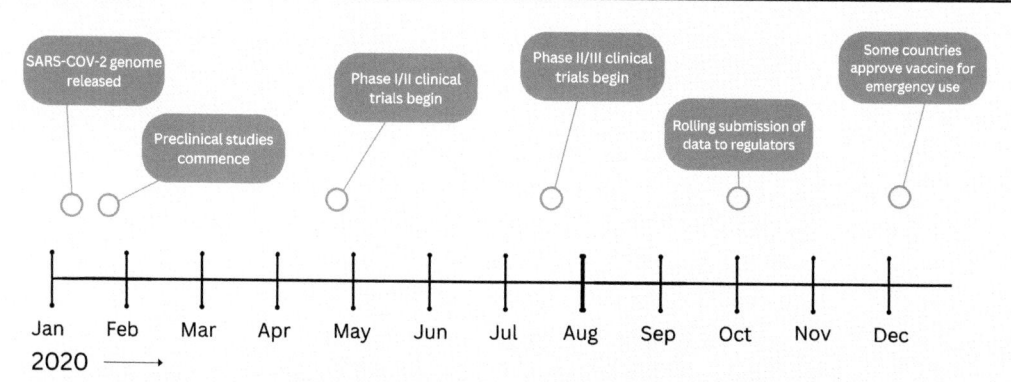

A VACCINE IN A YEAR
The drug firms Pfizer and BioNTech got their joint SARS-COV-2 vaccine approved less than eight months after trials started. The rapid turnaround was achieved by overlapping trials and because they did not encounter safety concerns.

Figure 6.5 The timeline for vaccine development by Pfizer and BioNTech. The rapid turnaround time was achieved by overlapping trials and there being fewer safety issues compared to previous vaccine development methods. Data: Principles of and Advances in Percutaneous Ablation, Ahmed, Brace, Lee, Goldberg. RSNA Radiology. February 1, 2011 https://doi.org/10.1148/radiol.10081634.

The slowest part of vaccine development is testing the vaccines for safety and efficacy on animals and then clinical trials in humans. With public investment of around $10 billion, the US Operation Warp Speed vaccine program made the development of vaccines faster than ever. This enormous investment made it possible for companies to take financial risks by running some tests at the same time. Figure 6.5 shows the timeline for COVID vaccine development by Pfizer and BioNTech. The rapid turnaround time was achieved by overlapping trials and there being fewer safety issues compared to previous vaccine development methods. These new efficient manufacturing processes can be extended to other diseases, thereby making vaccine access possibly for countries that are typically left behind. In fact, the WHO is helping to build facilities for vaccine development in several LMICs.

Thermal Ablation

Thermal ablation is the destruction of tissue through either heating or cooling the tissue to temperatures that cause cellular necrosis. The most commonly used forms of thermal ablation in the US are **radiofrequency ablation, microwave ablation**, and **cryoablation**. **Radiofrequency ablation** is the process of ablating cells using heat generated by electromagnetic waves in the radio frequency range. **Microwave ablation** is the process of ablating cells using heat generated by electromagnetic waves in the microwave range. As we will see, radio frequency and microwave ablation are not translatable for use in resource-constrained settings, as they require access to specialized providers called interventional radiologists, as well as expensive infrastructure. As

Thermal Ablation

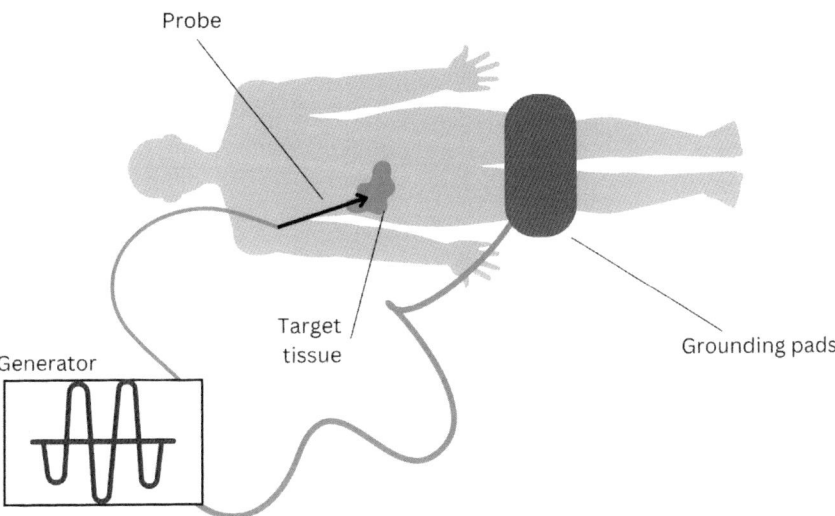

Figure 6.6 The basic components of a radio frequency ablation system. The first component is the probe, which is inserted into the tumor by an interventional radiologist. An interventional radiologist can choose between different probe geometries to ensure full coverage of the tumor. It uses waves between the probe and the grounding pad, creating heat around the tip of the probe, which causes cellular necrosis. Radio frequency ablation and microwave ablation have similar mechanisms of action.

a result, thermal ablation in LMICs is frequently performed through either **cryoablation** or **thermocoagulation**. **Cryoablation** is the process of ablating cells using cold temperatures generated by placing a supercooled probe directly in contact with the tissue. **Thermocoagulation** is the process of ablating cells using heat generated by placing a heated probe directly in contact with the tissue. Treatment of solid tumors would require the thermal probe to be inserted into the target area using image guidance. Therefore, these thermal ablation techniques are presently limited to superficial disease.

Radio frequency and microwave ablation systems are some of the most commonly used ablative technologies in the US. Figure 6.6 shows the basic components of a radio frequency ablation system. The first component is the probe, which is inserted into the tumor by an interventional radiologist. An interventional radiologist can choose between different probe geometries to ensure full coverage of the tumor. It uses waves between the probe and the grounding pad, creating heat around the tip of the probe, which causes cellular necrosis. Radio frequency ablation and microwave ablation have similar mechanisms of action.

As mentioned previously, a highly trained healthcare provider called an **interventional radiologist** is required to perform both radio frequency and microwave ablation. There are quite a few different decisions the interventional radiologist must make prior to and during a procedure, beginning with the placement of the probe within the tumor. Figure 6.7 shows the relationship

Figure 6.7

Relationship between probe placement, temperature, and time to cell death. The induced temperature decreases as the distance from the probe increases. A higher power will lead to higher temperatures near the probe tip. Higher temperature near the probe tip will lead to faster cell death and create a larger overall **ablative zone**. The lower the temperature, the longer it will take for the cells to die. For example, cells within tissue heated to 55 °C will die within a few seconds, whereas cells within tissue heated to 45 °C will take up to 15 minutes to die.

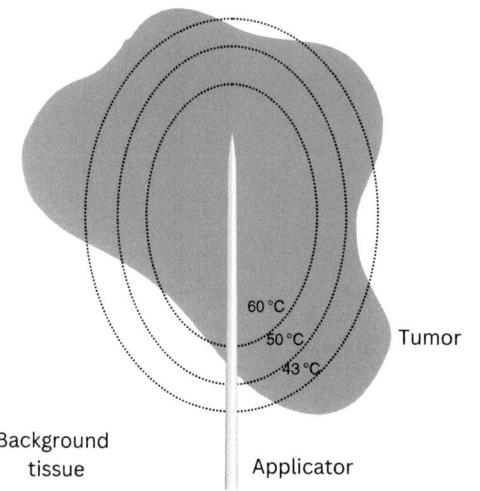

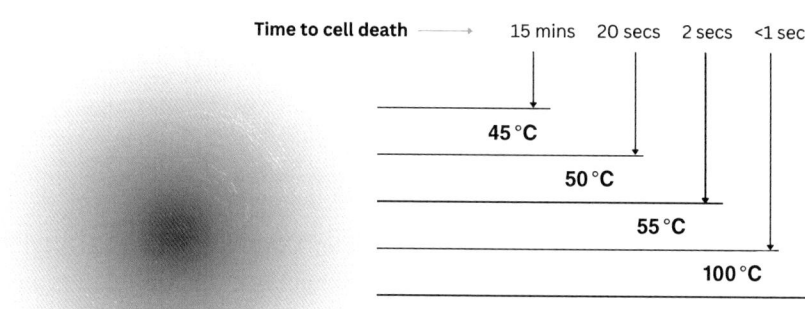

between probe placement, temperature, and time to cell death. The induced temperature decreases as the distance from the probe increases. A higher power will lead to higher temperatures near the probe tip. Higher temperature near the probe tip will lead to faster cell death and create a larger overall **ablative zone**. The lower the temperature, the longer it will take for the cells to die. For example, cells within tissue heated to 55 °C will die within a few seconds, whereas cells within tissue heated to 45 °C will take up to 15 minutes to die. In addition to the probe placement, the interventional radiologist must decide the amount of power that should be used, which will determine the size of the **ablative zone**.

How are radio frequency and microwave ablation currently used in the US? The most common use for these two ablation methods in the US is for liver cancer, or **hepatocellular carcinoma**. Liver cancer is one of the leading causes of death globally. While some liver cancers can be removed surgically, many are treated with ablative methods if they are in a sensitive region of the liver where surgery is not an option. Additionally, liver metastases (cancer within the liver that originated outside of the liver) are also frequently treated with radio frequency and/or microwave ablation. Other applications for radio frequency and microwave ablation in oncology include treatment of tumors on the kidney and metastatic lymph nodes.

Cryoablation is another commonly used technology in the US, and is performed by a number of different providers, including interventional radiologists, gynecologists, and dermatologists. Figure 6.8 shows the basic components of a cryoablation system. Cryoablation systems are simpler than radio frequency or microwave ablation systems, using compressed gas (typically CO_2 or N_2O) to cool a probe tip to ultracold temperatures. The probe tip is then placed in contact with the tissue to cool it and induce necrosis. As was the case with radio frequency and microwave ablation, the ablative zone is determined by the spread of temperatures within the tissue, which is inversely related to distance from the probe. Unlike radio frequency and microwave ablation, which could use both probe placement/geometry and power to establish the ablative zone, the ablative zone for cryoablation is only dictated by probe placement and the amount of time the probe is in contact with the tissue. Cryoablation is used in the US for similar indications as radio frequency and microwave ablation.

One of the most commonly used models for diffusion of heat through tissue is the Pennes model, which is represented mathematically in Equation 6.4, where k is the thermal conductivity, x, y, and z are the 3D coordinate space, ω_b is blood perfusion, ρ_b is the density, c_b is the specific heat, T_b is the arterial temperature, Q_{met} is the metabolic heat generation rate inside the tissue, and T is the unknown temperature. Though the specifics of solving the heat equation are beyond the scope of this textbook, it is useful to understand what the relative terms mean and how they relate to thermal ablation treatment. Suppose you want to know how the temperature will distribute throughout tissue during ablation; the first term in Equation 6.4 represents radiative heat, which is dependent on the thermal conductivity of the tissue; the second term represents conductive heat, which is affected by blood flow; the final term represents heat generated by metabolic activity of the cells:

$$k\left(\frac{\partial^2 T}{\partial x^2} + \frac{\partial^2 T}{\partial y^2} + \frac{\partial^2 T}{\partial z^2}\right) + \omega_b \rho_b c_b (T_b - T) + Q_{met} = 0. \quad (6.4)$$

Why is it important to consider the size of the ablative zone to ensure only the tumor is ablated? The ablative zone dictates the volume of necrosis that will be induced during an ablative procedure. If the ablative zone is too small, there will be residual tumor left that may continue to grow and potentially metastasize. Alternatively, if the ablative zone is too large, healthy tissue may be damaged, leading to undesirable side effects. Figure 6.9 shows a graphical representation of different zones of ablation. When tumor cells are ablated

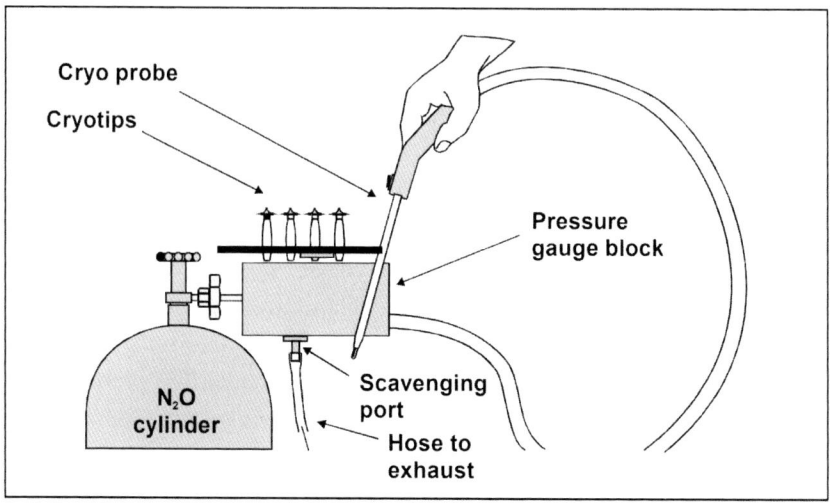

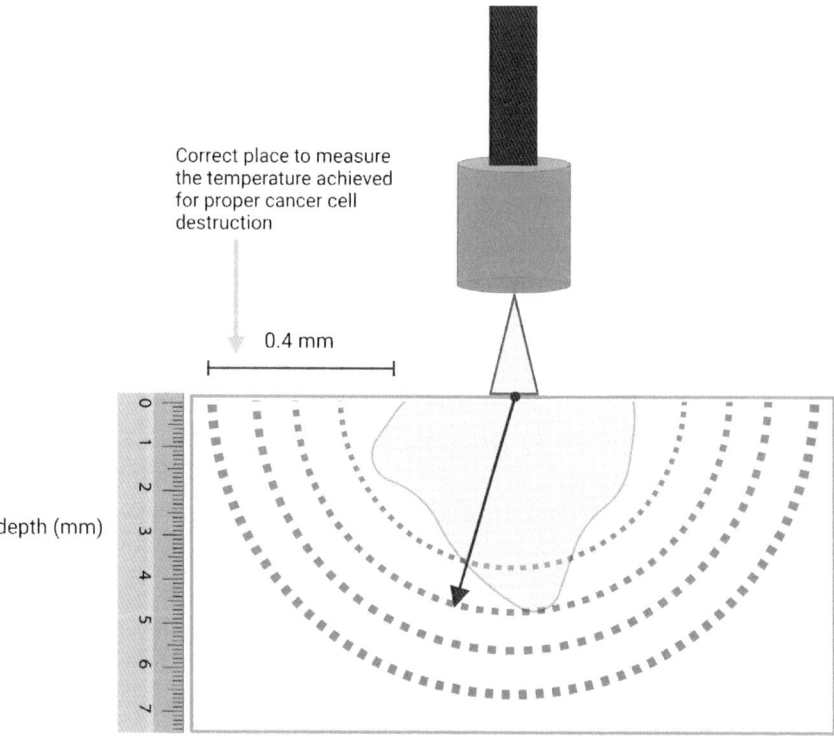

Figure 6.8 Basic components of a cryoablation system. Cryoablation systems are simpler than radio frequency or microwave ablation systems, using compressed gas (typically CO_2 or N_2O) to cool a probe tip to ultracold temperatures. The probe tip is then placed in contact with the tissue to cool it and induce necrosis. As was the case with radio frequency and microwave ablation, the ablative zone is determined by the spread of temperatures within the tissue, which is inversely related to distance from the probe.
Image from: (a) Amol Mehta, Rahmi Oklu, Rahul A. Sheth, "Thermal Ablative Therapies and Immune Checkpoint Modulation: Can Locoregional Approaches Effect a Systemic Response?", *Gastroenterology Research and Practice*, vol. 2016, Article ID 9251375, 11 pages, 2016. https://doi.org/10.1155/2016/9251375. Copyright © Centers for Disease Control and Prevention. (b) Created with BioRender.com.

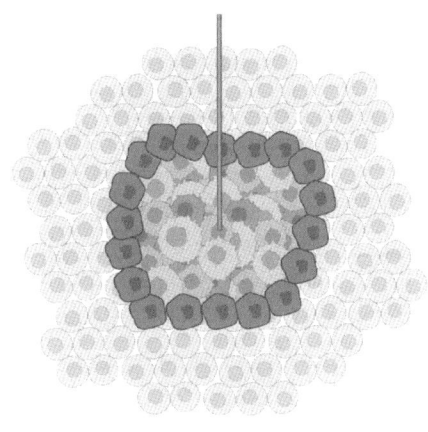
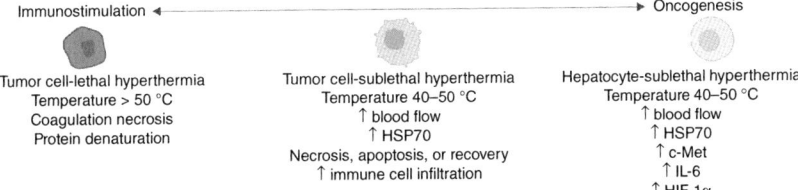

Figure 6.9 Graphical representation of different zones of ablation. When tumor cells are ablated with lethal hyperthermia, the result is cellular necrosis and stimulation of the immune system. Tumor cells that undergo sublethal hyperthermia can undergo either necrosis or apoptosis or potentially survive. Sublethal hyperthermia can also increase blood flow and expression of survival proteins, such as HSP70, which may cause tumor growth. Additionally, sublethal hyperthermia in healthy liver tissue can actually create an environment that promotes oncogenesis or conversion of healthy tissue into malignant tissue.
Source: Created with BioRender.com.

with lethal hyperthermia, the result is cellular necrosis and stimulation of the immune system. Tumor cells that undergo sublethal hyperthermia can undergo either necrosis or apoptosis, or potentially survive. Sublethal hyperthermia can also increase blood flow and expression of survival proteins, such as HSP70, which may cause tumor growth. Additionally, sublethal hyperthermia in healthy liver tissue can actually create an environment that promotes oncogenesis or conversion of healthy tissue into malignant tissue.

Example: Heat Transfer Through Tissue

Question: Explain how the following changes in variables would affect the distribution of heat within tissue during thermal ablation: (a) increase in the thermal conductivity of tissue, (b) decrease in the density of blood capillaries within a tumor, and (c) decreased metabolic activity within the tumor.

Answer: Each of these scenarios can be addressed using Equation 6.4. Because the sum of the terms in the equation must add to zero, any change in a variable will have to be compensated to maintain equilibrium. For scenario (a), an increase in the thermal conductivity of tissue would require a decrease in the derivatives with respect to temperature and x, y, z location, because an increase in thermal conductivity would not affect blood flow (term 2) or metabolic heat (term 3). The decrease in derivative would imply a smaller change in temperature over distance, resulting in an increase in ablative zone. For scenario (b), a decrease in the density of blood capillaries would make term 2 smaller. Because a decrease in capillaries would not affect metabolic heat, the only alternative to compensate for the reduction is to increase the derivatives in the first term, which would correspond to a decrease in ablation zone. For scenario (c), decreased metabolic activity within the tumor would not affect blood flow (term 2); therefore, the derivatives in the first term would have to increase, which would decrease the ablative zone.

Deeper Look: Trade-Off Between Excisional Treatment and Ablation for Cervical Precancers (Cervical Intraepithelial Neoplasia)

Almost 50 years ago, traditional treatments for cervical precancer were **cold knife conization (CKC)** (removal of tissue directly from the cervix) or **hysterectomy** (removal of the uterus). With the introduction of colposcopy in the 1970s, more conservative ablation treatments such as cryotherapy and laser ablation were adopted. However, with the introduction of **loop electrosurgical excision procedure (LEEP)** in the 1990s, ablative methods fell out of favor due to concerns that they undertreat occult cervical cancer or **carcinoma in situ** (Khan & Smith-McCune, 2014). The primary difference between LEEP and CKC is that LEEP removes less tissue.

Excisional techniques are more invasive and remove a portion of the cervix, whereas ablation is restricted to the treatment of the top layers of the cervix. There is a greater risk of preterm delivery with increasing length/volume of tissue removed (Castanon et al., 2014). Figure 6.10 shows the absolute risks of cervical intraepithelial neoplasia (CIN) treatment failure and preterm birth. Ablation has the highest treatment failure and lowest risk of preterm birth, and the opposite is observed for excisional techniques. A p-value less than 0.05 is considered to be statistically significant – that is, the findings are not due to chance (tests for statistical significance and p-values will be covered in greater detail in Chapter 7). Given the association between preterm risk and excision, a trend has been seen toward techniques that remove no tissue at all in women of reproductive age (Castanon et al., 2014). These patients are observed and only receive treatment if there is a high risk that precancerous disease will turn into cancer or there is inadequate information to determine the risk.

In many LMICs, the options for the treatment for cervical precancer are much like what was practiced in the US before 1990. Since LEEP is not readily available, if women have high-grade disease or cancer, either CKC or hysterectomy is performed when available. On the flip side, treatment for cervical precancers is either cryotherapy or thermal ablation. The former treatment approach, though effective, poses a high risk of preterm birth or no

	Any treatment failure	High-grade treatment failure	Preterm birth	Treatment worse than LLETZ
CKC	6·6% (5·4–8·5)	3·5% (2·2–5·6)	16·3% (12·7–20·6)	p<0·01
Laser conization	6·3% (4·8–8·3)	4·6% (2·3–8·9)	13·2% (10·0–17·3)	p=0·05 / p=0·10
Radical diathermy	16·7% (9·9–26·7)	11·2% (3·3–31·3)	13·9% (10·1–18·9)	
Laser ablation	16·2% (12·7–20·3)	11·2% (5·9–20·2)	8·3% (6·3–10·8)	p=1·00
Cold coagulation	11·0% (7·2–16·6)	4·8% (1·5–14·4)	5·5% (0·2–71·5)	
Cryotherapy	17·3% (13·2–22·6)	9·6% (4·2–20·4)	8·0% (2·9–20·0)	p=0·10 / p=0·05
LLETZ	10·2% (7·5–13·7)	5·3% (3·1–8·8)	10·5% (9·1–12·2)	p<0·01

Treatment better than LLETZ

Figure 6.10 Absolute risks of CIN treatment failure and preterm birth (Kilim plot). Ablation has the highest treatment failure and lowest risk of preterm birth, and the opposite is observed for excisional techniques. A *p*-value less than 0.05 is considered to be statistically significant – that is, the findings are not due to chance (tests for statistical significance and *p*-values will be covered in greater detail in Chapter 7). CIN, cervical intraepithelial neoplasia; CKC, cold knife conization; LLETZ, large loop excision of the transformation zone (the same as LEEP).
Image from: Oxidative stress-induced apoptosis of osteoblastic MC3T3-E1 cells by hydroxyapatite nanoparticles through lysosomal and mitochondrial pathways. Y. Jin, X. Liu, H. Liu, S. Chen, C. Gao, K. Ge, C. Zhang and J. Zhang, RSC Adv., 2017 7, 13010, DOI: 10.1039/C7RA01008G. Shared under the Creative Commons CC-BY license.

possibility for bearing children. The latter approach, though safer, can lead to high treatment failure. Conservative options such as following up on women of reproductive age to avoid unnecessary treatment or, when needed, the use of LEEP to minimize invasiveness are not feasible solutions in many settings. Therefore, there is a need for innovative approaches to address this ethical issue. Potential solutions can be created through chemical ablation techniques, which is the subject of the next section.

Radio frequency, microwave, and cryoablation are all widely used for treatment of cancer in the US; however, are all of these ablative therapies suitable for use in LMICs? The WHO uses the ASSURED criteria for assessing POCTs for disease screening and diagnosis. While there is not a direct equivalent to the ASSURED criteria for treatment choice, the same basic questions can be used for assessing therapies: Is the treatment affordable? Is the treatment user-friendly? Is the treatment rapid and robust? Is the treatment equipment free? Is the treatment deliverable to end users? Since sensitivity and specificity are specific to diagnostic technologies, the two "S's" can be replaced with a singular "S" for safety: Is the treatment safe?

Table 6.2 The application of the modified ASSURED criteria to radio frequency, microwave, and cryoablation

While radiofrequency and microwave ablation are safe, rapid, and robust, both have expensive startup costs to purchase the required equipment. Cryoablation, on the other hand, meets all of the modified ASSURED criteria with the exception of relying on equipment in the form of compressed gas tanks, which can be expensive and difficult to source.

ASSURED criteria	Radio frequency ablation	Microwave ablation	Cryoablation
Affordable	No	No	Yes
Safe	Yes	Yes	Yes
User-friendly	No	No	Yes
Rapid and robust	Yes	Yes	Yes
Equipment free	No	No	No
Deliverable	No	No	Yes

Table 6.2 shows the application of the modified ASSURED criteria to radio frequency, microwave, and cryoablation. While radio frequency and microwave ablation are safe, rapid, and robust, both have expensive startup costs to purchase the required equipment. Cryoablation, on the other hand, meets all of the modified ASSURED criteria with the exception of relying on equipment in the form of compressed gas tanks, which can be expensive and difficult to source. If radio frequency or microwave ablation were to be implemented in LMICs, they would be restricted to centralized health facilities that many people cannot access (i.e., not deliverable to end users). Cryoablation is still widely used for treatment of cervical precancers in LMICs. Unfortunately, high-grade cervical lesions often penetrate into the cervix beyond a depth of 3.4 mm, which is the treatment depth achievable with most CO_2-based cryoablation methods used in LMICs.

Since cryoablation does not achieve a deep enough ablative zone to treat high-grade cervical cancer lesions, are there any alternative technologies available? Thermocoagulation, mentioned at the beginning of this section, is another commonly used therapy for treatment of cervical precancer that is rapidly gaining popularity with the introduction of the thermocoagulator. Thermocoagulation is a form of thermal ablation that places a heated probe tip in contact with the tissue to be treated. Thermocoagulators are battery-operated to reduce their reliance on access to electrical outlets. Thermocoagulation has a deeper penetration depth than cryoablation with CO_2. However, the depth of treatment would still be restricted to superficial disease. Pictures of a thermocoagulator and cryotherapy system were shown in Chapter 3.

Chemical Ablation

One of the limitations of the ablative technologies described for use in LMICs (thermocoagulators and cryotherapy probes) in the previous section is their limited use in tumors seated deeper within the body. Technologies based on chemical ablation may be able to overcome some of these shortcomings. The major types of chemical ablation that will be discussed in this section are **photodynamic therapy** (PDT) and **ethanol ablation**. **Photodynamic therapy** is the use of a compound or drug to kill a cell after it is activated by light. **Ethanol ablation** is a process of inducing necrosis in cells by disrupting the cell membrane using ethanol.

Photodynamic therapy is becoming increasingly common as a chemical treatment of a variety of growths and abnormalities, including cancer. Figure 6.11(a) provides a visual overview of PDT. A photosensitive drug is administered systemically and allowed to accumulate within the tumor. Light is then used to activate the photosensitive drug within the tumor. Most drugs referred to as photosensitizers are activated to create **reactive oxygen species** (ROS), which leads to mitochondrial oxidative stress and cell death via apoptosis (Figure 6.11(b)). There are also indirect effects, including damage to blood vessels, which deprive tumor cells of oxygen and nutrients. Drug administration is typically performed intravenously, the same way most chemotherapy, molecular therapy, and immunotherapy drugs are administered. However, the drug that is administered is in an inactive form. After the drug is administered and accumulates within the tumor, light activation is required to set treatment in motion. Light activation is typically accomplished with a laser at a wavelength that will activate the drug. Finally, like other ablation techniques, PDT also stimulates the host immune system to attack the cancer cells.

Figure 6.12 shows a popular photosensitizer, protoporphyrin IX. The precursor to PpIX is 5-alvulolenicamino acid (5-ALA), a naturally occurring compound produced by plants. When administered into the body, ALA is converted into PpIX via biosynthesis pathways. These biosynthesis pathways are typically overactive in cancer cells, leading to increased accumulation of PpIX in tumor tissue compared to normal tissue. As a result, when red light interacts with the PpIX, it will create ROS to specifically kill the tumor cells.

One of the major advantages of photodynamic therapy over thermal ablation technologies is its specificity for killing tumor cells. Whereas thermal ablation will kill any cell that is heated or cooled beyond a certain temperature, photosensitizers can be used to specifically kill tumor cells through multiple mechanisms. First, though the drug can be absorbed by cells all over the body, photosensitizers typically accumulate at higher levels in tumors than in

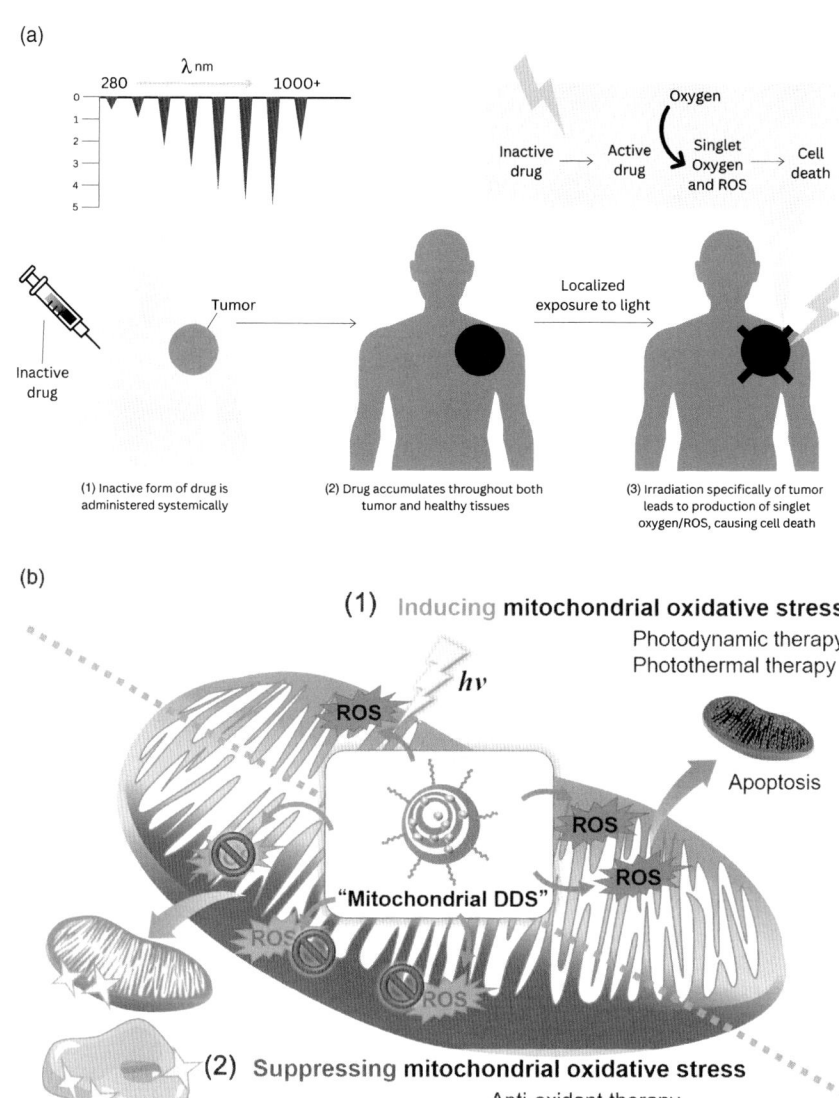

Figure 6.11

A visual overview of photodynamic therapy. A photosensitive drug is administered systemically and allowed to accumulate within the tumor. Light is then used to activate the photosensitive drug within the tumor. Most drugs are activated to create ROS when exposed to light, which leads to mitochondrial oxidative stress and consequently cell death via apoptosis.

Source: (b) Yamada et al.(2020) Shared under an open access CC BY license.

normal tissue. Second, the light source, which can be localized in the region where the cancer cells are, provides further specificity. Not only can photodynamic therapy be used for treatment, it can be used for imaging, particular in resource-constrained settings. As you learned in Chapter 5, cell phone cameras can be modified externally to perform fluorescence imaging. The addition of blue-light LEDs for fluorescence excitation and a red-light filter can allow a cell phone camera to be used for fluorescence imaging of PpIX, and a high-power LED can be used to provide sufficient activation for treatment. At present, the primary limitation of available photodynamic therapy is the depth

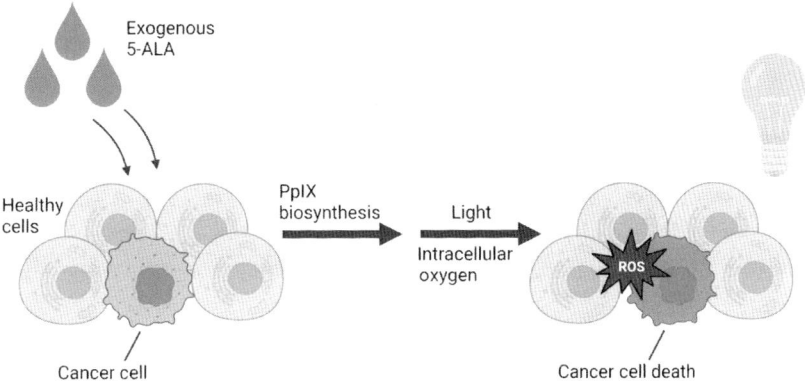

Figure 6.12 A popular photosensitizer, protoporphyrin IX. The precursor to PpIX is 5-alvulolenicamino acid (5-ALA), a naturally occurring compound produced by plants. When administered into the body, ALA is converted into PpIX via biosynthesis pathways. These biosynthesis pathways are typically overactive in cancer cells, leading to increased accumulation of PpIX in tumor tissue compared to normal tissue. As a result, when red light interacts with the PpIX, it will create ROS to specifically kill the tumor cells. Light only penetrates a few millimeters into the body and, as a result, only superficial lesions can be easily treated. Therefore, photodynamic therapy is well suited for treatment of skin lesions and pigmentation.
Source: Created with BioRender.com.

of penetration of the light and ability to target cells within one-third of an inch (approximately 1 cm) of the light source. Thus, large tumor masses cannot be treated with this technology.

The second type of chemical ablation that has seen prominent use is ethanol ablation. The initial site of application was in the treatment of inoperable hepatocellular carcinomas, in which surrounding liver tissue was too damaged to allow for surgical resection (Shiina et al., 1991; Sugira et al., 1983). In this capacity, ethanol ablation was widely used and led to five-year survival rates comparable to surgical resection (Ryu et al., 1997). While most commonly applied in the liver, ethanol ablation has also been successfully employed in treatment of cardiomyopathies (Sorajja et al. 2008), parathyroid (Solbiati et al., 1985) and pancreatic (Jurgensen et al., 2006) tumors, adrenal metastases (Artifon et al., 2007), and metastatic pelvic lymph nodes (DeWitt & Mohamadnejad, 2011).

Figure 6.13 shows an illustration of the percutaneous ethanol injection procedure in the liver. The procedure is fairly straightforward – a needle is inserted into the liver tumor under ultrasound guidance and ethanol is injected into the tumor through the needle to cause necrosis. The consumables used in the procedure, a syringe and ethanol, are also inexpensive to obtain and often on hand at clinics across all health system levels. Finally, the increased availability and adoption of affordable portable ultrasound systems, discussed in Chapter 5, makes percutaneous ethanol injection an exciting prospect for use in settings where surgical resection is unavailable.

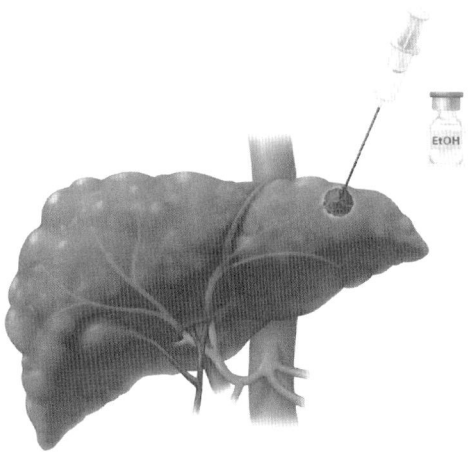

Figure 6.13 Illustration of ethanol ablation in the liver. The procedure is fairly straightforward – a needle is inserted into the liver tumor under ultrasound guidance and ethanol is injected into the tumor through the needle to cause necrosis. The consumables used in the procedure, a syringe and ethanol, are inexpensive to obtain and often on hand at clinics across all health system levels.
Source: http://www.magicray.ru/PDT_Photodynamic_therapy/Oncology_articles/PDT_for_skin_cancer_of_inconvenient_localizations.html.

How does ethanol ablation kill cells? Like the thermal ablation methods discussed in the previous section, ethanol ablation induces necrosis via cell membrane dehydration. Ethanol works by protein denaturation, leading to **coagulative necrosis**, **thrombosis** of small vessels, and formation of **fibrotic** and **granulomatous** tissue. **Coagulative necrosis** is a type of cell death that occurs when blood flow to cells stops or slows (ischemia). **Thrombosis** occurs when blood clots block blood vessels. **Granulomatous** inflammation is a histologic pattern of tissue reaction which appears following cell injury. It will be important to keep in mind how ethanol destroys cells later in this chapter, where the role of the immune system in ethanol ablation is discussed in greater detail.

Given that direct killing of cells by chemical ablation depends on contact between the chemical and the cells, diffusion of chemicals through tissue is one important consideration when designing an ablative therapy. Diffusion modeling using a two-compartment model is one way to investigate how the direct injection of a chemical into a tumor will affect chemical distribution. Figure 6.14 shows an example of a two-compartment model for ethanol diffusion in a tumor. Ethanol can be measured using an optical technique called Raman spectroscopy (discussed in Chapter 4) with a setup like the one shown in Figure 6.14. Ethanol is placed in a small dish underneath a polycarbonate membrane. A piece of tissue can be placed above

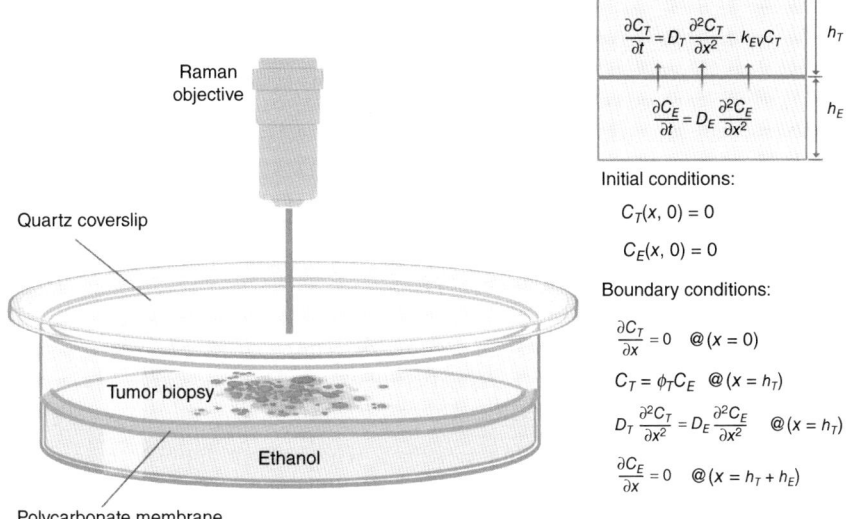

Figure 6.14 Example of a two-compartment model for ethanol diffusion in a tumor. Ethanol can be measured using a technique called Raman spectroscopy with a setup like the one shown here. Ethanol is placed in a small dish underneath a polycarbonate membrane. A piece of tissue can be placed above the membrane. Over time, ethanol will diffuse through the polycarbonate membrane into the tissue, based on the equations and boundary conditions shown. Here, C_T is the ethanol concentration in the tumor, C_E is the ethanol concentration below the polycarbonate membrane, D_T and D_E are the diffusion coefficients in the tumor and ethanol, and h_T and h_E are the thickness of the tumor and ethanol layers. Source: Created with BioRender.com.

the membrane. Over time, ethanol will diffuse through the polycarbonate membrane into the tissue, based on the equations and boundary conditions shown in Figure 6.14. Here, C_T is the ethanol concentration in the tumor, C_E is the ethanol concentration below the polycarbonate membrane, D_T and D_E are the diffusion coefficients in the tumor and ethanol, and h_T and h_E are the thickness of the tumor and ethanol layers. Though solving the diffusion equation is beyond the scope of this text, it is useful for understanding how chemicals diffuse through tissue.

The major shortcoming of ethanol ablation is the unpredictable nature of ethanol distribution after it is injected into the tissue, owing to leakage away from the site of interest. Ethanol leakage beyond the tumor can lead to adverse side effects when surrounding healthy tissue is damaged. It is effective for an encapsulated tumor, like hepatocellular carcinoma, which is surrounded by liver tissue made firm by underlying disease (cirrhotic liver). The alcohol diffuses throughout the tumor but is prevented from diffusing into the normal liver parenchyma by the tumor capsule and surrounding cirrhotic parenchyma. Unfortunately, ethanol ablation is less effective for treating other types of tumors since they are often firm tumors surrounded by normal liver tissue.

> **Example: Fluid Diffusion Through a Tumor**
>
> Question: Given that ethanol distribution is one of the main shortcomings of ethanol ablation, a biomedical engineer hypothesizes that increasing the viscosity (a measure of how much internal friction is present in a liquid) of the injected ethanol may reduce ethanol leakage outside of the tumor. Explain, using the diffusion equations, why an increase in viscosity would limit diffusion.
>
> Answer: An increase in viscosity would be akin to decreasing the diffusion coefficient, as the liquid will move more slowly through the system. Based on the diffusion equations, there is a linear relationship between the change in concentration over time and the diffusion coefficient of the liquid, therefore, a liquid with a higher viscosity would have a lower change in concentration over time, which would limit diffusion.

The first section of this chapter discussed how vaccines can be used to induce an immune response against a particular antigen. Figure 6.15 shows the effect of ablative therapy on the body's immune system. When a cell undergoes necrotic death following ablation, cellular debris is left behind. Antigen presenting cells, such as dendritic cells, will clear the cellular debris and present the debris to the immune system. During this process, TAAs or tumor antigens can stimulate **CD3+ T cells** (immune cells involved in activating both **CD8+ cytotoxic T cells** and **CD4+ T helper cells**) in the immune system to attack the tumor. As was the case with vaccines, the immune system will recognize the TAAs as a foreign entity since they do not occur in healthy cells. After immune recognition, T cells and B cells specific to the TAAs will be activated and can fight off any residual tumor cells that were not successfully treated.

As mentioned previously, ablative therapies can activate the immune system to actively fight against the cancer. One question that arises is whether antitumor immune response is localized only to the ablated tumor or if it is systemic. The idea that a local treatment like ablation can induce a systemic antitumor immune response to treat cancer at a distant site (i.e., metastases) is referred to as the **abscopal effect**. Figure 6.15 illustrated how local treatment with ablation can activate the immune system. The activated immune cells have the potential to leave the tumor and survey the rest of the body for the presence of cancer cells, which they can then attack.

Figure 6.16 shows an example of the abscopal effect using a modified formulation of ethanol ablation. When ethanol is injected into the primary tumor, TAAs are released into the surrounding environment, which are used to train

Chemical Ablation

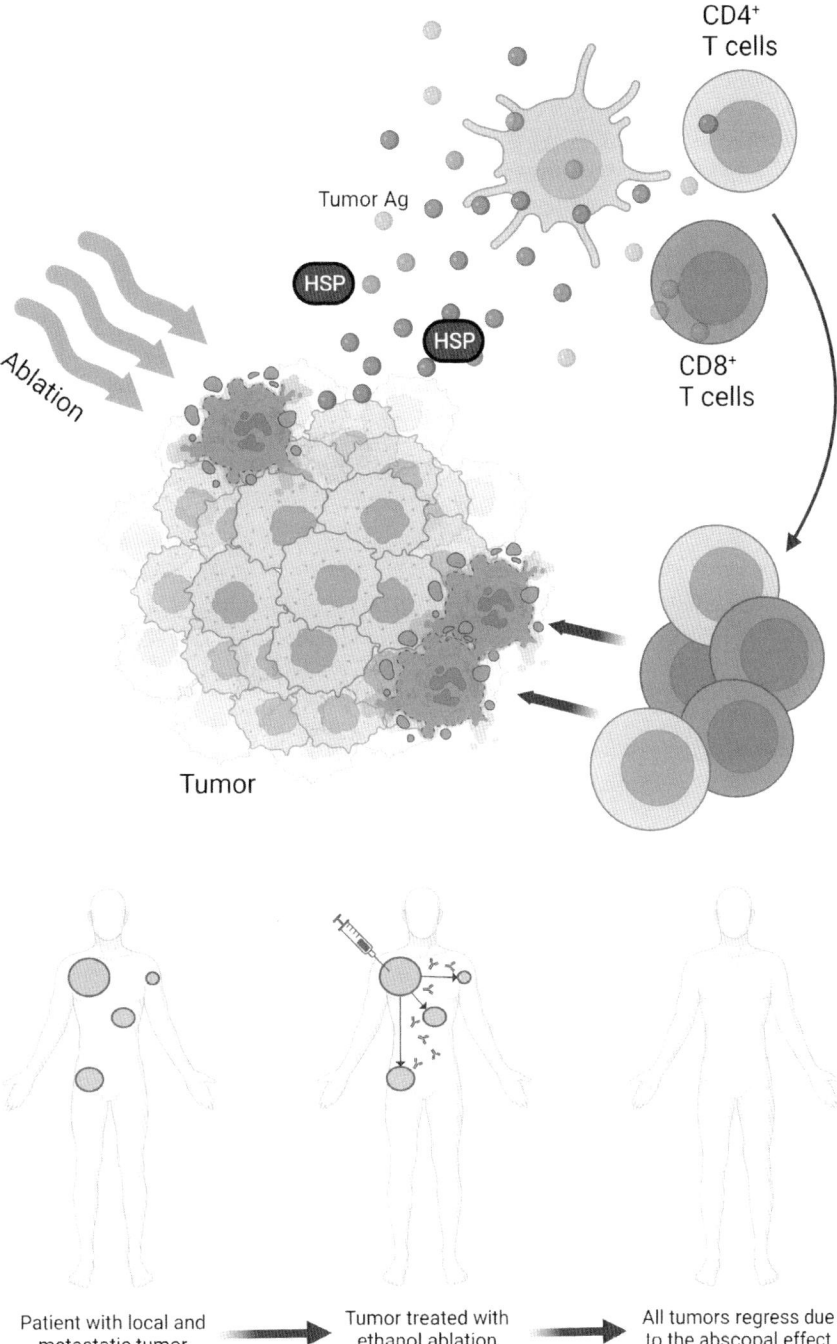

Figure 6.15 The effect of ablative therapy on the body's immune system. When a cell undergoes necrotic death following ablation, cellular debris is left behind. Antigen presenting cells, such as dendritic cells, will clear the cellular debris and present the debris to the immune system. During this process, TAAs or tumor Ags can stimulate T cells (CD4, CD8) in the immune system to attack the tumor.
Source: Created with BioRender.com.

Figure 6.16 Example of the abscopal effect using a modified formulation of ethanol ablation. When ethanol is injected into the primary tumor, TAAs are released into the surrounding environment, which are used to train the body's immune cells to recognize the tumor in a highly specific manner. In addition to fighting and destroying the primary tumor, the immune cells can survey the rest of the body for metastases that share the same TAAs as the primary tumor. The immune cells can then attack these metastases in the same manner as the primary tumor, even though there was no direct ablation at the metastatic sites.
Source: Created with BioRender.com.

the body's immune cells to recognize the tumor in a highly specific manner. In addition to fighting and destroying the primary tumor, the immune cells can survey the rest of the body for metastases that share the same TAAs as the primary tumor. The immune cells can then attack these metastases in the same manner as the primary tumor, even though there was no direct ablation at the metastatic sites.

Deeper Look: The Dual Role of Ethanol for Tumor Therapy

A simple method has been developed to dramatically improve the efficacy of ethanol ablation using polymer-assisted delivery of ethanol with ethyl cellulose. Ethyl cellulose is an inert, ethanol-soluble polysaccharide that is frequently used as a coating for medical pills. It is "generally regarded as safe" by the US Food and Drug Administration (FDA). Figure 6.17 shows the benefits of combining ethanol with the ethyl cellulose polymer. A petri dish containing a liquid mixture of ethanol and ethyl cellulose (a) turns into a gel upon the addition of water (b). The cotton-like gel formed as a result of the liquid-to-solid phase change in aqueous media (tissue) occludes pores and vessels that ethanol could leak through (c). Sequestering ethanol in the region of interest increases delivery efficiency and reduces off-target systemic toxicity (Morhard et al., 2017).

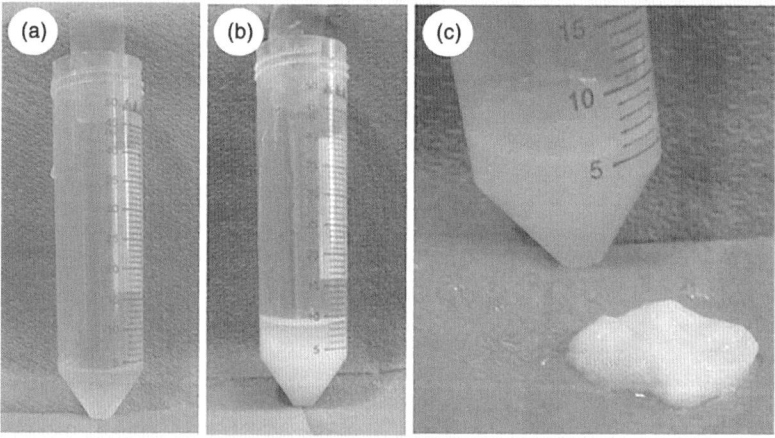

Figure 6.17 The benefits of combining ethanol with the ethyl cellulose polymer. A petri dish containing a liquid mixture of ethanol and ethyl cellulose (a) turns into a gel upon the addition of water (b). The cotton-like gel formed as a result of the liquid-to-solid phase change in aqueous media (tissue) occludes pores and vessels that ethanol could leak through (c). Sequestering ethanol in the region of interest increases delivery efficiency and reduces off-target systemic toxicity.
Source: Dompmartin et al. (2011).

Looking Ahead

The cost of basic surgical care would outstrip the GDP of many of the countries where these resources are lacking. Therefore, disruptive innovations that reimagine current screening, diagnosis, and treatment paradigms are critical to the mitigation of the growing cancer burden in LMICs. There has been tremendous effort to develop early detection technologies (Chapters 4 and 5), but without effective treatment these technologies will not reap dividends. The best solution is vaccination, and it is indeed exciting that there are preventive vaccines for liver and cervical cancer. In the absence of vaccines, ablation is a powerful way to address the limited access to surgery and radiation, with the potential to bolster the systemic immune response. Ablation is already accepted as a treatment solution for solid tumors in the US, but using energy-based devices that are difficult to sustain in locations with limited infrastructure.

The translation of alternative therapies such as ablation to LMICs is urgent. As of 2015, a majority of the world's population – over five billion people – did not have access to surgery (Jain & Puranik, 2022). Further, while 90 percent of the world's population resides in LMICs, approximately 30 percent have access to radiotherapy facilities. In fact, approximately 15 countries do not have a single radiation therapy machine (International Atomic Energy Agency, 2003). Although chemotherapy is becoming more common in LMICs (Price et al. 2012), it remains largely inaccessible due to cost (Bazargani et al., 2014; Ruff et al., 2016). As a result, long-term cancer survival rates in LMICs are approximately 20 percent in comparison to over 50 percent in HICs (Economist Intelligence Unit, 2009). The fact that ablation therapy is already having impact in cervical precancer treatment suggests that this is a viable approach for cancer treatment, with the added benefit of eliciting an antitumor immune response. This technology can impact both local and systemic disease.

Using an augmented version of a low-cost chemical solution such as ethanol can replace surgery and bolster systemic therapies. Given that these types of solutions are no longer the standard of care in HICs, there is a high bar for demonstrating the safety and efficacy of these approaches in rigorous clinical trials and likely an onerous regulatory process that requires substantial resources to apply for. Clinical trials will be discussed in the next chapter. This problem has to be addressed so that simple, low-cost, and effective therapies can reach patients who urgently require alternatives to conventional treatments without the attendant costs that make drugs, for example, prohibitively expensive for cancer treatment.

SUMMARY

Anticancer vaccines and ablative technologies offer a beacon of hope for bringing life-saving therapies to areas of the globe that need them the most. Preventive vaccines, such as the HPV and hepatitis B vaccines, work by training the body's immune system to recognize and eliminate the virus before it has a chance to entrench itself within the body. When vaccines are not available, cancer control is achieved through surgery, radiation, or chemotherapy – or a combination of each. Cancer ablation is emerging as an attractive alternative to surgery as it can be performed, in some cases, with limited infrastructure and training. The two main cancer ablation methods are thermal ablation and chemical ablation. Though they have different mechanisms of action, both methods induce cell death via cell necrosis, which is important for immune system activation.

The two most commonly used ablative methods for increasing the temperature within a tumor in the US are radio frequency and microwave ablation. Both technologies use electromagnetic radiation to heat the tip of a probe that is placed within the tumor. The heated tip then heats the surrounding tissue, leading to necrosis. Conversely, cryoablation uses either CO_2 or N_2O to create a supercooled probe tip that cools the surrounding tissue. Cryoablation is more amenable for use in LMICs than either radio frequency or microwave ablation; however, its dependence on hard-to-supply gas tanks and limited penetration depth render it a nonideal solution. The invention of thermocoagulation, which uses a heated probe to induce necrosis at depths greater than cryoablation, is improving access to thermal ablation for treatment of cervical precancers in LMICs.

The thermocoagulator and cryoablation strategies are excellent options for treatment of superficial lesions; however, they are not able to treat solid tumors that are not readily accessible from outside the body. Chemical ablation is an alternative to thermal ablation that may be better suited for treatment of solid tumors. The two most commonly used chemical ablation technologies are PDT and ethanol ablation. Photodynamic therapy uses photosensitizing drugs that are activated by light to create ROS to treat tumors. The limited penetration of depth of light through tissue, however, limits the application of PDT to superficial lesions. Ethanol ablation can be performed very simply under image guidance with ultrasound to access tumors located deeper within the body. While ethanol ablation was originally pioneered for treatment of liver tumors, it eventually fell out of favor due to unpredictable distribution in tissue leading to off-target side effects. Increasing the retention of ethanol within the tumor by using agents such as the polymer ethyl cellulose can help overcome off-target leakage in tissue. In addition to their ability to achieve local control, ablative technologies can induce a potent antitumor immune response to help treat and prevent metastases.

PROBLEMS

Cancer Prevention and Treatment

1. What is the role of each of the following cells in vaccine-induced immunity? Dendritic cells, B cells, Th cells, cytotoxic T lymphocytes.
2. Why will an individual who already has the HPV virus not benefit from the vaccine?
3. List two benefits of using an inactivated virus to make a vaccine.
4. List the three benefits of mRNA vaccines over previously developed approaches that make it particularly attractive for wide-scale dissemination.
5. What is the key difference between the Moderna and Johnson and Johnson vaccines for COVID-19?
6. A key goal of immunization programs is to protect as many people as possible. Practitioners have long recognized that achieving total vaccination among the entire population is difficult, if not impossible. Some people may be unable to be vaccinated due to illness or a compromised immune system, while still others may choose not to vaccinate due to religious beliefs or skepticism of science. Herd immunity relies on the fact that populations with higher rates of protected individuals are more protected. How does herd immunity achieve this goal?
7. The hepatitis B vaccine has the potential to greatly reduce liver cancer, as many liver cancer cases are caused by sustained hepatitis B infection. Assuming R_o for hepatitis B is 1.5, the prevalence of hepatitis B among vaccinated people is 0.5 percent, and the prevalence of hepatitis B among unvaccinated people is 30 percent, what percentage of the population must be vaccinated to see a downward trend in hepatitis B cases?
8. The FDA, European Medicines Agency, and other regulatory agencies around the world are evaluating monoclonal antibodies for use as a therapy to treat COVID-19. How does the monoclonal antibody treat COVID-19?
9. What are three different ways in which cells die during cancer therapy and which form of cell death is most effective in eliciting an antitumor immune response?

Thermal Ablation

10. A liver tumor is thermally ablated for 20 seconds – the temperature at the core, intermediate, and outer regions is 100, 55 and 25 °C, respectively. In which regions does cell death occur?
11. What are two reasons that it is important to consider the size of the ablative zone?

12. A patient has a cervical lesion that is determined to be a cancer. Would CO_2 cryoablation be effective at treating this lesion? Why or why not?
13. A biomedical engineer is attempting to improve heat distribution within a tumor during thermal ablation. Using the heat equation, explain how the injection of a paste with a higher thermal conductivity than the tumor would help increase the size of the ablative zone.

Chemical Ablation

14. Why is photodynamic therapy more specific than thermal ablation?
15. CT imaging is an excellent way to image ethanol distribution in tissue; the units are Hounsfield units. If ethanol shows up brighter on a CT image than the surrounding tissue, would it have a higher or lower level of Hounsfield units? Would higher ethanol concentrations show up as brighter or darker?
16. The graphs in Figure 6.18 show how the concentration of ethanol in tissue changes over time for two different formulations: (1) ethanol only and (2) ethanol with an additive that increases the viscosity. Which graph corresponds to ethanol only and which to ethanol with the additive? Explain your rationale using the diffusion equations.

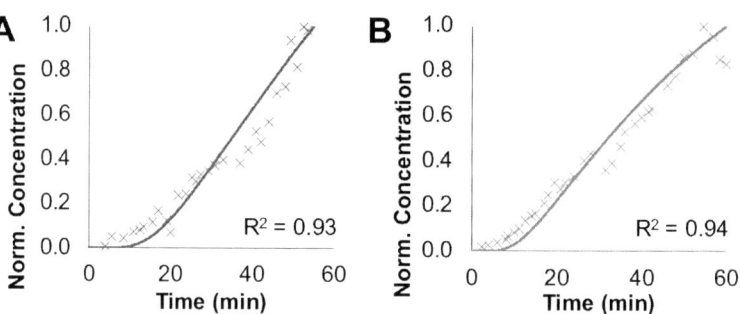

Figure 6.18

Consider two different scenarios below:
1. A woman with stage III liver cancer.
2. A woman with cervical precancer.
17. Which application will photodynamic therapy be most useful for? Why?
18. Which application will ethanol therapy be most useful for? Why?
19. What is an advantage and a disadvantage of covering an ablative zone larger than the tumor?
20. What are three similarities between the immune response following a vaccine and the immune response following ablation?

REFERENCES

Abou-Ghali, A., Stiban, J. 2015. Regulation of ceramide channel formation and disassembly: insights on the initiation of apoptosis. *Saudi Journal of Biological Sciences*, 22(6), 760–772. ISSN 1319-562X, https://doi.org/10.1016/j.sjbs.2015.03.005

Artifon, E. L., Lucin, A., Sakai, P., et al. 2007. EUS-guided alcohol ablation of left adrenal metastasis from non-small-cell lung carcinoma. *Gastrointestinal Endoscopy*, 66(6), 1201–1205.

Bazargani, Y. T., de Boer, A., Schellens J., et al. 2014. Selection of oncology medicines in low- and middle-income countries. *Annals of Oncology*, 25(1), 270–276.

Castanon, A., Landy, R., Brocklehurst, P., et al. 2014. Risk of preterm delivery with increasing depth of excision for cervical intraepithelial neoplasia in England: nested case-control study. *BMJ*, 349.

DeWitt, J., & Mohamadnejad, M. 2011. EUS-guided alcohol ablation of metastatic pelvic lymph nodes after endoscopic resection of polypoid rectal cancer: the need for long-term surveillance. *Gastrointestinal Endoscopy*, 74(2), 446–447.

Dompmartin, A., Blaizot, X., Théron, J. et al. 2011. Radio-opaque ethylcellulose-ethanol is a safe and efficient sclerosing agent for venous malformations. *Eur Radiol* 21, 2647–2656. https://doi.org/10.1007/s00330-011-2213-4.

Economist Intelligence Unit. 2009. Breakaway: the global burden of cancer-challenges and opportunities, a report from the Economist Intelligence Unit [Online]. Available: https://graphics.eiu.com/upload/eb/EIU_LIVESTRONG_Global_Cancer_Burden.pdf (accessed April 16, 2024).

International Atomic Energy Agency. 2003. Millions of cancer victims in developing countries lack access to life-saving radiotherapy [Online]. Available: www.iaea.org/newscenter/pressreleases/millions-cancer-victims-developing-countries-lack-access-life-saving-radiotherapy (accessed April 16, 2024).

Jain, S., & Puranik, A. 2022. General surgery: requirements, rationale, and robust results. *The Surgery Journal*, 8(4), e342–e346.

Jurgensen, C., Schuppan, D., Neser, F., et al. 2006. EUS-guided alcohol ablation of an insulinoma. *Gastrointestinal Endoscopy*, 63(7), 1059–1062.

Khan, M. J., & Smith-McCune, K. K. 2014. Treatment of cervical precancers: back to basics. *Obstetrics & Gynecology*, 123(6), 1339–1343.

Morhard, R., Nief, C., Barrero Castedo, C., et al. 2017. Development of enhanced ethanol ablation as an alternative to surgery in treatment of superficial solid tumors. *Scientific Reports*, 7(1), 8750.

Price, A. J., Ndom, P., Atenguena, E., et al. 2012. Cancer care challenges in developing countries. *Cancer*, 118(14), 3627–3635.

Rosa, S. S., Prazeres, D. M., Azevedo, A. M., & Marques, M. P. 2021. mRNA vaccines manufacturing: challenges and bottlenecks. *Vaccine*, 39(16), 2190–2200.

Ruff, P., Al-Sukhun, S., Blanchard, C., et al. 2016. Access to cancer therapeutics in low- and middle-income countries. *American Society for Clinical Oncology Educational Book*, 35, 58–65.

Ryu, M., Shimamura, Y., Kinoshita T., et al. 1997. Therapeutic results of resection, transcatheter arterial embolization and percutaneous transhepatic ethanol injection in 3225 patients with hepatocellular carcinoma: a retrospective multicenter study. *Japanese Journal of Clinical Oncology*, 27(4), 251–257.

Shiina, S., Tagawa, K., Unuma, T., et al. 1991. Percutaneous ethanol injection therapy for hepatocellular carcinoma: a histopathologic study. *Cancer*, 68(7), 1524–1530.

Solbiati, L., Giangrande, A., De Pra, L., et al. 1985. Percutaneous ethanol injection of parathyroid tumors under US guidance: treatment for secondary hyperparathyroidism. *Radiology*, 155(3): 607–610.

Sorajja, P., Valeti, U., Nishimura, R. A., et al. 2008. Outcome of alcohol septal ablation for obstructive hypertrophic cardiomyopathy. *Circulation*, 118(2), 131–139.

Sugiura, N. T. K., Ohto, M., Okuda, K., & Hirooka, N. 1983. Percutaneous intratumoral injection of ethanol under ultrasound imaging for treatment of small hepatocellular carcinoma. *Acta Hepatology Japan*, 21(920).

Yamada, Y, Takano, Y, Satrialdi, Abe J, Hibino, M, Harashima H. 2020. Therapeutic strategies for regulating mitochondrial oxidative stress. *Biomolecules*, 10(1):83. https://doi.org/10.3390/biom10010083.

7 From Technology to Translation

The twentieth century was clearly marked by dramatic changes in medical practice, with new methods to examine experimental designs implemented over the course of the century. The emergence of evidence-based practice was followed by the need for standardized procedures to assess the efficacy of tests and therapies, and guidelines for protecting the patients involved. Ultimately, standardized clinical trials became critical in answering questions that scientific investigations could not. Therefore, it is critical for any researcher working on medical innovations to understand and appreciate the design, testing, and interpretation of clinical data.

Clinical trials are essential to informing providers and patients of the safety and efficacy of an intervention. This information is also necessary for approval to manufacture and sell a medical device or drug. The regulatory body that oversees this process in the US is the Food and Drug Administration (FDA). The FDA has a set of guidelines of what documents manufacturers must submit in order for a device or drug to be approved. The greater the risk of a particular technology or medicine, the more data is required, largely in the form of clinical studies that are well designed to accurately inform the safety and efficacy compared to an existing solution or a placebo. The study design must also be conducted on ethical grounds that consider the risks to the populations tested and to not exploit vulnerable populations.

The goal of this chapter is to discuss methods to rigorously evaluate devices and drugs to demonstrate clinical benefit over the status quo. The type of data collected, numerical vs. categorical, impacts the type of statistical tool that is needed for hypothesis testing. Ultimately, to design definitive clinical investigations, it is essential to know how many patients to enroll to reach a meaningful conclusion. Enrolling a small number of patients may introduce bias, whereas enrolling more patients than are needed to answer the question will be a waste of resources. In this chapter you will learn how to interpret data collected from technologies to inform decision outcomes.

LEARNING OBJECTIVES

Basic Concepts for Statistical Analysis
- Methods for visualizing data, specifically histograms and box plots;
- calculation of key metrics for summarizing data, such as the mean, median, and standard deviation;
- the selection of the appropriate types of tests for describing statistical significance or similarity.

Determining Statistical Significance
- An understanding of the null and alternative hypotheses for statistical testing;
- calculation of statistical differences and similarities between groups;
- calculation of and interpretation of confidence intervals.

Calculation of Key Metrics for a Clinical Study
- Calculation of power calculation to determine the sample size for a clinical study;
- explain the difference between type I and type II errors;
- definition of different types of clinical trials, including randomization and blinding.

Basic Concepts for Statistical Analysis

One of the most important concepts for accurate interpretation of research or clinical data is hypothesis testing, to answer the question: Are the differences observed between a new test or drug from the standard of care real or did it occur by chance? Statistical analysis is the primary method for testing a hypothesis. A control group is made up of study participants who do not receive the intervention (they undergo the standard tests and treatments), while participants who are exposed to the intervention are part of the experimental group. The statistical tests determine whether or not experimental and control groups are statistically different from one another.

The type of analysis that is required to determine if two groups are different from each other depends on whether the data is categorical or numerical and is illustrated below using breast cancer as an example. Categorical data, as the name suggests, can be divided into **ordinal** (e.g., small, medium, and large lesion sizes) or **nominal** (e.g., fatty, fibrous, or glandular tissues) categories. Numerical data, on the other hand, involves numbers and can be divided into **continuous** (e.g., age of the patient) or **discrete** (e.g., the number of tumors in a mammogram) categories. To reiterate, ordinal categories are a way of describing data based on orders or positions, while nominal categories are a way of describing data without using a quantitative value; continuous

Basic Concepts for Statistical Analysis

data has an infinite number of possible values, while discrete data has a finite number of possible values.

Before beginning to analyze data with statistical tests, it is first helpful to visualize the data. Figure 7.1 shows different ways to visualize data. Two common ways to visualize data include histograms and box plots (also called box and whisker plots). Histograms show the different possible occurrences of a variable on the x-axis and the number of occurrences on the y-axis. Box plots also show the distribution of the data; however, box plots are more useful when comparing several data sets to each other. For example, in a subset of breast cancer patients, a histogram could be used to show the number of patients of different ages. Keeping with the breast cancer and age example, a box plot could be used to compare the distribution of ages for women with HER2+, ER+, and TNBC. Histograms can be used for both categorical numerical inputs, whereas box plots are appropriate for the representation of numerical data. Histograms may not accurately display the distribution shape if the data size is too small; in this case, box plots are preferable.

In addition to visualizing data, it is important to understand how to define different characteristics and attributes of data. One of the most commonly used summary parameters for a data set is the mean. The population mean or μ is described by Equation 7.1, where N is the number of samples and x is a specific sample within that distribution. When performing statistical analysis, it is important to distinguish populations from samples. When a clinical trial is being performed, the collected data is a sample from a larger population (e.g., breast cancer patients enrolled in a clinical trial is a sample of the larger population of all breast cancer patients). As a result, when researchers discuss

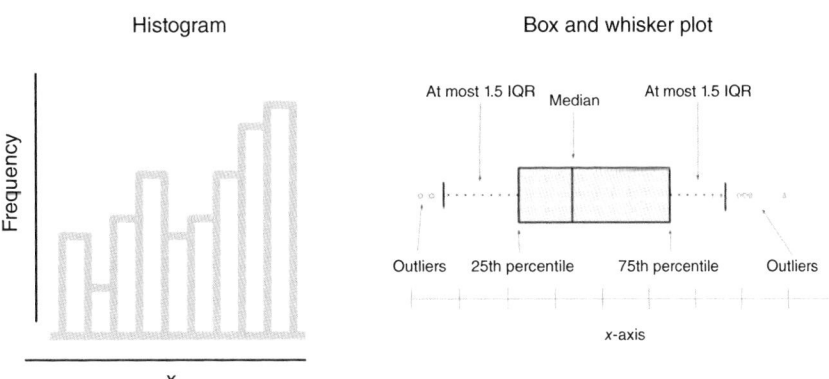

Figure 7.1 Different ways to visualize data. Two common ways to visualize data include histograms and box plots (also called box and whisker plots). Histograms show the different possible occurrences of a variable on the x-axis and the number of occurrences on the y-axis. Box plots also show the distribution of the data; however, box plots are more useful when comparing several data sets to each other.

the mean of their data, they are referring to the sample mean $\underline{x}$, which can be calculated using Equation 7.2.

While the mean is a helpful summary parameter, it does not contain any information about the spread of the data. For example, the average tumor size among six patients could be 2 cm because all six patients had a 2 cm tumor, or because three patients had a 1 cm tumor and three patients had a 3 cm tumor. While both of these samples have an average of 2 cm, the spread of the data within the population is different. Standard deviation is a metric for calculating the spread of data. The population standard deviation (σ) and corresponding standard error (SE) is shown in Equation 7.3, where μ is the population mean, x is the sample value, and N is the number of samples. The sample standard deviation (s) and corresponding SE is shown in Equation 7.4, where N is the number of samples, x is the sample value, and $\underline{x}$ is the sample mean. It is important to note the difference between σ and SE. While the former corresponds to the spread of the data around the mean of a single sample of size N, the SE corresponds to the spread of the data around multiple means where each mean is calculated from different samples of size N.

$$\mu = \sum_{i=1}^{N} \frac{x_i}{N}, \tag{7.1}$$

$$\underline{x} = \sum_{i=1}^{N} \frac{x_i}{N}, \tag{7.2}$$

$$\sigma = \sqrt{\frac{\sum_{i=1}^{N}(x_i - \mu)^2}{N}}, \sigma_{\underline{x}} = \frac{\sigma}{\sqrt{N}}, \tag{7.3}$$

$$s = \sqrt{\frac{\sum_{i=1}^{N}(x_i - \underline{x})^2}{N-1}}, SE = \frac{s}{\sqrt{N}}. \tag{7.4}$$

Another important concept to introduce at this stage is the normal distribution. Figure 7.2 shows a normal distribution. The normal distribution is a bell-shaped curve and can be described by a mean and standard deviation. The area under the curve for a normal distribution is always 1. In order for a distribution to be normal, the first, second, and third standard deviations encompass 68.3, 95.5, and 99.7 percent, respectively, of the area under the curve. The second standard deviation, which accounts for 95 percent of the data, is an important benchmark for a number of statistical tests. The standard normal distribution is a normal distribution with a mean of zero and standard deviation of 1.

Another important parameter that is a part of many statistical tests is the z-score. A z-score is used to report on how many standard deviations above

Basic Concepts for Statistical Analysis

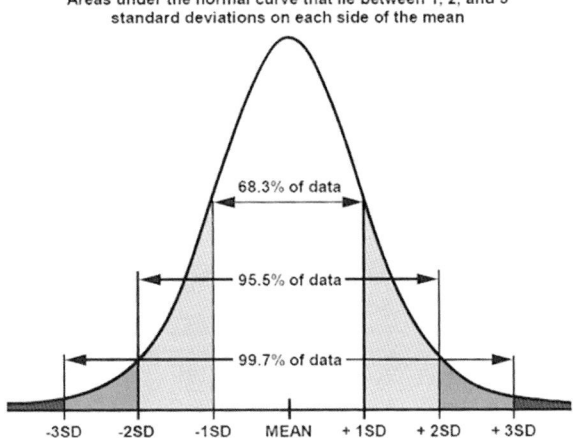

Figure 7.2 Normal distribution. The normal distribution is a bell-shaped curve and can be described by a mean and standard deviation. The area under the curve for a normal distribution is always 1. In order for a distribution to be normal, the first, second, and third standard deviations encompass 68.3, 95.5, and 99.7 percent, respectively, of the area under the curve.

or below the population mean a given sample within the population is. The z-score is calculated using Equation 7.5, where z is the z-score, x is the sample value, $\underline{x}$ is the sample mean, and s is the standard deviation of the sample. Z-scores range from −3 standard deviations (which would fall to the far left of the normal distribution curve) up to +3 standard deviations (which would fall to the far right of the normal distribution curve). In order to calculate a z-score, you need to either know the population mean (μ) and standard deviation (σ) or the sample mean $(\underline{x})$ and standard deviation (s), as shown in Equation 7.5:

$$z = \frac{x - \underline{x}}{s}. \tag{7.5}$$

Experiments and clinical trials are designed to test whether two or more groups are different from each other. When evaluating the differences between sample or population distributions, it is important to determine the **statistical significance** of the test result. Statistical significance is the likelihood that the difference in a particular variable between two groups is real and not due to random chance. In other words, the statistical significance of a test establishes whether or not the test result should be believed. Table 7.1 summarizes the tests needed to demonstrate statistical significance or similarity. Different statistical tests are needed for numerical and categorical data. Further, the data that is compared within a subject before and after an intervention versus data that is compared between groups of patients require different statistical methodologies for analysis. Each of these tests will be elaborated on in the next few paragraphs.

Table 7.1 Tests to demonstrate statistical significance or similarity

Different statistical tests are needed for numerical and categorical data. The data that is compared within a subject before and after an intervention versus data that is compared between groups of patients require different statistical methodologies for analysis.

Type of data	Numerical	Categorical
Subcategories	Continuous and discrete	Ordinal and nominal
Statistical test	Parametric t-test (1 comparison) ANOVA (>1 comparison)	Nonparametric Wilcoxon rank-sum test (1 comparison) Kruskal–Wallis (>1 comparison)
Summary statistics	Mean, standard deviation	Median, upper, and lower quartiles

Statistical tests are performed on **summary statistics** of the data set (e.g., mean, minimum, maximum, standard deviation, etc.). It is important to consider the different assumptions a statistical test makes about the data prior to determining which test to use. The two main categories of tests are parametric tests and nonparametric tests. The difference between **parametric tests** and **nonparametric** tests is the assumption of normality – parametric tests assume the data set is normally distributed, while nonparametric tests do not. For continuous data that is normally distributed, a parametric test would be appropriate for testing whether two groups are different.

If the averages of a variable (for example, white blood cell count) between two independent groups are compared (for example, breast cancer patients with and without chemotherapy), an unpaired **t-test** is used; for comparisons within a group (blood cell count within a patient before and after chemotherapy), a paired t-test is used. If the averages of a variable from more than two groups are being compared, an **analysis of variance (ANOVA)** is used to determine whether any of the groups are different from one another. Importantly, an ANOVA only establishes that the mean of at least one or more groups is different from the mean of one or more other groups. As a result, a secondary test, called a **post hoc test**, must be performed after an ANOVA to determine which groups are different from each other.

If the data is categorical, it is described by median (middle value), upper and lower quartiles (the top quarter and bottom quarter range of the data set). In the case of categorical data, nonparametric tests (no assumptions made about distributions) are used. If a variable (for example, lesion size) is compared between two independent groups (patients with and without chemotherapy), a **Wilcoxon rank-sum** test is used. The Wilcoxon signed-rank test is used for comparison of a variable (lesion before or after chemotherapy) within a patient. A **Kruskal–Wallis** test is used (the nonparametric equivalent of an ANOVA) if more than two groups are being compared. As was the case with an ANOVA, a post hoc test must be performed in order to determine which groups are different from each other.

If more than two groups are being compared, why is an ANOVA or Kruskal–Wallis test used rather than simply performing multiple t-tests or Wilcoxon rank-sums? As you learned above, a statistical test tells you how likely it is that the difference between two groups is real. An important subtlety here is that there is always a chance that the difference between the two groups is random (i.e., the two groups are actually the same even though the test said they were different).

When comparing two groups to each other, the chance is low that the statistical test found the incorrect result. However, as more and more groups are compared to each other, the chance increases that the statistical test result may be incorrect for one or more of the tests, a phenomenon called **multiple comparison bias**. A multi-comparison test like ANOVA or Kruskal–Wallis protects against multiple comparison bias by comparing all of the groups together at one time to establish that at least one group is different from at least one other group. By performing the multi-comparison test first, the likelihood that any testing of pairs of data within the larger group leads to an incorrect test result is reduced.

While the previously discussed statistical tests can determine whether the means are significantly different between the groups, different analyses are required to provide evidence that there is agreement rather than disagreement between groups. Demonstrating that there is no statistical difference between the two groups only indicates that there is a lower probability that the two samples are different from each other; however, this does not constitute proof that the groups are the same. To test agreement between two groups that are described by categorical results (for example, the number of patients who are diagnosed with breast cancer using two different imaging modalities), the percentage agreement can be calculated.

To compare the agreement between two sets of continuous data (e.g., white blood cell count after chemotherapy by two different assays), correlation tests can be used to examine the relationship of two results (white blood cell count). On the other hand, a Bland–Altman test can be used to assess the difference between the results of two different types of tests. Similarity tests yield similar results – for example, when a particular variable (e.g., white blood cell count) is statistically insignificant before and after an intervention (e.g., chemotherapy). Correlation tests and Bland–Altman tests will be described in more detail later in the chapter.

Deeper Look: What Do Error Bars Mean?

Error bars can be calculated in different ways and may be showing different things (e.g., standard deviation, confidence interval) – they cannot be interpreted as being the same. It is important to understand the differences between them. The next question is whether the data is independent (for between-subject comparisons) or paired (for within-subject comparisons). For paired data, the error bars are not relevant. Figure 7.3 shows the three common types of error bars: standard deviation (σ or s as noted earlier or SD as used here), standard error or SE, and confidence intervals (CI). Data is shown for two samples of size $n=10$ along with the p-value of the difference in sample means. In Figure 7.3(a) the different error bars appear the same for different p-values, while in Figure 7.3(b) they appear different for the same p-values. p-values < 0.05 reflect statistical significance. In general, a gap between bars does not ensure significance, nor does overlap rule it out – it depends on the type of bar (Krzywinski and Altman, 2013). Both CIs and p-values will be discussed in greater detail in the next section.

Error bars based on SD inform us about the spread of the data around the mean. Standard deviation reflects the variation of the data and not the error in the measurement. When SDs of two populations overlap, the differences are likely not statistically significant or are just at the border of being significant (as shown in Figure 7.3(b)). When SDs don't overlap, it may suggest that the difference is probably statistically significant (Figure 7.3(a)). However, neither are conclusive without a statistical test.

Unlike SD, SE reflects the uncertainty in the mean and its dependency on the sample size. As sample size increases, SE decreases. With a very large sample size, the SE tends toward 0. When the SE error bars overlap, the difference between two means is not statistically significant $(p > 0.05)$. In order to reach a p-value ≤ 0.05, the SE bars are separated by about at least 1 SE.

The CI is defined as a specified probability that a value lies within. The size of the CI depends on n; two useful approximations for the CI are 95% CI $\approx 4 \times$ SE ($n = 3$) and 95% CI ≈ 2 SE ($n > 15$). If the CI error bars do not overlap, the group means are significantly

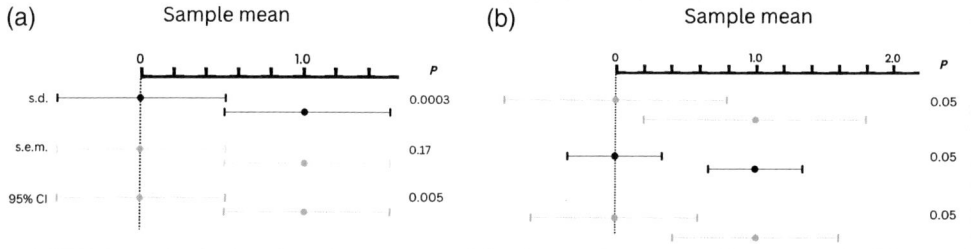

Figure 7.3 Three common types of error bars: standard deviation (SD), standard error (SE), and confidence intervals (CI). Data is shown for two samples of size $n = 10$ and the p-value of the difference in sample means. In (a) the different error bars appear the same for different p-values, while in (b) they appear different for the same p-values.

> different. However, if the two 95 percent CI error bars do overlap, statistical significance or lack of it cannot be concluded. Which one should you choose? The SD are the most intuitive and the CI are the most explicit. Whichever error bar is chosen, it needs to be explicitly defined.

Determining Statistical Significance

The previous section alluded to the idea of statistical significance as a determinant for whether two groups are the same or different. This section will look more closely at some of the statistical tests mentioned in the previous section, as well as how to perform them to establish statistical significance by a **difference test**, **a similarity test**, or the **CI calculations**. Prior to describing these different tests, it is important to cover the concept of degrees of freedom. **Degrees of freedom** (df) are the number of independent values that a statistical analysis can estimate (i.e., the number of values that are free to vary as you estimate parameters). If one constraint is placed on a variable, the df = 1, if it is 2, df = 2, etc. Degrees of freedom are relevant to statistical calculations and will be discussed further in the context of the t-test and ANOVA test.

What do these different degrees of freedom mean? Suppose we have two groups $(k=2)$ that we want to compare. If we know the mean of one of the groups and the grand mean, the other group must have a specific value such that (group mean 1 + group mean 2) / 2 = grand mean (this example assumes equal cell sample sizes, but unequal cell sample sizes would not change the number of degrees of freedom). Therefore, for a two-group design, df1 = 1. For a three-group design $(k=3)$, using the same process we would come to the conclusion that df1 = 2. Therefore, for a one-way ANOVA the general formula is df1 = k −1. The second term, df2, is the total number of observations in all cells within a group (n) minus the degrees of freedom lost because the cell means are set by the number of groups, k : df2 = $n - k$. Say we have 150 participants across four conditions; we will have df2 = 150 − 4 = 146.

Difference test: To interpret the results of a statistical test, it is important to understand the underlying principle of *why* statistical tests are carried out in the first place: That is, is there a significant difference between two groups? We form two potential answers to the question, also called **hypotheses**. Hypotheses are the expected outcomes after a test. For example, a hypothesis could be "The sample mean of group 1 is greater than the sample mean of group 2." The *null hypothesis* (H_0) states that there will be no statistical difference between the two groups (e.g., the white blood cell count of patients with and without chemotherapy are not different). The *alternative*

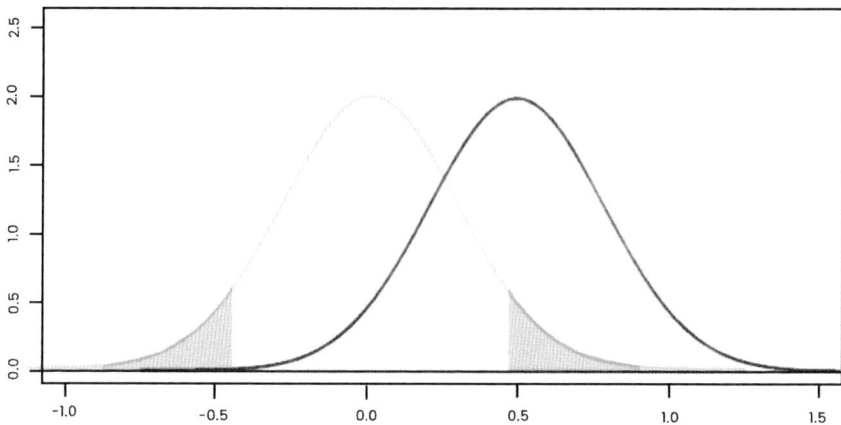

Figure 7.4 Null and alternative distribution groups. The gray curve corresponds to the null distribution and the black curve corresponds to the alternative distribution. The shaded area corresponds to an area outside two SD of the mean and is referred to as the significance level, α. It will be important to keep in mind that forming the null and alternative hypotheses for a statistical test is critically important, as they establish what will be tested and what test should be used.

hypothesis (H_1) states that there is a statistical difference between the distribution of white blood cell counts between groups. It will be important to keep in mind that forming the null and alternative hypotheses for a statistical test is critically important, as they establish what will be tested and what test should be used.

Figure 7.4 illustrates null and alternative distribution groups. The gray curve corresponds to the null distribution and the black curve corresponds to the alternative distribution. The shaded area corresponds to an area outside two SD of the mean and is referred to as the significance level, α. The significance level, α, sets the standard for how extreme the measured values must be to reject a null hypothesis; by convention it is set at 0.05, corresponding to an area that is two SD from the mean (recall that one SD is 68.3 percent, the second is 95.5 percent, and the third is 99.7 percent). In other words, α is the probability below which a null hypothesis is rejected when it is *actually* true. The α value gives us the probability of a type I error. For example, when α is 0.05 = 1/20, a true null hypothesis will be rejected 1 in 20 times.

The other number that is part of a test of significance is a *p*-value. While α corresponds to the *level of significance* at which the null hypothesis is rejected, the *p*-value corresponds to the *smallest level of significance* at which the null hypothesis would be rejected. If the *p*-value is less than or equal to α, the null hypothesis is rejected, and the result is statistically significant. In other words, we can rule out that this is a chance occurrence. As an example, if the null distribution is the white blood cell count distribution of patients with chemotherapy, and the alternative distribution is the white blood cell count distribution of patients without chemotherapy, we can reject the null hypothesis if the

Determining Statistical Significance

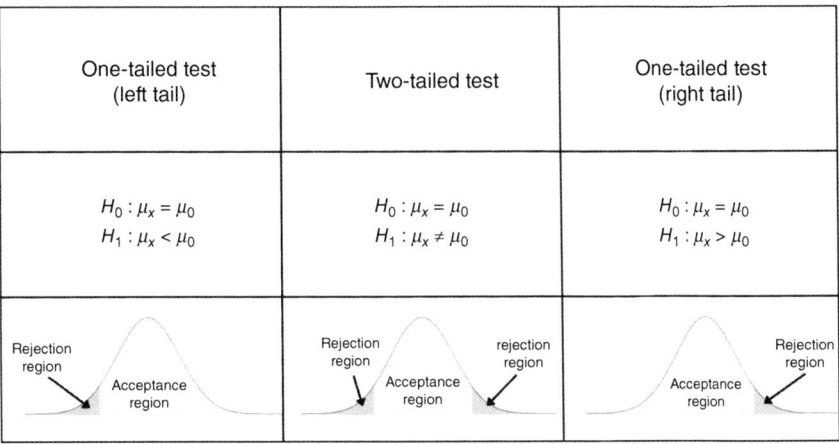

Figure 7.5 Three alternative hypotheses that can be tested with a *t*-test. The first two alternative hypotheses are tested by a one-tailed test, as shown on the left and right sides, by only testing one side of the distribution. The third alternative hypothesis is tested by a two-tailed test as shown in the middle.
Source: Adapted from Ibe (2014).

p-value is less than 0.05. If the *p*-value is greater than α, the null hypothesis is *not* rejected, even though the result is not statistically significant.

***Detailed explanation of the* t-test:** A *t*-test is used to determine if the difference between the means of two sample distributions is statistically significant. Figure 7.5 shows the two different types of *t*-tests and three alternative hypotheses that can be tested. One of three alternative hypotheses can be tested against the null hypothesis that the two means are not different: (1) the mean of group 1 is larger than that of group 2; (2) the mean of group 1 is smaller than that of group 2; (3) the mean of group 1 is either larger or smaller than that of group 2. Figure 7.5 shows three alternative hypotheses that can be tested with a *t*-test. The first two alternative hypotheses are tested by a one-tailed test, as shown on the left and right sides, by only testing one side of the distribution. The third alternative hypothesis is tested by a two-tailed test, as shown in the middle. Keeping with the chemotherapy example, a one-tailed test can test significance in one direction only (the white blood cell count of patients after chemotherapy is less than *or* greater than that of patients without chemotherapy), whereas a two-tailed test tests for significance in both directions. The *p*-value threshold for a one-tailed test is 0.05, whereas for a two-tailed test it is 0.025 (split between the two tails), as shown in the shaded regions. In other words, it is more difficult to achieve statistical significance with a two-sided test than a one-sided test.

How do you determine whether to perform a one-tailed vs. a two-tailed *t*-test? The answer lies in what the biologically possible outcomes are and what the study is trying to determine. For example, if a study is testing whether a new chemotherapy lowers white blood cells more or less than an established chemotherapy, a two-tailed test would be used because the possible outcomes are that white blood cell counts are lowered more or less with the new chemotherapy. Conversely, if a study is testing whether more frequent dosing with a chemotherapy decreases white blood cell counts more than less frequent dosing, a one-tailed test would be used because the only possible outcome is that white blood cell counts are lowered more.

The formula for the two-tailed t-test (for samples with a normal distribution), shown in Equation 7.6, is the ratio of the difference in group means and the SE. In this formula, t is the t-value statistic, $\overline{x_1}$ and $\overline{x_2}$ are the means of the two groups being compared (white blood cell count in patients before and after cancer therapy), S_p is the pooled SD (defined in Equation 7.7), n_1 and n_2 are the sample size for each group, and s is the SD. A larger t-value shows that the difference between group means is greater than the pooled SE:

$$t = \frac{\overline{x_1} - \overline{x_2}}{\sqrt{s_p^2 \left(\frac{1}{n_1} + \frac{1}{n_2} \right)}}, \qquad (7.6)$$

$$S_p = \sqrt{\frac{(n_1 - 1)s_1^2 + (n_2 - 1)s_2^2}{n_1 + n_2 - 2}}. \qquad (7.7)$$

The calculated t-value can be compared to the values in a t-table chart to determine if the t-value is greater than what would be expected by chance. If so, the null hypothesis can be rejected to conclude that the two groups are in fact different. The t-table is a matrix in which the top row corresponds to the p-value (e.g., 0.05), and the left-most column, the degrees of freedom, is the sum of the samples in all groups – # groups ($n_1 + n_2 - 2$). To determine the level of significance of a t-statistic for a significance level of 0.05 for a two-tailed t-test, the t-statistic will range from 12.71 (1 df) to 1.98 (100 df).

Example: *t*-Test Calculation

Question: A physician is testing two different therapies for breast cancer to see which one performed the best at reducing tumor volume before surgery. Tumor volumes (in millimeters) were measured three months after beginning therapy. The results are summarized in the table below. Is there a statistical difference in mean tumor volume between the two therapies?

Therapy 1 (x_1)	Therapy 2 (x_2)
16.6	20.1
15.9	19.5
17.0	18.0
18.3	18.7
16.0	21.5

Answer: The null hypothesis is that the two population means are equal, while the alternative hypothesis is that the two population means are not equal. Because we are comparing the mean values across two groups, a t-test is most appropriate. The pooled SD and the t-statistic are obtained using Equations 7.6 and 7.7. In order to do so, we first need to calculate the means and SD for the two groups using Equations 7.2 and 7.4. The math below is for Therapy 1, and the same method can be used for Therapy 2:

$$\underline{x_1} = \sum_{i=1}^{N} \frac{x_i}{N} = \frac{16.6 + 15.9 + 17.0 + 18.3 + 16.0}{5} = 16.76,$$

$$s_1 = \sqrt{\frac{\sum_{i=1}^{N}(x_i - \underline{x})^2}{N-1}}$$

$$= \sqrt{\frac{(16.6 - 16.76)^2 + (15.9 - 16.76)^2 + (17.0 - 16.76)^2 + (18.3 - 16.76)^2 + (16 - 16.76)^2}{5 - 1}}$$

$$= 0.97,$$

$\underline{x_2} = 19.56,$

$s_2 = 1.34.$

Now we are ready to calculate the pooled SD using Equation 7.7:

$$S_p = \sqrt{\frac{(n_1 - 1)s_1^2 + (n_2 - 1)s_2^2}{n_1 + n_2 - 2}} = \sqrt{\frac{(5-1)(0.97)^2 + (5-1)(1.34)^2}{5 + 5 - 2}}.$$

$$= 1.17$$

Lastly, we can calculate the t-statistic using Equation 7.6:

$$t = \frac{\underline{x_1} - \underline{x_2}}{\sqrt{s_p^2 \left(\frac{1}{n_1} + \frac{1}{n_2}\right)}} = \frac{16.76 - 19.56}{\sqrt{1.17^2 \left(\frac{1}{5} + \frac{1}{5}\right)}} = -3.77.$$

The final step is to look up the critical t-statistic in a table based on the number of degrees of freedom (the sum of the samples in all group – # groups), 5+5−2=8, which is 2.306. Since the t-value magnitude is greater than 2.306 (i.e., 3.77 > 2.306) (see a portion of the *t*-statistic table below) we can reject the null hypothesis and conclude the means are statistically different.

df/p	0.40	0.25	0.10	0.05	0.025	0.01	0.005	0.0005
1	0.324920	1.000000	3.077684	6.313752	12.70620	31.82052	63.65674	636.6192
2	0.288675	0.816497	1.885618	2.919986	4.30265	6.96456	9.92484	31.5991
3	0.276671	0.764892	1.637744	2.353363	3.18245	4.54070	5.84091	12.9240
4	0.270722	0.740697	1.533206	2.131847	2.77645	3.74695	4.60409	8.6103
5	0.267181	0.726687	1.475884	2.015048	2.57058	3.36493	4.03214	6.11688
6	0.264835	0.717558	1.439756	1.943180	2.44691	3.14267	3.70743	5.9588
7	0.263167	0.711142	1.414924	1.894579	2.36462	2.99795	3.49948	5.4079
8	0.261921	0.706387	1.396815	1.859548	2.30600	2.89646	3.35539	5.0413
9	0.260955	0.702722	1.383029	1.833113	2.26216	2.82144	3.24984	4.7809
10	0260185	0.699812	1.372184	1.812461	2.22814	2.76377	3.16927	4.5869

Detailed explanation of ANOVA: Now that we have covered how to perform calculations for a *t*-test, we will look at how an ANOVA works. An ANOVA test is used when comparing the means between more than two groups and only provides information that at least one group is statistically different from one other group. A post hoc test is needed to determine which groups are different from one another (e.g., a *t*-test). The underlying idea behind an ANOVA is that if the sample means from multiple groups are different, then the variance within each sample group will be smaller than the variance if all sample groups are combined. One-way means the ANOVA has one independent variable. Two-way means the test has two independent variables. The ratio of variance between samples to variance within samples is referred to as the *F* ratio and is calculated as shown in Equation 7.8:

$$F = \frac{Variance_{between}}{Variance_{within}}. \quad (7.8)$$

Let's first look at how to calculate the variance between groups. The variance between groups is a measure of how different the means from each group are from the grand mean. The **grand mean** is the mean of all samples combined, regardless of which group they came from. Equation 7.9 shows the equation for calculating the variance between groups. In this equation, *n* represents the number of samples within each group, k represents the total number of groups, x_i is the sample mean for each group, and $\bar{\bar{x}}$ is the grand mean:

$$Variance_{between} = \frac{\sum_{i=1}^{k} n_i (x_i - \bar{\bar{x}})^2}{k-1}. \tag{7.9}$$

Next, we will calculate the variance within groups. The variance within groups is a measure of how different each sample within a group is from the group mean. Equation 7.10 shows how to calculate the variance within groups. In this equation, n represents the number of samples within each group, k represents the total number of groups, x_j is the sample value, x_j is the sample mean for each group, and N is the total number of samples across all groups:

$$Variance_{within} = \frac{\sum_{i=1}^{k} \sum_{j=1}^{n_i} (x_j - x_j)^2}{N-k}. \tag{7.10}$$

Once the F ratio has been calculated, the critical F ratio at a given significance level (usually $p = 0.05$) can be determined using a look-up table. Each F ratio will have a different critical value that depends on the number of groups (k) and the total number of samples (N). The ratio is typically in terms of degrees of freedom (df1 and df2). For an ANOVA, df1 = $k - 1$ and df2 = $N - k$.

Example: ANOVA Calculation

Question: A physician is testing four different therapies for breast cancer to see which one performed the best at reducing tumor volume before surgery. Tumor volumes (in millimeters) were measured 3 months after beginning therapy. The results are summarized in the table below. Is there a statistical difference in mean tumor volume between the four therapies?

Therapy 1	Therapy 2	Therapy 3	Therapy 4
18.5	19.0	16.6	20.1
17.9	20.9	15.9	19.5
19.2	18.2	17.0	18.0
16.5	17.8	18.3	18.7
17.4	18.1	16.0	21.5

Answer: The null hypothesis is that the four population means are equal, while the alternative hypothesis is that the four population means are not equal. Because we are comparing the mean values across more than two groups, an ANOVA test is most appropriate for use; therefore, we need to calculate the variance between groups and within groups using

Equations 7.9 and 7.10. Beginning with the variance between groups, we need to calculate the mean for each group and the grand mean. The mean for each group can be found by summing the total volumes (shown in bold) and dividing by the number of samples to get the mean (shown in bold and italics):

Therapy 1	Therapy 2	Therapy 3	Therapy 4
18.5	19.0	16.6	20.1
17.9	20.9	15.9	19.5
19.2	18.2	17.0	18.0
16.5	17.8	18.3	18.7
17.4	18.1	16.0	21.5
89.5	**94**	**83.8**	**97.8**
17.9	***18.8***	***16.76***	***19.56***

The grand mean can be calculated by finding the mean of all the means:

$$\bar{\bar{x}} = \frac{(17.9 + 18.8 + 16.76 + 19.56)}{4} = 18.255.$$

Now the variance between can be calculated using Equation 7.9, where $k=4$ because there are four groups and $n=5$ for each group:

$$Variance_{between} = \frac{\sum_{i=1}^{k} n_i (x_i - \bar{\bar{x}})^2}{k-1}$$

$$= \frac{5(17.9-18.255)^2 + 5(18.8-18.255)^2 + 5(16.76-18.255)^2 + 5(19.56-18.255)^2}{4-1}$$

$$= 7.27.$$

Applying the same principles to Equation 7.10 gives the variance within groups as:

$$Variance_{within} = 1.35.$$

Finally, we can calculate the F ratio using Equation 7.8:

$$F = \frac{Variance_{between}}{Variance_{within}} = \frac{7.27}{1.35} \approx 5.39.$$

Using the look-up table shown below (just the portion of the F table that corresponds to this example) for $df1 = k-1 = 3$ and $df2 = N - k = 16$, we find that the critical value for F at a p-value of 0.05 is 3.24. Because 5.39 is larger than the critical value of 3.24, there is a significant difference between the mean tumor volumes.

/	df1 = 1	2	3	4	5
df2 = 1	161.4476	199.5000	19.1643	224.5832	230.1619
2	18.5128	19.0000	19.1643	19.2468	19.2964
3	10.1280	9.5521	9.2766	9.1172	9.0135
4	7.7086	6.9443	6.5914	6.3882	6.2561
5	6.6079	5.7861	5.4095	5.1922	5.0503
6	5.9874	5.1433	4.7571	4.5337	5.0503
7	5.5914	4.7374	4.3468	4.1203	3.9715
8	5.3177	4.4590	4.0662	3.8379	3.6875
9	5.1174	4.2565	3.8625	3.6331	3.3258
10	4.9646	4.1028	3.7083	3.4780	3.3258
11	4.8443	3.9823	3.5874	3.3567	3.2039
12	4.7472	3.8853	3.4903	3.2592	3.1059
13	4.6672	3.8056	3.4105	3.1791	3.0254
14	4.6001	3.7389	3.3439	3.1122	2.9582
15	4.5431	3.6823	3.2874	3.0556	2.9013
16	4.4940	3.6337	3.2389	3.0069	2.8524

The ANOVA test makes three assumption: (1) The responses for each factor level have a normal population distribution; (2) these distributions have the same variance; and (3) the data are independent. One of the main advantages of nonparametric tests (i.e., rank-sum and Kruskal–Wallis) over parametric tests, such as ANOVA, is that they do not make any assumptions about the distribution of the data. However, because of this it can be more difficult to obtain a significant p-value than with a parametric test.

Detailed explanation of Wilcoxon rank-sum: A rank-sum test, also called a Wilcoxon rank-sum test or Mann–Whitney U-test, ranks all of the data regardless of group in ascending order from lowest to highest, assigning a rank of 1 to the lowest data point and increasing the rank by 1 for each data point that follows. The ranks are then compared between the two groups to determine statistical significance. The Wilcoxon rank-sum tests whether or not the median between two groups is different.

The rank-sum test uses a test statistic, as was the case with a t-test (t-score) and ANOVA (F ratio), which is referred to as U. There are two

U values calculated, as shown in Equations 7.11 and 7.12, where n is the number of samples in each group and R is the sum of the ranks for each group. The smaller of the two U values is used to determine the p-value, which can be found using a look-up table. Within the look-up table, if U is smaller than the value shown for the given sample size, then the difference is considered significant. The reason the U must be lower than the critical value is that smaller U values indicate more separation between the two groups. Importantly, Equations 7.11 and 7.12 do not use any information about the distribution of the samples (i.e., there are no sample means, SD, etc.):

$$U_1 = n_1 n_2 + \frac{n_1(n_1+1)}{2} - R_1, \qquad (7.11)$$

$$U_2 = n_1 n_2 + \frac{n_2(n_2+1)}{2} - R_2. \qquad (7.12)$$

Example: Wilcoxon Rank-Sum Calculations

Question: A physician is testing two different therapies for breast cancer to see which one performed the best at reducing tumor volume before surgery. Tumor volumes (in millimeters) were measured 3 months after beginning therapy. The results are summarized in the table below. Is there a statistical difference in median tumor volume between the two therapies?

Therapy 1	Therapy 2
16.6	20.1
15.9	19.5
17.0	18.0
18.3	18.7
16.0	21.5

Answer: The null hypothesis is that the two population medians are equal, while the alternative hypothesis is that the two population medians are not equal. Because we are comparing the median values across two groups, a rank-sum test is most appropriate for use; therefore, we need to calculate U_1 and U_2 using Equations 7.11 and 7.12. In order to calculate U_1 and U_2, we need to first assign ranks to each data point and then sum them:

Therapy 1		Therapy 2	
Volume	Rank	Volume	Rank
16.6	3	20.1	9
15.9	1	19.5	8
17.0	4	18.0	5
18.3	6	18.7	7
16.0	2	21.5	10
	16		**39**

Now we can calculate U_1 and U_2 using $n_1 = n_2 = 5$:

$$U_1 = 5 \times 5 + \frac{5(5+1)}{2} - 16,$$
$$= 24$$
$$U_2 = 5 \times 5 + \frac{5(5+1)}{2} - 39.$$
$$= 1$$

The smaller of the two is U_2; therefore, 1 will be used as the critical value in the look-up table to determine the p-value. For $n_1 = n_2 = 5$, the critical value is 2. Since 1 is less than 2, there is a statistical difference between the median volumes for each group.

Detailed explanation of Kruskal–Wallis: A Kruskal–Wallis test is the nonparametric version of an ANOVA. As was the case with ANOVA, a Kruskal–Wallis test is used when comparing the median between more than two groups, and only provides information that at least one group is statistically different from one other group. A post hoc test is needed to determine which groups are different from one another (e.g., a Wilcoxon rank-sum test). The test statistic for a Kruskal–Wallis test is denoted by H. Equation 7.13 shows how to calculate H, where N is the total number of samples across all groups, k is the number of groups, R is the sum of the ranks for each group, and n is the number of samples in each group. Once H has been calculated, the critical H value can be determined using a look-up table. If H is greater than the critical value, the result is significant:

$$H = \left(\frac{12}{N(N+1)} \sum_{j=1}^{k} \frac{R_j^2}{n_j} \right) - 3(N+1). \quad (7.13)$$

Example: Kruskal–Wallis Test

Question: A physician is testing four different therapies for breast cancer to see which one performed the best at reducing tumor volume before surgery. Tumor volumes (in millimeters) were measured 3 months after beginning therapy. The results are summarized in the table below. Is there a statistical difference in median tumor volume between the four therapies?

Therapy 1	Therapy 2	Therapy 3	Therapy 4
18.5	19.0	16.6	20.1
17.9	20.9	15.9	19.5
19.2	18.2	17.0	18.0
16.5	17.8	18.3	18.7
17.4	18.1	16.0	21.5

Answer: The null hypothesis is that the four population medians are equal, while the alternative hypothesis is that the four population medians are not equal. Because we are comparing the median values across more than two groups, a Kruskal–Wallis test is used. We need to calculate H using Equation 7.13. In order to calculate H, we need to first assign ranks to each data point and then sum them:

Therapy 1		Therapy 2		Therapy 3		Therapy 4	
Volume	Rank	Volume	Rank	Volume	Rank	Volume	Rank
18.5	13	19.0	15	16.6	4	20.1	18
17.9	8	20.9	19	15.9	1	19.5	17
19.2	16	18.2	11	17.0	5	18.0	9
16.5	3	17.8	7	18.3	12	18.7	14
17.4	6	18.1	10	16.0	2	21.5	20
	46		62		24		78

Now we are ready to plug into Equation 7.13 using $N = 20$ and $n = 5$, since there are 20 total samples and 5 samples in each group:

$$H = \left(\frac{12}{N(N+1)} \sum_{j=1}^{k} \frac{R_j^2}{n_j} \right) - 3(N+1) = \frac{12}{20(20+1)} \left(\frac{46^2}{5} + \frac{62^2}{5} + \frac{24^2}{5} + \frac{78^2}{5} \right) - 3(20+1).$$
$$= 9.11$$

Now that we have H, we can use a look-up table to see whether 9.11 is above or below the critical value corresponding to a p-value of 0.05. The number of degrees of freedom is the number of comparison groups minus 1, which is 3. Using a look-up table, we find the critical value for H is 7.81. Because $9.11 > 7.81$, we can reject the null hypothesis and establish that there is a statistical difference between the median volumes.

	Area in the right tail									
	0.999	0.995	0.990	0.975	0.950	0.900	0.100	0.050	0.025	0.010
Degrees of freedom										
1	0.000	0.000	0.000	0.001	0.004	0.016	2.706	3.841	5.024	6.635
2	0.002	0.010	0.020	0.051	0.103	0.211	4.605	5.991	7.378	9.210
3	0.024	0.072	0.115	0.216	0.352	0.584	6.251	7.815	9.348	11.345
4	0.091	0.207	0.297	0.484	0.711	1.064	7.779	9.488	11.143	13.277
5	0.210	0.412	0.554	0.831	1.145	1.610	9.236	11.070	12.833	15.086
6	0.381	0.676	0.872	1.237	1.635	2.204	10.645	12.592	14.449	16.812

Deeper Look: *p*-Hacking in Statistical Testing

p-hacking is the relentless analysis of data (intentional or unintentional) in order to discover patterns that could be presented as statistically significant, when in reality there is no underlying effect. Figure 7.6 shows a cartoon of a man fishing as an analogy for *p*-hacking: *p*-hacking is fishing for *p*-values in a data ocean which will lead to the pot of gold. It is not always nefarious. In most cases, it is a human tendency to find evidence that confirms what we already believe to be true, referred to as confirmation bias. *p*-hacking is driven by a system that provides incentives and/or pressure to get statistically significant results. For example, if a clinical trial of a drug that cost millions of dollars to develop is being carried out for regulatory approval (such as from the FDA), achieving statistically significant results is essential in order to get the drug to market. The magnitude of the bias for the use of *p*-hacking is not yet established; however, it is estimated to be sufficiently high to warrant concern.

Psychologists Uri Simonsohn, Joseph Simmons, and Leif Nelson demonstrated the problem in what is now a classic paper, "False-positive psychology," published in 2011. They originally used the phrase "researcher degrees of freedom" to describe the little decisions that scientists make when designing a study, collecting data, and analyzing results. Simonsohn gave a talk at a psychology conference in 2012, at which he used the term *p*-hacking for the

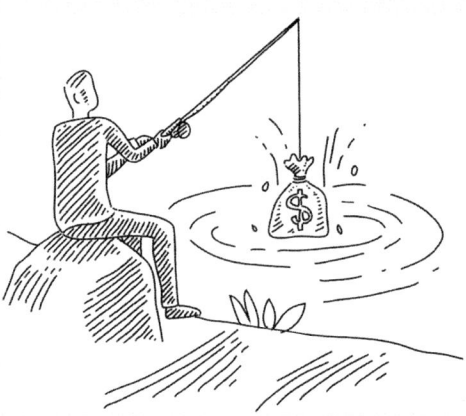

Figure 7.6 A cartoon of a man fishing as an analogy for *p*-hacking. *p*-hacking is fishing for *p*-values in a data ocean which will lead to the pot of gold.
Source: ©LEOcrafts/DigitalVision Vectors/Getty Images.

first time. The phrase made its debut in a paper the team published in 2014, where they wrote that "*p*-hacking can allow researchers to get most studies to reveal significant relationships between truly unrelated variables."

There are many ways to manipulate clinical studies to achieve statistically significant findings. For example, when conducting a clinical study it is important to pre-specify the sample size (e.g., number of patients, specimens, test runs, etc.). Under ideal settings this would be done based on the use of power calculations to ensure that the planned study has a reasonable chance of finding a real positive if one exists. One way to achieve statistically significant findings is to enroll a few patients and analyze the results, then enroll a few more and repeat the analysis. Once the desired results are achieved, the enrollment can be halted. There is no real penalty to stopping enrollment early if statistically significant results are achieved. Researchers can also modify variables such as what kind of patients to enroll, what age range, how long they will be followed, what parameters will be measured, and at what points in time, etc.

p-hacking is difficult to detect and it cannot be easily eliminated. There are, however, some measures to control for this. With respect to clinical trials, registries such as www.clinicaltrials.gov and www.alltrials.net are intended to provide transparency in the conduct and reporting of clinical trials. Investigators are supposed to "register" their studies in advance, including critical features of study design and an analysis plan. Any deviation from the predefined study plan would have to be disclosed and justified when presenting the study results. If used as intended, deviations from the registered and reported study details would be evident, and a red flag for potential *p*-hacking.

Similarity test: The degree of similarity between two variables can be quantified with two different methods – the correlation between the two tests or the difference between the two. Figure 7.7 shows a correlation plot and a difference plot. The correlation plot shows the linear relationship

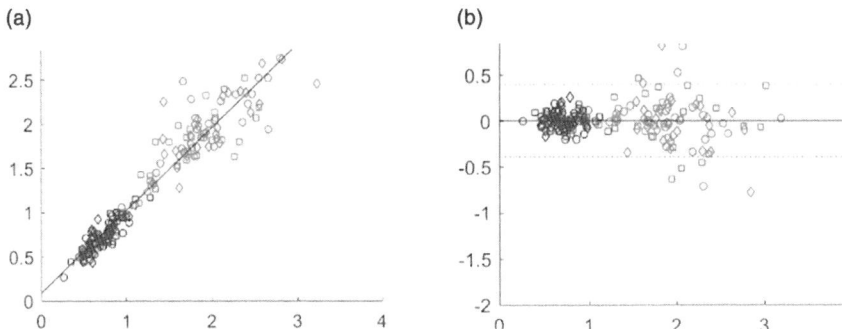

Figure 7.7 Correlation plot (a) and difference plot (b). The correlation plot shows the linear relationship between two variables, which are plotted on the x-axis and y-axis. A difference plot, also called a Bland–Altman plot, shows the difference between the two. Both types of plots are applied to relationships of variables within a subject.

between two variables, which are plotted on the *x*-axis and *y*-axis. A difference plot, also called a Bland–Altman plot, shows the difference between the two. Both types of plots are applied to relationships between variables within a subject.

Detailed explanation of the Pearson correlation coefficient: The most common measure of correlation is the **Pearson correlation coefficient**, which reflects the linear relationship between two sets of data and can be calculated using Equation 7.14, where r is the Pearson coefficient, x_i and y_i are scores associated with the two variables being compared within the same subject, $\underline{x}$ and $\underline{y}$ are the means of the two variables, and n is the number of subjects. The formula used to calculate a correlation coefficient returns a value between −1 and 1, where 1 indicates a perfect positive relationship and −1 indicates a perfect inverse relationship. The statistical significance of a Pearson correlation can be tested using a *t*-statistic calculated using Equation 7.15 (where r is the Pearson correlation and n is the number of subjects), and the significance level determined using the *t*-table as described earlier:

$$r = \frac{\sum_{i=1}^{n}(x_i - \underline{x})\left(y_i - \underline{y}\right)}{\sqrt{\sum_{i=1}^{n}\left(x_i - \underline{x}\right)^2}\sqrt{\sum_{i=1}^{n}\left(y_i - \underline{y}\right)^2}}, \quad (7.14)$$

$$t = r\sqrt{\frac{n-1}{1-r^2}}. \quad (7.15)$$

Detailed explanation of the Bland–Altman plot: The most common measure of similarity is the Bland–Altman plot, which reflects the relationship between the difference of two variables, and their means. The bias between the two tests is measured by the mean of the differences, across all data points, as shown in Equation 7.16, where d_i corresponds to the difference between each sample and $\underline{d}$ to the average difference for all samples. The limit of agreement between the two tests is defined by a limit of agreement of 95 percent, as shown in Equation 7.17, where s is the SD (Equation 7.4). The 95 percent limit of agreement states that the differences between the two groups are within two SD of the difference distribution:

$$\underline{d} = \frac{1}{n}\sum_{i=1}^{n} d_i, \qquad (7.16)$$

$$\underline{d} \pm 1.96 \times s. \qquad (7.17)$$

The correlation and similarity tests are not able to tell the difference between dependent (y) and independent (x) variables. For example, there might be a high correlation or small difference between the independent variable smoking and the dependent variable lung cancer. The results would be the same value if the variables x and y were switched for the calculation, indicating that lung cancer causes smoking, which is untrue and illogical. In other words, the above tests indicate a relationship between x and y. They do not indicate whether there is an actual causal relationship or agreement between the two variables.

Confidence interval: This bounds a range of values which is likely to contain the population parameter of interest. A 95 percent CI, for example, corresponds to a range of values that is within two SD of the mean. In other words, if the same population is sampled on numerous occasions, the resulting intervals would bracket the true population parameter in approximately 95 percent of cases. Confidence stated at a $1-\alpha$ level can be thought of as the inverse of a significance level, α. In the same way that t-tests can be one- or two-tailed, CIs can be one- or two-sided. A two-sided CI brackets the population parameter from above and below. A one-sided CI brackets the population parameter either from above or below and furnishes an upper or lower bound to its magnitude. The CI is related to the SE. It is calculated as $t \times SE$, where t is the value of the Student's t-distribution for a specific α (most commonly 0.05). Its value is often rounded to 1.96 (its value with a large sample size).

Detailed explanation of confidence intervals: The CI for data following a normal distribution is shown in Equation 7.18, where CI is the confidence interval, $\underline{x}$ is the sample mean, Z is the critical value of the z-distribution (defined by Equation 7.5), s is the sample SD, and n is the sample size. The value of Z is set based on what CI is being calculated and must be looked up each time. The most common CI is 95 percent, for which $Z = 1.96$. When applying Equation 7.18 to calculate a CI, the resulting CI will be in terms of the z-space rather than the r-space. Z can be related to the Pearson correlation r using Equation 7.19. In order to convert the bounds back to the r-space, Equation 7.19 is inverted into Equation 7.20. The sample SD s is estimated based on the sample size n using Equation 7.21:

$$CI = \underline{x} \pm Z \frac{s}{\sqrt{n}}, \tag{7.18}$$

$$z = 0.5 \ln \frac{1+r}{1-r}, \tag{7.19}$$

$$r = \frac{e^{2z} - 1}{e^{2z} + 1}, \tag{7.20}$$

$$s = \frac{1}{\sqrt{n-3}}. \tag{7.21}$$

Example: Correlation Coefficient Calculation

Question: A dietician wants to know if there is a correlation between the age and weight of women who are on estrogen therapy. She has data from six patients, shown in the table below. What is the Pearson correlation between age and weight? Is the relationship positive or negative?

Patient #	Age (x)	Weight (y)	xy	x^2	y^2
1	40	78	3,120	1,600	6,084
2	21	70	1,470	441	4,900
3	25	60	1,500	635	3,600
4	31	55	1,705	961	3,025
5	38	80	3,040	1,444	6,400
6	47	66	3,102	2,209	4,356
Total	202	409	13,937	7,280	28,365

Answer: The correlation coefficient for the relationship between age and weight is calculated using Equation 7.14:

$$r = \frac{\sum_{i=1}^{n}(x_i - \underline{x})(y_i - \underline{y})}{\sqrt{\sum_{i=1}^{n}(x_i - \underline{x})^2}\sqrt{\sum_{i=1}^{n}(y_i - \underline{y})^2}}.$$

To use Equation 7.14, we need to calculate the sample means for x and y:

$$\underline{x} = \sum_{i=1}^{N} \frac{x_i}{N},$$

$$\underline{y} = \sum_{i=1}^{N} \frac{y_i}{N}.$$

Plugging in from the table, we get $\underline{x} = \dfrac{202}{6} = 33.7$ and $\underline{y} = \dfrac{409}{6} = 68.2$.
Plugging into Equation 7.14 and simplifying results:

$$r = \dfrac{\sum_{i=1}^{n}(x_i - 33.7)(y_i - 68.2)}{\sqrt{\sum_{i=1}^{n}(x_i - 33.7)^2}\sqrt{\sum_{i=1}^{n}(y_i - 68.2)^2}}.$$
$$= 0.35$$

Because the value of $r > 0$, the correlation is positive.

Example: Bland–Altman Analysis

Question: The weight used for the Pearson correlation calculation was taken as the mean of two measurements taken with different scales (data shown below). The dietician wants to confirm that the two scales have a high level of agreement. What is the bias and limits of agreement between the two scales?

Scale 1	Scale 2	Average
78.2	77.8	78
70.4	69.6	70
59.9	60.1	60
54.2	55.8	55
79.7	80.3	80
66.7	65.3	66

Answer: To calculate the bias and limits of agreement, we can perform a Bland–Altman analysis. To calculate the bias, we first need to calculate the difference between each set of measurements:

Scale 1	Scale 2	Difference
78.2	77.8	78.2 − 77.8 = 0.4
70.4	69.6	70.4 − 69.6 = 0.8
59.9	60.1	59.9 − 60.1 = −0.2
54.2	55.8	54.2 − 55.8 = −1.6
79.7	80.3	79.7 − 80.3 = −0.6
66.7	65.3	66.7 − 65.3 = 1.4

Next, we can calculate the mean of the differences to get the bias using Equation 7.16:

$$\bar{d} = \frac{0.4 + 0.8 + (-0.2) + (-1.6) + (-0.6) + 1.4}{6} = 0.033.$$

To calculate the limit of agreement, we need to calculate the SD using Equation 7.4:

$$s = \sqrt{\frac{(0.4-0.033)^2 + (0.8-0.033)^2 + (-0.2-0.033)^2 + (-1.6-0.033)^2 + (-0.6-0.033)^2 + (1.4-0.033)^2}{6-1}}$$

$$= 1.07$$

Finally, we can calculate the limits of agreement using Equation 7.17:

$$\text{upper limit} = 0.033 + 1.96 \times 1.07 = 2.13,$$

$$\text{lower limit} = 0.033 - 1.96 \times 1.07 = -2.06.$$

Example: Confidence Interval Calculation

Question: The dietician from the previous example also wants to calculate the 95 percent CI for the Pearson correlation using the same data. What is the 95 percent CI?

Answer: To calculate the CI, first the Pearson correlation r needs to be converted into the z-space using Equation 7.19:

$$z = 0.5 \ln \frac{1 + 0.35}{1 - 0.35} = 0.37.$$

The sample SD, s, must also be calculated using Equation 7.21:

$$s = \frac{1}{\sqrt{6-3}} = 0.58.$$

The z calculated in the above equation corresponds to x in Equation 7.18. The CI in the z-space can now be calculated as:

$$\text{CI} = 0.37 \pm 1.96 \frac{0.58}{\sqrt{6}} = 0.37 \pm 0.46.$$

Therefore, the upper and lower limits are:

$$\text{upper limit} = 0.37 + 0.46 = 0.83,$$

$$\text{lower limit} = 0.37 - 0.46 = -0.09.$$

Remember that the upper and lower limits are still in the z-space and need to be converted back to the r-space using Equation 7.20:

$$r_{\text{upper}} = \frac{e^{2\times 0.83}-1}{e^{2\times 0.83}+1} = 0.68,$$

$$r_{\text{lower}} = \frac{e^{2\times -0.09}-1}{e^{2\times -0.09}+1} = -0.09.$$

Therefore, the 95 percent CI for the Pearson correlation is –0.09 to 0.68.

Difference tests, similarity tests, and CIs are all useful ways to establish whether or not two groups are different from one another. Difference tests typically test the null hypothesis that two or more groups have the same sample mean. Similarity tests typically test the null hypothesis that two or more groups have a different sample mean. Finally, CIs are used to establish the boundaries for significance for multiple groups.

Calculation of Key Metrics for a Clinical Study

Clinical studies are an important step in the validation of a medical technology or drug. The previous section covered some of the basic principles that underlie statistical testing. This next section builds upon the previous section by exploring the experimental designs that can be used with these statistical tests, with a particular focus on clinical trial design. Before delving into the complexities of clinical trial design, the different summary metrics and the importance of sample size calculations will be described.

Summary metrics: Let us begin with diagnostic technologies. The first step is to compare the performance of a new medical diagnostic technology to a gold standard. In addition, a longer-term outcome also needs to be measured if possible, as that is what is most relevant to a patient and a physician. For a diagnostic technology, the performance of the test could directly impact treatment. For example, if the technology correctly identifies all patients that need treatment but also incorrectly identifies 50 percent of patients for treatment when they are negative for the disease, the consequence would be overtreatment and potential morbidity to the patient. If the case is the opposite, this would lead to undertreatment and increased morbidity and potentially mortality. In both cases, the patient and the healthcare system would incur additional costs with minimal benefit.

There are also short-term and long-term metrics for drugs. Depending on the mechanism of action of the drug, surrogate metrics for efficacy could be used, such as decrease in expression of a biomarker within the tumor (e.g., decrease in HER2 expression in a breast tumor following treatment with a HER2 inhibitor like trastuzumab). When testing the safety of the drug, adverse events can be evaluated. For example, a new drug could have the same efficacy as another drug but with fewer side effects. Long-term outcomes could include overall survival (OS), progression-free survival (PFS), or disease-free survival (DFS). **Overall survival** is the length of time from either the date of diagnosis or the start of treatment for a disease that patients diagnosed with the disease are still alive. **Progression-free survival** is the length of time during and after the treatment of a disease that a patient lives with the disease, but it does not get worse. **Disease-free survival** is the measure of time after treatment during which no sign of the disease is found. This term can be used for an individual or for a group of people within a study.

Though sensitivity, specificity, negative predictive value, and positive predictive value were introduced in Chapter 2, we will cover them again here as they are relevant to the performance of short-term metrics for both devices and drugs. **Sensitivity** (Equation 7.22) is the ability of a test to correctly identify the presence of a disease (true positive rate), whereas test **specificity** (Equation 7.23) is the ability of the test to correctly identify the absence of a disease (true negative rate):

$$\text{Sensitivity} = \frac{\text{\# of true positives}}{\left(\text{\# of true positives} + \text{\# of false negatives}\right)} \times 100, \quad (7.22)$$

$$\text{Specificity} = \frac{\text{\# of true negatives}}{\left(\text{\# of true negatives} + \text{\# of false positives}\right)} \times 100. \quad (7.23)$$

It is important to introduce two additional terms – **positive and negative predictive values**. The positive predictive value (PPV, Equation 7.24) is the probability that subjects identified as having the disease by the test truly have the disease. The negative predictive value (NPV, Equation 7.25) is the probability that subjects who are identified as not having the disease by the test truly do not have the disease:

$$\text{PPV} = \frac{\text{true positive}}{\left(\text{true positive} + \text{false positive}\right)} \times 100, \quad (7.24)$$

$$\text{NPV} = \frac{\text{true negative}}{\left(\text{true negative} + \text{false negative}\right)} \times 100. \quad (7.25)$$

Sample size calculation: Clinical testing is needed to show the true benefit of a test. Clinical studies consider an input – the test or intervention, and an output – which is some measure of health outcome that the intervention is supposed to affect – for example, the sensitivity and specificity of a test. One of the most common questions that needs to be answered when designing a clinical study is the number of patients to enroll. If the study is too small, it will not be able to answer the question posed or will answer the question incorrectly, which is unethical. However, studies cannot be infinitely large as resources would be wasted if fewer patients would have sufficed. A good analogy is a coin toss example. If a coin is tossed 10 times and lands 10 times on heads, it will be considered biased because the probability of observing such a series is very low for a coin (analogous to a small sample size). However, if the same series of 10 tails in a row appears as part of 10,000 tosses with the same coin, it is more likely to be seen as a random fluctuation in the long series of tosses (large sample size).

The sample size of a clinical study is determined by performing a calculation that assesses the study's **statistical power** for testing the difference or similarity between endpoints between two or more groups. Statistical power refers to the probability that a statistical measure will reject the null hypothesis when it is false. The study needs to be appropriately "powered" so as to not underestimate the sample size, and at the same time be within a range that can be supported by available resources. Two terms that serve as an important metric for a power calculation are **type I** and **type II errors**. Table 7.2 shows a table of true positives, false positives (type I error), true negatives, and false negatives (type II error). As described earlier, a type I error (α) rejects the null hypothesis when it is true. A type II error (β) occurs when the null hypothesis is not rejected when it is indeed false. A type I error is referred to as a false positive because the alternative hypothesis is accepted when it should not be. A type II error is referred to as a false negative because the alternative hypothesis is rejected when it should not be.

Table 7.2 A table of true positives, false positives (type I error), true negatives, and false negatives (type II error)

As described earlier, a type I error (α) rejects the null hypothesis when it is true. A type II error (β) occurs when the null hypothesis is not rejected when it is indeed false.

		Null hypothesis is	
		True	False
Decision about null hypothesis	Don't Reject	Correct inference (true negative) (probability = $1 = \alpha$)	Type II error (false negative) (probability = β)
	Reject	Type I error (false positive) (probability = α)	Correct inference (true positive) (probability = $1 - \beta$)

Example: Type I Error Calculation

Question: Two drugs are being compared for effectiveness in treating the same condition. Drug 1 is very affordable but Drug 2 is extremely expensive. The null hypothesis is "Both drugs are equally effective," and the alternative is "Drug 2 is more effective than Drug 1." What would be the type I error? What are the implications of a type I error for patients?
Answer: In this situation, a type I error would be deciding that Drug 2 is more effective when in fact it is no better than Drug 1 but would cost the patient much more money. That would be undesirable from the patient's perspective, so a small significance level is warranted.

In a clinical trial the goal is to use a power calculation to determine the appropriate sample size so that the outcome results will have a significant (positive) result – that is, a p-value of less than the specified significance level (usually $\alpha = 0.05$). It is neither practical nor feasible to study the whole population, therefore the sample is a set of participants that adequately represent the population from which they are drawn. This ensures that true inferences about the population can be made from the results obtained. Sample sizes smaller than those informed by a power calculation may not be able to detect the precise difference between study groups. Moreover, the results of the study cannot be generalized to the population, as this sample will be unable to represent the target population.

In a power calculation, the "power" of the study is equal to $1-\beta$, where β is the type II error rate. For a β of 0.2, power = 0.8, indicating that there is a one in five chance (i.e., 20 percent) that the null hypothesis is accepted when there is a real difference between two groups (alternative hypothesis). The parameter α is typically 0.05, or a 5 percent chance that the null hypothesis is rejected. Shown below is the sample size calculation for comparison of two proportions (e.g., sensitivity and specificity relative to a fixed benchmark or between two tests), though there are additional formulas for sample size estimations for differences in the means of two groups.

The formula for calculation of sample size for two proportions (level of significance = 5 percent, power = 80 percent, type of test = two-sided) is shown in Equation 7.26. These α and β values are typically what are used in a power calculation:

$$n = \frac{(Z_{\frac{\alpha}{2}} + Z_{\beta})^2 \left[\left(p_1(1-p_1) \right) + p_2(1-p_2) \right]}{(p_1 - p_2)^2}, \qquad (7.26)$$

where n is the total sample size needed for the study; p_1 is the proportion of subjects impacted by test A; p_2 is the proportion of subjects impacted by test B; $p_1 - p_2$ is the clinically significant difference (difference in sensitivity [specificity]); $Z_{\alpha/2}$ depends on level of significance (for 5 percent this is 1.96); and Z_β depends on power (for 80 percent this is 0.84).

This sample size estimation formula will provide the number of evaluable subjects required to achieve the desired statistical significance for a given hypothesis. However, more subjects need to be enrolled to account for potential dropouts. If n is the sample size required as per the formula, and if d is the dropout rate, then adjusted sample size $N = n/(1-d)$. The expected difference in sensitivity or specificity between two groups is usually determined from previous trials. If this information is not available, it can be obtained from previously published literature.

Example: Power Calculation

Question: A placebo-controlled randomized trial proposes to assess the effectiveness of Drug A in relieving nausea in cancer patients receiving chemotherapy. A previous study showed that the proportion of subjects with a reduction in nausea by Drug A is 50 percent, and a difference of 16 percent between the treatment and placebo is acceptable. The researchers want to use this as the basis for designing the trial. What is the total sample size needed in order to test this expected difference?

Answer: To calculate the sample size, plug the given values into Equation 7.26:

$$n = \frac{(1.96+0.84)^2 \left[0.5(1-0.5)+0.34(1-0.34)\right]}{(0.5-0.34)^2} = 145.3.$$

Therefore, 146 patients would be required per group, resulting in a sample size of 292 patients.

Now that summary parameters and the concept of statistical power have been introduced, we will take a look at the different types of clinical trials. There are two overarching types of clinical studies: retrospective and prospective. **Retrospective** studies look back at data after it has been collected to look for possible trends and differences. **Prospective** studies generate new data to test a specific hypothesis. Retrospective studies are often used to generate hypotheses that can be tested in a prospective study.

Retrospective study: When performing a sample size calculation, often the input is obtained from a retrospective study. For example, if a new medical imaging technology has been developed for detecting cervical precancer, the initial studies in humans would likely be used to test the sensitivity and specificity of the device with the informed consent of study participants. After the study is completed, the data is compared to pathology, the gold standard to separate the two tissue types. The variables measured are tested for significance

Calculation of Key Metrics for a Clinical Study

or similarity as described earlier. The statistical difference of the variable or variables is considered significant if the *p*-value is less than 0.05. Next a score will be calculated for each sample labeled positive or negative based on a classification algorithm (the focus of next two chapters). The scores can then be compared to ground truth to determine sensitivity and specificity.

Prospective study: The sensitivity and specificity of the test in a retrospective study can serve as the basis for the sample size calculation in a prospective study. In a prospective clinical investigation, the algorithm from above is applied to new data as it is collected. The results from the optimized algorithm classify the samples as positive or negative and they are then compared to pathology results. This process emulates the realistic use of the algorithm in a clinical practice. If the prospective study includes only one test, the sample size will be based on the expected difference in sensitivity and/or specificity (using pathology as the ground truth) that is at least as good as that observed in the retrospective study. If the prospective study involves two tests on the same patient (e.g., comparison of two devices, both of which are compared to the ground truth), then the sample size will be used to achieve a difference in sensitivity and/or specificity between the two tests based on a paired comparison within a patient.

Randomized controlled trials (RCT): One approach to study a new drug or performance of a new medical technology is to do a single-arm study where the intervention is performed on everyone in the study and historical data of a comparable sample size is used to compare the new test/drug and existing test/drug. The problem with this approach is that temporal spacing between the existing and new clinical study can confound the results. For example, if the existing test was performed on a population prior to the COVID-19 pandemic and the new test on patients who could be affected by the COVID-19 virus, there might be underlying differences in the two populations that could confound the results of the trial. **Randomized controlled trials** reduce confounders such as time by randomly assigning study participants to either the experimental or control group within the same population. This is considered the most rigorous way of reducing bias. There are several different approaches for RCTs. It is most effective to compare the existing and new tests or drugs at the same time. Randomization in RCTs typically utilizes a computer program that randomly assigns subjects into either the test arm or standard of care arm. This is the most basic RCT.

Randomized controlled trials can assign randomization across individuals or across clusters. Clusters typically include a population of subjects rather than an individual subject. A **cluster randomized trial** (CRT) might be preferred when the target of the intervention is a collective or system rather than a particular subject (e.g., a patient), when there is potential for bias (subjects in the control group within the same setting might learn about the new intervention and want aspects of it applied to them), or in cases where longitudinal monitoring of individual patients would be impractical.

Block randomization is designed to randomize subjects into groups that result in equal sample sizes, controlling for the factor that might significantly influence the results. This method is used to ensure a balance in sample size across groups over time (e.g., Block 1 contains patients aged 18–25; Block 2 contains patients aged 26–40, etc.). Blocks are small and balanced, with predetermined group assignments, where the numbers of subjects in each group is always similar. Blocks are best used in smaller increments as researchers can more easily control balance. Within each block, the "test" is assigned randomly such that an equal number of people within each block receive the treatment versus the placebo or standard of care.

The stratified randomization method addresses the need to control and balance the influence of covariates (other characteristics or factors influencing a statistical relationship). This method can be used to achieve balance among groups in terms of subjects' baseline characteristics (covariates). In a stratified randomization, the entire population of subjects is grouped into smaller sections (strata) by a similar characteristic, as is done in block randomization. After the first strata are divided, subjects are again stratified into smaller groups from which they are randomly assigned to a treatment group.

If a particular characteristic is of fundamental importance (i.e., will have a measurable influence on the outcome) it needs to be accounted for in the randomization, in order to **control for bias**. For example, if age may affect the performance of a particular test or drug, it is important that the distribution of ages within the experimental and control groups are comparable, so that the results are not attributable to a difference in age between the two groups. In other words, controlling for bias helps ensure that the only difference between the experimental and control groups is the test or drug being investigated.

Blinding is used to ensure that there are no differences in the way each group is assessed or managed, and therefore minimizes bias. A clinical trial is called single-blinded when only one party is blinded, usually the participants. If both participants and study staff are blinded, the study is double-blinded. Triple-blinded studies extend to blinding to the data analysis. A trial in which no blinding is used and all parties are aware of the treatment groups is called open-label or unblinded.

Figure 7.8 summarizes the clinical trial randomization and blinding processes. Block randomization is designed to randomize subjects into groups that result in equal sample sizes, controlling for the factor that might significantly influence the results (e.g., age). Stratified randomization is used to achieve balance among groups in terms of subjects' baseline characteristics (covariates). Blinding is used to help prevent bias during the trial and/or analysis. For an unblinded study, all participants, study staff, and data analysts

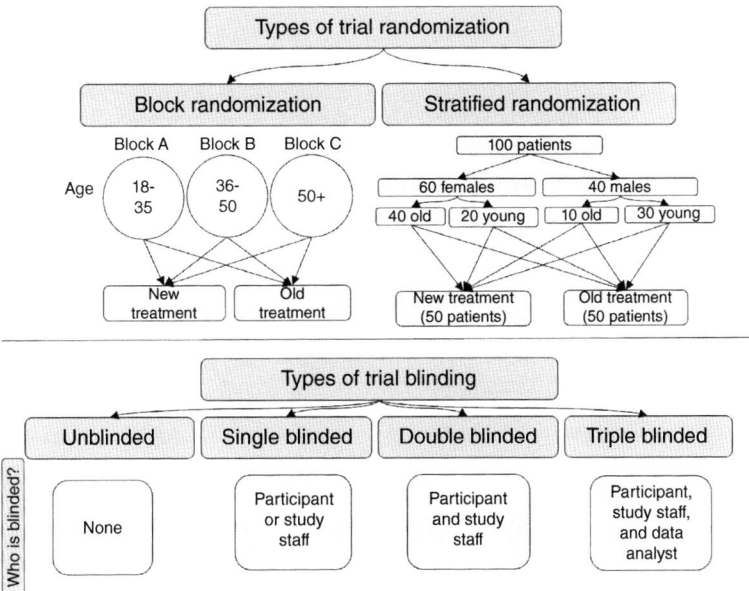

Figure 7.8 Clinical trial randomization and the blinding process. Block randomization is designed to randomize subjects into groups that result in equal sample sizes, controlling for the factor that might significantly influence the results (e.g., age). Stratified randomization is used to achieve balance among groups in terms of subjects' baseline characteristics (covariates). Blinding is used to help prevent bias during the trial and/or analysis. In an unblinded study, all participants, study staff, and data analysts know which group participants were assigned to.

know which group participants were assigned to. For a single-blinded study, only one group of people (e.g., study participants or study staff) are blinded to which group the participants were assigned to. For a double-blinded study, both study participants and study staff are blinded to which group the participants were assigned to. Finally, for triple-blinded studies, everyone – including data analysts – are blinded to the participants' group.

Deeper Look: Double Standards for Standard of Care?

Many new drugs confer only a small benefit over existing treatments; therefore, a large number of human subjects are required to measure relative improvements with statistical significance. Recruiting a sufficient number of patients remains a major bottleneck for medical research, and companies have turned to LMICs to conduct trials because it is easier to recruit a statistically significant number of human subjects over a shorter period of time. Moreover, operational costs in developing countries are low and there are large pools of "treatment-naive" patients, whereas in wealthier countries the use of too much medication generates the risk of drug–drug interactions. Further, a major benefit of conducting human subject studies in LMICs is that it is easy to enroll patients who are willing to participate, particularly if they are poor.

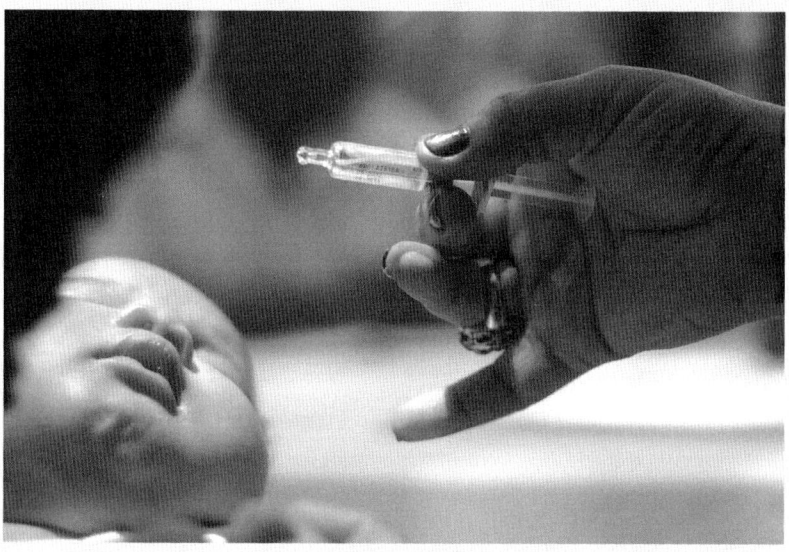

Figure 7.9 An infant receiving a vaccine for the rotavirus. The vaccine is given as a liquid straight into the baby's mouth for them to swallow. The clinical trial, which was conducted in India, enrolled approximately 6,800 infants between March 11, 2011, and November 5, 2012, in rural and urban areas of the country. The experimental vaccine was given by injection in three doses at 6–7 weeks, 10 weeks or older, and 14 weeks or older. Two-thirds of the infants received the vaccine, and one-third received saltwater placebo injections. The trial results showed that, as with the two available oral rotavirus vaccines, the new vaccine was effective in preventing severe rotavirus-induced gastroenteritis and hospitalizations due to such infections.
Source: ©HECTOR RETAMAL/Staff/AFP/Getty Images.

One of the important considerations in any clinical trials, including those in LMICs, is the definition of placebo. A true placebo is an inert substance that would have no negative or positive effect on the patient and therefore serves as an ideal control to which to compare a new intervention. However, the use of placebo, or no treatment, is acceptable in studies *only* when no current proven intervention exists, *or* is necessary to determine the efficacy or safety of an intervention under the condition that the patients who receive no treatment will not be subject to any risk or irreversible harm.

An example of a clinical trial where these basic ethical guidelines were not enforced was during the testing of an experimental vaccine to against a very common, potentially life-threatening viral infection called rotavirus (Figure 7.9) (Bhandari et al., 2014). [2] Rotavirus infection is one of the leading causes of gastroenteritis and death in children worldwide. The benefit of the new vaccine, if efficacious, is that it would prevent the rotavirus infection altogether as compared to two existing vaccines that were highly effective in preventing serious rotavirus infections in infants and young children, but not the rotaviral infection itself.

Why were saltwater injections used when there were two effective vaccines that could have been used in the control group? Large clinical trials of both vaccines, RotaTeq and Rotarix, demonstrated that they were highly effective in preventing rotavirus-induced gastroenteritis – including the most severe cases – and the need for hospitalization. These trials enrolled infants in both developed countries (including the US and multiple European nations) and developing countries (including Costa Rica, Guatemala, South Africa, Malawi, Ghana, Kenya, Mali, Bangladesh, and Vietnam) (Carome, 2014).

The reason for not choosing either of these vaccines in the control group were two-fold. The first reason was that even though these vaccines demonstrated approximately 85–90 percent efficacy in clinical trials in the US, Europe, Australia, and Latin America, they showed lower efficacy in Asia and Africa. In addition, these vaccines had not undergone clinical trials in India and were of unknown efficacy there. This could have been addressed by performing the trials of these two effective vaccines in India. However, the second reason was that trials using an active comparator would be expensive (the trial in India enrolled 6,800 participants; a trial using a nonplacebo design would require a substantially larger number of participants).

Given the availability of two highly effective rotavirus vaccines at the time the India study was initiated, the failure to provide infants with one of these two vaccines instead of a placebo violated international ethical standards for conducting human research. Saltwater placebo injections did not represent the "best current proven intervention" available at the time the India trial began, given the proven efficacy of the alternative vaccines. There was no compelling scientific reason for placebo use, exposing subjects to risk of a potentially fatal infection, and there was an active treatment available to design a scientifically and ethically sound clinical trial. The rotavirus vaccine study in which infants received a placebo would never have been permitted in the US.

Clinical studies and the regulatory pathway: The FDA defines medical devices as any tool that treats a patient without medication. Because the definition of "medical device" is so broad in the eyes of the FDA, the agency divides devices into different classes. A device's class determines what kind of testing it needs to go through for approval. Class I devices are products like latex gloves, bandages, and other everyday items. They are generally exempt from testing; 47 percent of medical devices fall under this category, and 95 percent are exempt from regulatory testing. Examples of exempt devices include bedpans, mercury thermometers, and manual stethoscopes. Class II devices do require regulation and include items such as some pregnancy test kits and powered wheelchairs. These are devices that pose a higher risk to patients, so it is important that they are formally tested before being approved. Knee prosthesis and single-use scalpels also fall under this category. Class III devices carry the highest risk for patients. They usually sustain or support life or are implanted in the body. An insulin pen or a stent are two examples of Class III devices.

Table 7.3 shows clinical trial classification. Device trials only have a pilot and pivotal trial, whereas drug studies have phase I, II, and III trials. For drugs and devices that require post-market approval (PMA), additional clinical data

Table 7.3 Clinical trial classification

Device trials only have a pilot and pivotal trial, whereas drug studies have phase I, II, and III trials. For drugs and devices that require PMA, additional clinical data is required.

Clinical trial classification	
Device studies	**Drug studies**
Pilot: Small study (10–30 patients with the condition) to determine preliminary safety and performance	**Phase I:** Small study (20–100 healthy volunteers or people with condition) to determine preliminary safety and dosage
Pivotal: Larger study (150–300 patients with the condition) to determine efficacy and adverse effects	**Phase II:** Larger study (up to several hundred people with the condition) to determine efficacy and adverse effects
Post-approval: Post-approval study to collect long-term data	**Phase III:** *(Sometimes known as pivotal study)* Even larger study (up to thousands of people with the condition) to determine efficacy and monitor adverse effects
	Phase IV: Post-marketing study to collect long-term data

Source: https://premier-research.com/perspectivesmedical-devices-vs-drug-trial.

is required. The shortest and least resource-intensive regulatory process is 510(k) premarket notification. Medical devices that are equivalent in safety and efficacy to a similar technology, a predicate device that is 510(k) cleared, are eligible for this process. Devices that do not have a predicate need to undergo extensive clinical studies. If the medical device for which approval is sought does not have a predicate, then clinical studies are required. After that phase, the manufacturer may submit the device for PMA, which is significantly more expensive and longer than a 510(k) process. Typically, devices do not need to undergo an RCT like a drug, as no therapeutic effect needs to be determined. Table 7.3 shows clinical investigations for medical devices that are not eligible for 510(k) clearance.

Example: Determining the Phase of a Clinical Trial

Question: A physician has read research on a drug called Avastin, which has previously been used to successfully treat brain tumors. One side effect of Avastin is a reduction in inflammation via mechanisms that work differently from steroids. The physician is

> intrigued by these findings and would like to perform a study on patients with brain tumors to see how Avastin affects inflammation compared to steroid use. What phase clinical trial would be most appropriate?
>
> Answer: Because Avastin has previously been used in patients with brain tumors and has been shown to be safe and effective, there is little rationale to perform a phase I trial. Because the physician is interested in a new indication for using Avastin and comparing it to an existing drug, a phase II trial to get initial data on efficacy would be most suitable.

Looking Ahead

Statistical testing is foundational to establishing safety and efficacy of new interventions. The availability of tools to evaluate different types of data (continuous, discrete) and different sample sizes (which might deviate from a normal distribution) facilitate tailoring of the test to the question in hand. With the development of new technologies and therapies to address gaps in access to healthcare on a global scale, it will become increasingly important to understand how to design and implement appropriate clinical trials that are backed by these statistical tools. This is not only important with respect to generating interpretable results; it also aids in the optimization of sample size such that it does not defeat the purpose of the investigation by being too small, or significantly increases clinical costs by wasting unnecessary resources.

As described in Chapters 4–6, we are making significant headway in bringing care directly to the patient, thereby increasing the number of patients that can have access to care. This, coupled with data analytics, can further extend the reach of these tools, particularly in under-resourced settings, whether these are in the US or half-way around the world. One of the challenges, however, is the regulatory process. Developing brand new innovations in the US comes at a cost. If there is not a previous device or drug that can serve as a predicate, the regulatory process can be extremely onerous, significantly increasing time and cost. So this is an important consideration as hundreds of thousands of dollars – or even more – could be spent getting a product to market. This suggests that the development of "me too" solutions that have a predicate will have the greatest impact in the short term.

Clinical trials benefit patients when it leads to an action that benefits the patient. This is where data analytics plays a significant role. In other words, it is not sufficient to observe if a test or drug works; it is also important to determine how to act on it. This is where four questions arise: What happens? Why did it happen? What will happen in the future? And what action will be taken in response to it? Referring back to the Pocket Colposcope described in Chapter 5, a clinical study that compares the sensitivity and specificity is only the first step in validating a technology. Using that information to design a prediction model that can inform treatment is ultimately where the impact lies. Algorithms that can leverage the observations to create explainable results can pave the way for prediction and ultimately prescription of the solution, addressing the gap in expertise that is far too common in the economically most disadvantaged countries. This is the subject of the next chapter.

SUMMARY

This chapter has covered a wide range of statistical methods to analyze and interpret experimental and clinical data. Statistical tests are performed on summary statistics of the data set (e.g., mean, minimum, maximum, SD). There are different assumptions that each type of test makes about the data used for the test. The two main categories of tests are parametric and nonparametric tests. The difference between these is the assumption of normality – parametric tests assume the data set is normally distributed, while nonparametric tests do not.

Statistical tests revolve around testing null and alternative hypotheses. The null and alternative hypotheses are mutually exclusive (there is no overlap) and collectively exhaustive (there are no other possibilities). As a result, if a statistical test rejects the null hypothesis, then the alternative hypothesis must be true. If the results are not statistically significant, that does not necessarily translate to similarity. Separate tests are available to determine if two sets of results show similarity. Confidence intervals measure the degree of uncertainty or certainty in a sampling method. It essentially translates to confidence that most of the samples are reflective of the true population.

One important aspect of statistical testing is determining the sample size for a clinical study. This type of calculation is referred to as a power calculation. The study needs to be appropriately "powered" in order to not underestimate the sample size, and at the same time be within a range that can be supported by available resources.

There are two overarching types of clinical studies: retrospective and prospective. Retrospective studies look back at data after it has been collected to look for possible trends and differences. Prospective studies generate new data to test a specific hypothesis. Retrospective studies are often used to generate hypotheses that can be tested in a prospective study. Randomized controlled trials are the true tests of the performance of an intervention as they allow comparison of the new solution to the standard of care in an unbiased manner. They are essential to approval by the US FDA, particularly for new drugs and devices.

PROBLEMS

Basic Concepts for Statistical Analysis

1. You get data from the US Census Bureau on the median age distribution of women who should undergo screening for cervical cancer in your city, and you decide to display it graphically. Which is the better choice for this data, a bar graph or a histogram?
2. The box plot in Figure 7.10 represents the distribution of antibody levels in the blood for patients participating in a trial for a new cancer therapy.

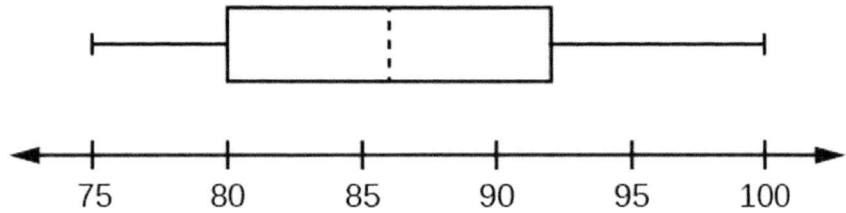

Figure 7.10

   a. What is the median for this data?
   b. What are the first and third quartiles for this data, and how do you know?
   c. What is the range for this data?
3. Six patients who undergo an experimental therapy have the following survival outcomes: 10, 11, 15, 15, 17, 22.
   a. Compute the mean and SD for this data.
   b. What number is two SD above the mean of this data?
   c. Calculate the z-score for this data.
4. A researcher repeatedly draws samples of $n = 100$ from a population of patients who have been screened for breast cancer, and calculates a mean of 75 and an SD of 5.
   a. What is the expected distribution of the sample means?
   b. What is the SE of the mean?
   c. What is the z-score for a sample mean of 76?
   d. What is the z-score for a sample mean of 74?
   e. What sample mean corresponds to a z-score of 1.5?
   f. If you decrease the sample size to 50, will the SE of the mean be smaller or larger? What would be its value?
5. A sample size of 60 is drawn from a population of smokers with a mean of 70 and an SD of 9.
   a. What range of values would you expect would include 68 percent of the sample mean?
   b. If you increased the sample size to 100, what range would you expect to contain 68 percent of the sample mean?

6. A medical assistant sampled the blood pressures of 20 randomly selected patients with high blood pressure before and after they received a dose of a new medicine.
   a. Are these numerical or categorical data?
   b. Which test should she run?
   c. If the null hypothesis is true (there is no difference), then what additional tests could she run to determine if there is a relationship between the results?
7. What kind of data is the amount of money spent on a wellness visit to the clinic?
   a. Continuous – numerical
   b. Continuous – discrete
   c. Categorical – ordinal
   d. Categorical – nominal

Determining Statistical Significance

8. A medical manufacturer wants to determine if a high-level disinfection of a surgical instrument tool for 10 minutes is equivalent in removing contaminants compared to 20 minutes. The test is run approximately 50 times using each disinfection protocol.
   a. What is the manufacturer's hypothesis?
   b. How will they test it?
   c. If the results show a p-value of 0.043, what should they conclude?
9. Suppose we are interested in the correlation between last year's weight and this year's weight for a group of cancer patients.
   a. If the correlation between last year's weight and this year's weight is 1, does it follow that everyone in the group had the same weight in both years? Will this information give us any help in predicting what their weight is this year?
   b. Suppose that the correlation between last year's weight and this year's weight is 0. If we know what patients weighed last year, will this information give us any help in predicting what their weight is this year?
   c. The data below shows the actual weights in the prior and current year. What is the correlation coefficient and is it statistically significant? What is the 95 percent confidence interval?

Person	Weight last year	Weight this year
A	150	150
B	160	165
C	130	125
D	180	185
E	110	125

10. The data below show the consumption of alcohol (X, liters per person per year, 14 years or older) and the death rate from cirrhosis, a liver disease (Y, death per 100,000 population) in 15 countries (each country is an observation unit).

Country	Alc. consumption	Death rate from Cirrhosis	x^2	y^2	xy
France	24.7	46.1	610.09	2,125.21	1,138.67
Italy	15.2	23.6	231.04	556.96	358.72
Germany	12.3	23.7	151.29	561.69	291.51
Australia	10.9	7	118.81	49	76.3
Belgium	10.8	12.3	116.64	151.29	132.84
US	9.9	14.2	98.01	201.64	140.56
Canada	8.3	7.4	68.89	54.76	61.42
England	7.2	3.0	51.84	9	21.6
Sweden	6.6	7.2	43.56	51.84	47.52
Japan	5.8	10.6	33.64	112.36	61.48
Netherlands	5.7	3.7	32.49	13.69	21.09
Ireland	5.6	3.4	31.36	11.56	19.04
Norway	4.2	4.3	17.64	18.49	18.06
Finland	3.9	3.6	15.21	12.96	14.04
Israel	3.1	5.4	9.61	29.16	16.74
Total	134.2	175.5	1,630.12	3,959.61	2,419.61

   a. Draw a scatter plot to show the association, if any, between these two variables. Can you draw any conclusion/observations without doing any calculation?
   b. Calculate the Pearson correlation coefficient and the level of significance and the 95 percent CI.
   c. Form the regression line by calculating the estimate intercept and slope; if the model holds, what would be the death rate from cirrhosis for a country with an alcohol consumption rate of 11.0 liters per person per year.

11. A radiologist hypothesizes that a new imaging system is comparable to an existing system to diagnose breast cancer. They are interested primarily in whether the size calculated for breast tumors is comparable between the two systems. They have a different radiologist assess the tumor diameter

from seven patients who were imaged with both systems. The data is shown below. Calculate the bias and limits of agreement.

Original system	New system
1.2 cm	1.4 cm
0.8 cm	0.7 cm
2.3 cm	2.4 cm
1.7 cm	1.5 cm
3.1 cm	3.4 cm
2.5 cm	2.2 cm
1.6 cm	1.7 cm

12. Consider a phase II clinical trial designed to investigate the effectiveness of a new drug to reduce symptoms of asthma in children. A total of $n=10$ participants are randomized to receive either the new drug or a placebo (5 in each arm). Participants are asked to record the number of episodes of shortness of breath over a one-week period following receipt of the assigned treatment. The data are shown below.
    a. What is the null hypothesis and the alternative hypothesis? Is this categorical or numeric data?
    b. What type of statistical test would be appropriate?
    c. Would a paired or unpaired test be used?

Placebo	7	5	6	4	12
New drug	3	6	4	2	1

Calculation of Key Metrics for a Clinical Study

13. Explain why it would not be possible to use random assignment to study the health effects of smoking.
14. A researcher offers free treatment to patients who take part in her research studies. What is an ethical problem with this method of recruiting subjects?
15. An oncologist wants to test a new blood test for the diagnosis of pancreatic cancer. He wants the test to have a sensitivity of at least 70 percent and a specificity of 90 percent. The existing test has a sensitivity of 50 percent and a specificity of 90 percent.
    a. How many patients does the oncologist need to be 95 percent sure his test is at least 10, 20, and 30 percent more sensitive than the existing test?
    b. How does the sample size change with increase in sensitivity difference?

16. Suppose a study was performed to assess the relationship between lung cancer risk and diet (vegetarian/nonvegetarian). Subjects were randomized by dietary group. Based on a pilot study, the researchers want to demonstrate that 75 percent of the population in the nonvegetarian group has high risk of lung cancer, whereas only 25 percent of the vegetarian group has high risk for lung cancer.
    a. What is the sample size needed for this study for a level of significance of 0.05 and a power of 0.8?
    b. Can you name one potential factor that could confound the interpretation of the results? Remember, for a factor to be a confounder, it must be associated with both lung cancer and with being vegetarian.
    c. What randomization approach would you use to reduce bias and why?
17. The percentage of HER2 subtypes of patients diagnosed with breast cancer is determined using two different molecular tests. The first test has a false positive rate of 40 percent, whereas the second test has a false positive rate of 20 percent. What fraction of patients will benefit from Herceptin (a drug to treat HER2-positive breast cancer) using the test with a 40 percent false positive rate and what percentage will benefit from the test with a 20 percent false positive rate?
18. A statistician is interested in the number of patients who complete a COVID test at home or in a clinic. He randomly assigns 100 individuals from a largely Spanish-speaking population into one of two groups: the first is given a home test while the second is given a clinic test. He records the number of patients who complete the test in each group. Identify the following components of this study:
    a. population
    b. sample size
    c. input variable
    d. intervention
    e. response variable.
19. A physician is interested in knowing how many times a patient visits her clinic in one week. She decides to ask every tenth patient on a specified day to complete a short survey including information about how many times they have visited the clinic in the past week. What kind of a sampling design is this?
    a. cluster
    b. stratified
    c. simple random
    d. systematic.
20. A pulse oximeter is developed to measure the oxygen saturation in cancer patients. The company applies to the FDA to get approval to market this device. If a predicate device is available to which the new device can be compared, what type of application would the manufacturer submit? If a predicate device is not available, what type of approval would the manufacturer seek? What is the difference with respect to demonstrating safety and efficacy between the two scenarios?

REFERENCES

Bhandari, N., Rongsen-Chandola, T., Bavdekar, A., et al. 2014. Efficacy of a monovalent human-bovine (116E) rotavirus vaccine in Indian infants: a randomised, double-blind, placebo-controlled trial. *The Lancet*, 383(9935), 2136–2143.

Carome, M., 2014. Unethical clinical trials still being conducted in developing countries. *Huffington Post* (October 3, 2014).

Ibe, O. C. 2014. *Fundamentals of Applied Probability and Random Processes*, 2nd ed., Academic Press, New York.

Krzywinski, M., & Altman, N. 2013. Error bars: the meaning of error bars is often misinterpreted, as is the statistical significance of their overlap. *Nature Methods*, 10, 921–923.

Simmons, J. P., Nelson, L. D., & Simonsohn, U. 2011. False-positive psychology: undisclosed flexibility in data collection and analysis allows presenting anything as significant. *Psychological Science*, 22(11), 1359–1366.

Simonsohn, U., Nelson, L. D., & Simmons, J. P. 2014. P-curve: a key to the file-drawer. *Journal of Experimental Psychology: General*, 143(2), 534.

8 Making Decisions Using Data Analytics

We have previously discussed the shift from traditional to precision medicine and its importance in advancing therapies specific to a disease and, more recently, to a patient. Patient-level precision depends on the generation and analysis of large amounts of data. For example, when researchers investigate responses to a particular cancer therapeutic, they can use the "omics" techniques discussed in Chapter 2 to quantify expression levels of hundreds of thousands of genes and proteins to identify differences between patients who responded and did not respond to therapy. The information generated can then be used to predict which patients are likely to respond to treatment with a particular therapy. With the vast amounts of data generated during "omics" studies, it is impossible to gain insights without using data analytics, specifically machine learning.

Why is machine learning important in extending healthcare to a broader population? Figure 8.1 shows the number of health professionals in countries stratified by the sociodemographic index (SDI). The SDI is a summary measure that identifies where countries or other geographic areas sit on the spectrum of development, on a scale from 0 to 1. Compared to high-SDI countries, where nurses, midwives, and physicians make up the bulk of the health workforce, low- and lower-middle-SDI countries mainly rely on nurses and midwives (Peiffer-Smadja et al., 2020). Further, within a given region there are significantly more midwives and nurses compared to physicians. If community health providers can be trained to make effective decisions with supportive tools, healthcare can become more accessible and have a broader reach to impact more lives (Peiffer-Smadja et al., 2020). For example, as discussed in Chapter 3, currently healthcare providers without formal medical training perform cervical cancer screening using the unaided eye. Owing to variability in the skill levels of the providers, the inherent subjectivity, and the lack of magnification, there is a high level of variability in the performance of visual inspection with acetic acid (VIA). Using a device like the Pocket Colposcope, or for that matter a smartphone, equipped with a machine learning algorithm has the potential to bring the capabilities of a real expert into the hands of less experienced providers, and at the same time reduce subjectivity.

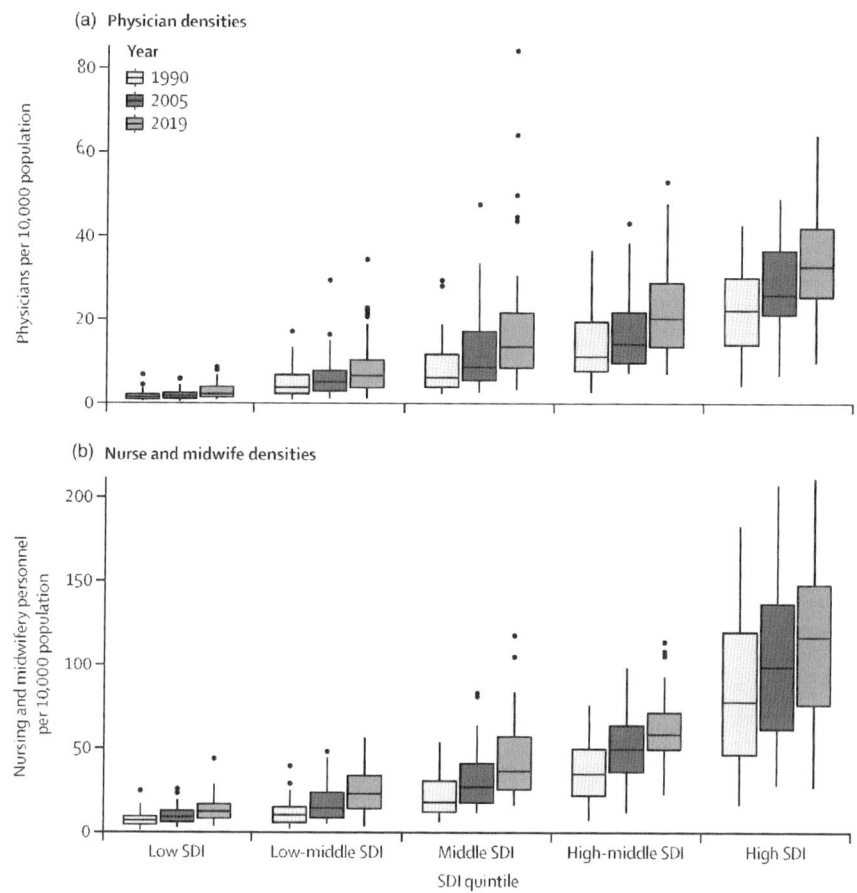

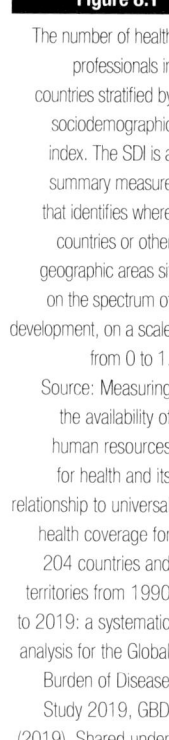

Figure 8.1

The number of health professionals in countries stratified by sociodemographic index. The SDI is a summary measure that identifies where countries or other geographic areas sit on the spectrum of development, on a scale from 0 to 1. Source: Measuring the availability of human resources for health and its relationship to universal health coverage for 204 countries and territories from 1990 to 2019: a systematic analysis for the Global Burden of Disease Study 2019, GBD (2019). Shared under an open access CC BY license.

This chapter will cover the different types of data analytics techniques that fall under the umbrella of machine learning. **Machine learning** describes the design of algorithms that learn from an example data set in order to make accurate predictions on new, or "unseen," data. The goal is to optimize a task's performance on a *new* data set as opposed to creating a "best fit" model on the example data set. In an ideal scenario, **machine learning** uses a rules framework to replicate clinical decision-making comparable to that of an expert physician. There are three distinct components to consider when using data analytics for healthcare. First, there is the data itself, which can come in multiple different formats. Next, there is the pace at which data is being generated and the corresponding storage capacity. Finally, there are the different methods for analyzing the data. All three are integral to effective development of algorithms for healthcare. This chapter will specifically focus on analytical methods for classification, while the next chapter will be dedicated to artificial neural networks (ANN) and convolutional neural networks (CNN).

LEARNING OBJECTIVES

Data Analytics for Classification
- The purpose of a data analytics model and the basic steps;
- the basic components of a machine learning model;
- the different types of machine learning, including supervised, unsupervised, and reinforcement learning.

Supervised and Unsupervised Learning
- Underlying principles of linear regression (for continuous outputs) and logistic regression algorithms (for discrete outputs) and the difference between the two;
- the principles of Bayesian theorem and decision tree networks, which leverage *a priori* information to strengthen decision-making;
- the principles of support vector machine and clustering algorithms, both of which categorize objects into one or more classes based on features.

Dimension Reduction and Generalization
- Differences between linear discriminant analysis and principal component analysis;
- the process by which principal component analysis leads to dimension reduction;
- the purpose of training and validation when developing a robust, generalizable algorithm.

Data Analytics for Classification

What is the goal of analyzing data for healthcare applications? In general, clinicians and researchers are ultimately interested in making predictions about how a patient is likely to respond to a particular therapy, whether it be for cancer, cardiovascular disease, or a bacterial infection. In order to adequately make predictions about the future, there must be data from the past that can be used to look for patterns, which is where data analytics comes into play. What exactly is data analytics? Figure 8.2 shows a data analytics model. Data analytics can be divided into four parts: What is happening (descriptive analytics), why it is happening (diagnostic analytics), what is likely to happen (predictive analytics), and what should be done (prescriptive analytics) (Qayyum, 2020). In healthcare, we are particularly interested in predictive and prescriptive analytics, as they tie back to the primary goal of predicting outcomes.

In the previous chapter, tests of statistical significance were described that can be used to identify whether measured endpoints are actually different between two or more groups. Similar to the goal of identifying whether two groups are different, the overall goal of a machine learning algorithm is to look for patterns within the data that can be used to divide the data into distinct groups. Figure 8.3 shows an example of a machine learning model. The key features of the model

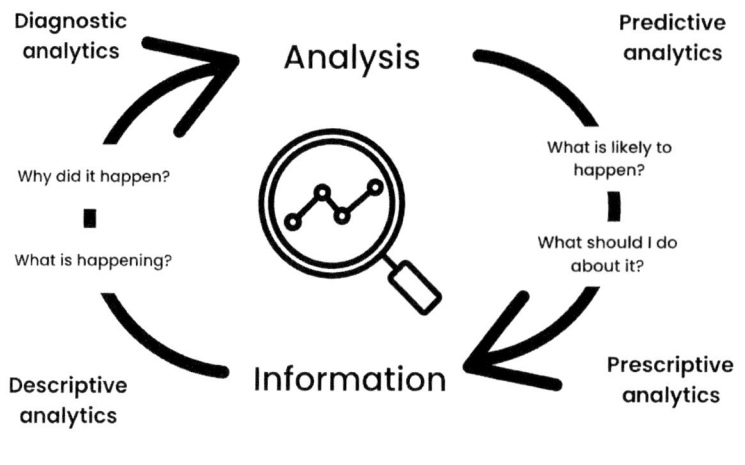

Figure 8.2

Data analytics model. Data analytics can be divided into four parts: What is happening (descriptive analytics), why it is happening (diagnostic analytics), what is likely to happen (predictive analytics), and what should be done (prescriptive analytics) (Qayyum, 2020).

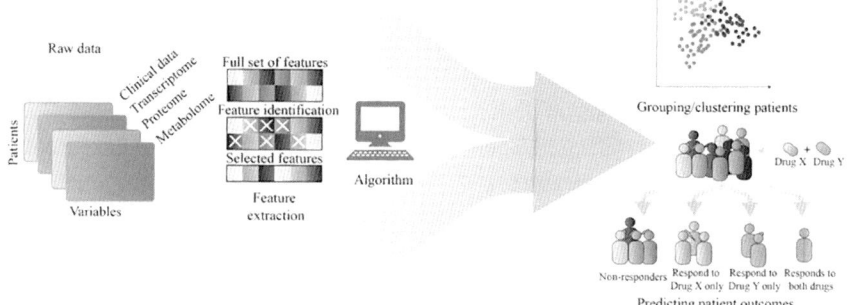

Figure 8.3

Example of a machine learning model. The key features of the model are inputs, a method of simplifying the number of variables into their salient features, and a classification technique used to analyze the extracted features. Inputs are the data that is introduced into the machine learning algorithm. They can be *raw* inputs (e.g., images straight from the image-capture device) or *preprocessed* inputs (e.g., images that have been cropped or converted into grayscale).
Source: Looking beyond the hype: Applied AI and machine learning in translational medicine, Toh, Dondelinger, Wang. eBioMedicine VOLUME 47, P607-615, SEPTEMBER 2019. DOI: https://doi.org/10.1016/j.ebiom.2019.08.027 © 2019 The Authors. Published by Elsevier B.V. Shared under CC BY-NC-ND 1.0.

are inputs, a method of simplifying the number of variables into their salient features, and a classification technique used to analyze the extracted features. Inputs are the data that is introduced into the machine learning algorithm. They can be *raw* inputs (e.g., images straight from the image-capture device) or *preprocessed* inputs (e.g., images that have been cropped or converted to grayscale).

Features are characteristics of the input data that may be used by the algorithm to help sort, distinguish, or classify the inputs. For example, mean blood pressure may be a feature from a patient's chart that can serve as an input into an algorithm that identifies patients that are at risk for cancer. Classification is a common machine learning task in which the algorithm learns to assign at least one label to each instance of the input data. For example, an algorithm can learn to assign a label of "skirt" or "pants" to an image that shows an article of clothing. In the case shown in Figure 8.3, the raw data consists of four categories: clinical data, transcriptome data, proteome data, and metabolome data. From these data, there are features that are selected as relevant for classification. The algorithm then takes the features and assigns the original patients into classes based off of the features (Toh et al., 2019).

Deeper Look: How Do Physicians Make Decisions in an Uncertain World?

The expectation in algorithm development is that good decisions can be made when there is sufficient data that is representative of the population it is being designed for. In reality, there are varying degrees of uncertainty that the algorithm may not capture. This could include uncertainty due to limited resources and/or a large volume of patients in the waiting room, necessitating quick decisions. How would algorithms take all of this into account? Presumably they would need to be adaptive.

In this deeper look, we will consider what rules physicians use. In situations where there are different levels of resources and uncertainty, providers often use informal problem-solving that can quickly and efficiently lead to solutions. These cognitive shortcuts are known as **heuristics**. By simplifying difficult decisions, providers determine a course of action for resource constrained tasks.

This idea is based on the theory of **bounded rationality** conceived by Nobel laureate Herbert Simon. In 1957, he conceptualized an idea in response to rational choice theory. Rational choice theory posits that consumers would make optimized economic decisions, as it was in their self-interest to do so. In other words, consumer would always choose the optimal choice. Bounded rationality is the theory that consumers have limited rational decision-making, driven by three main factors: cognitive ability, time constraints, and imperfect information. For example, when ordering at a restaurant, customers will make suboptimal decisions if they feel rushed by the waiter. This is the premise of heuristic decision-making.

An area of heuristics referred to as **fast-and-frugal heuristics** was introduced in 2003. Like other heuristics, fast-and-frugal trees are built around three questions: What heuristics do physicians use to make decisions? Which environments will it perform well in? And can the heuristics aid in decision-making? Figure 8.4 shows an example of a

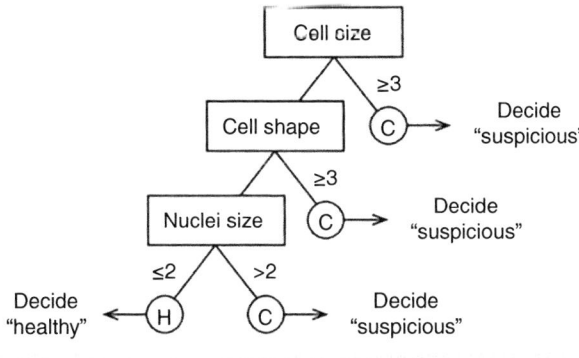

Figure 8.4

An example of a fast-and-frugal heuristics model to identify disease on a pathology slide. Three variables are used to make a decision: cell size, cell shape, and nuclear size.

> fast-and-frugal heuristics model to identify disease on a pathology slide. Three variables are used to make a decision: cell size, cell shape, and nuclear size. Fast-and-frugal heuristics sequentially orders cues, where every cue has two branches and one branch is an exit point (Martignon et al., 2003). The final cue in the sequence will have two exit points to ensure that a decision is always made.

There are three different types of learning that are commonly used: supervised, unsupervised, or reinforcement learning. **Supervised learning** algorithms are those in which labeled data is provided as inputs that the model uses to learn to make accurate predictions (i.e. assign correct labels) to future unlabeled data. In **unsupervised learning**, unlabeled data is fed into the algorithm, and the algorithm, instead of making precise predictions, explores the structures within the data to uncover common patterns, such as with clustering methods. In **reinforcement learning**, the algorithm is either rewarded or penalized based on which action, of a subset of actions, it decides to take. It learns to modify its actions in order to maximize its net rewards until a predefined threshold is met.

Generally, the type of learning that is used depends on the raw data available for training the algorithm. **Training** describes the process in which the algorithm iteratively runs through the training data to optimize its parameters to improve overall performance metrics. **Validation** involves the use of independent data that can be used to test the algorithm and in doing so serve as a feedback loop to continue optimization. It can either train for a certain number of iterations or train until performance metrics fail to improve. In order to train the algorithm, the input data needs to have labels that designate the category to which each data point belongs. For example, if the goal of the algorithm is to determine whether a patient with breast cancer is likely to respond to a particular treatment, the samples in the training data should be **labeled** as either responders or nonresponders. The supervised learning should then be able to train a classifier to recognize the patterns associated with each label. In future scenarios, the supervised learning algorithm can then be used to make predictions on unlabeled data and assign them into the appropriate class. **Class** describes the specific category each prediction is assigned. The number of classes in the output reflects the level of classification required. For example, binary classification may predict whether an image is an animal or not an animal, multiclass classification may differentiate between a dog, cat, or bird, and multi-label classification can go a step further, such as identifying black dog, white cat, etc.

> **Example: How Many Classes Can Patients Diagnosed with Breast Cancer be Assigned To?**
>
> Question: Patients with breast cancer can undergo testing for several different receptors, including the estrogen receptor (ER), progesterone receptor (PR), and human epidermal growth factor receptor (HER2). For each receptor, a patient can be positive or negative. How many different ways could these patients be grouped into classes based on receptor status? If there are targeted treatments for patients who are ER+/PR+/HER2- and ER-/PR-/HER2+, how many useful classes are there?
>
> Answer: There are three receptors, each of which can be positive or negative. As a result, there are eight possible classes (2 ER × 2 PR × 2 HER2):
>
> ER+/PR+/HER2+
> ER+/PR+/HER2−
> ER+/PR−/HER2+
> ER+/PR−/HER2-
> ER−/PR+/HER2+
> ER−/PR+/HER2−
> ER−/PR−/HER2+
> ER−/PR−/HER2−
>
> If there are only targeted treatments for patients with ER+/PR+/HER2− and ER−/PR−/HER2+, there would be three useful classes: ER+/PR+/HER2−, ER−/PR−/HER2+, and all other groups lumped together.

Supervised learning can be expressed mathematically as a function (f) that converts input (X) into output (Y) using the available data. The output (Y), also referred to as the label, can be a number or a category. For instance, if we are predicting the price of a drug, then the output is a number as opposed to finite categories. If we are predicting whether a patient responds or does not respond to a drug, the output is a category. For **supervised learning**, the input data X used to train the algorithm (i.e., the data used to generate the function f) must have a corresponding label Y, otherwise there is no method to find the function relating X to Y.

While supervised learning is useful for making predictions about future data, data analytics can also be used to look for patterns within existing data using **unsupervised learning**. For example, patient characteristics like age, height, and weight could be used to create clusters that might correspond to high, medium, or low risk of developing heart disease. We say "might" because the data does not have a known label for whether or not the person has heart disease. The results from the unsupervised learning method could be a precursor to a supervised learning model, identifying key variables to use in a decision-making algorithm.

Reinforcement learning is a machine learning approach where the algorithm can choose from a subset of actions and is either rewarded or penalized depending on how its decisions impact the target variables. The goal of reinforcement learning algorithms is to make a series of decisions that can optimize long-term rewards. This method is particularly beneficial in that the algorithm, given the necessary computing resources, can quickly run through many iterations of the problem, each with different decisions and outcomes, faster than is humanly possible. Reinforcement learning can be used to implement dynamic treatment regimens for patients with long-term illnesses or conditions, drug discovery and development, and adaptive and personalized interventions in health management – for example, exercise and weight management regimes for diabetic patients (Yu et al., 2019).

Figure 8.5 summarizes the different types of machine learning. In supervised learning, the algorithm is trained on data that has labels (for example, an image of a normal or diseased condition based on pathology). Once trained on this

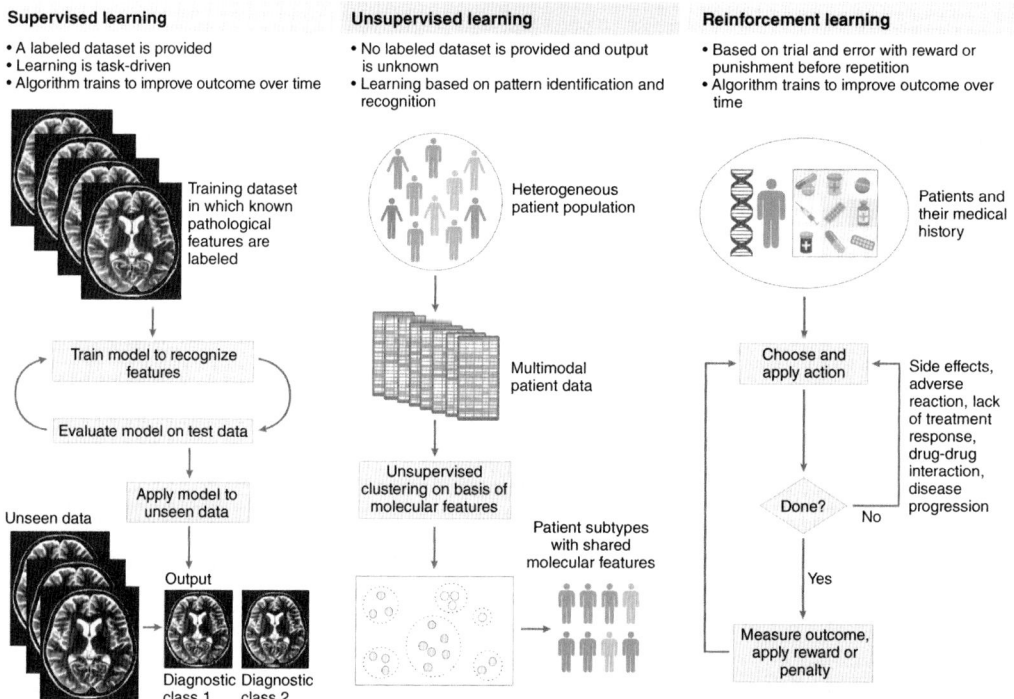

Figure 8.5 Summary of different types of machine learning. In supervised learning, the algorithm is trained on data that has labels. Once trained on this knowledge, it predicts the labels for a new set of unseen data. Unsupervised learning is the instance where analyses are performed to cluster the data in order to identify patterns that can give further insight into the data. Reinforcement learning is based on a feedback loop where the intervention is continually updated based on the response (Myszczynska et al., 2020).

Source: Myszczynska et al. (2020).

knowledge, it predicts the labels for a new set of unseen data. Unsupervised learning is the instance in which analyses are performed to cluster the data to identify patterns that can give further insight into the data (e.g., identify subsets of patients who have a particular genetic mutation or anomaly and then relate that back to patient characteristics). Reinforcement learning is based on a feedback loop where the intervention is continually updated based on the response. For example, if a patient has a symptom, the physician might introduce an intervention to address that symptom. Based on how the patient responds, the physician will make the next decision and so on (Myszczynska et al., 2020).

While machine learning as a field began in the mid 1950s, its application in healthcare did not begin until the 1970s. The first artificial intelligence application for healthcare was an expert system called MYCIN, named after the suffix for the most commonly used antibiotics at the time it was created, developed in the early 1970s by scientists at Stanford University. As is the case with all expert systems, MYCIN was a rules-based framework for decision-making initially used to select antibiotic type and dosage for patients with bacterial infections. MYCIN consisted of around 600 rules that it used to make a diagnosis and treatment recommendation. MYCIN worked by asking physicians a series of yes/no questions (inputs), which it then ran through its framework to determine a list of possible diagnoses and recommended treatments (outputs). The outputs also included a probability and confidence level for each diagnosis and recommended treatment.

Supervised and Unsupervised Learning

Figure 8.6 shows different types of supervised learning and unsupervised learning methods. Machine learning comprises supervised, unsupervised, and reinforcement learning. Within supervised learning, there are decision trees, ordinary least squares regression, logistic regression, Bayesian classifiers, and support vector machines (SVM). Within unsupervised learning, clustering is the most commonly used approach, along with dimension reduction methods such as principal component analysis (PCA). We will discuss PCA in detail later in the chapter. With respect to reinforcement learning, there are positive and negative reinforcement methods. Each of the sub-algorithms are described in greater detail below.

Reinforcement learning is briefly described here; however, a detailed description is beyond the scope of this chapter. **Positive reinforcement learning** is defined as an event that occurs because of specific behavior. It increases the strength and frequency of the behavior and positively impacts the action taken by the agent. **Negative reinforcement learning** is defined as strengthening behavior that occurs because of a negative condition that should have been avoided or stopped. What are the potential benefits

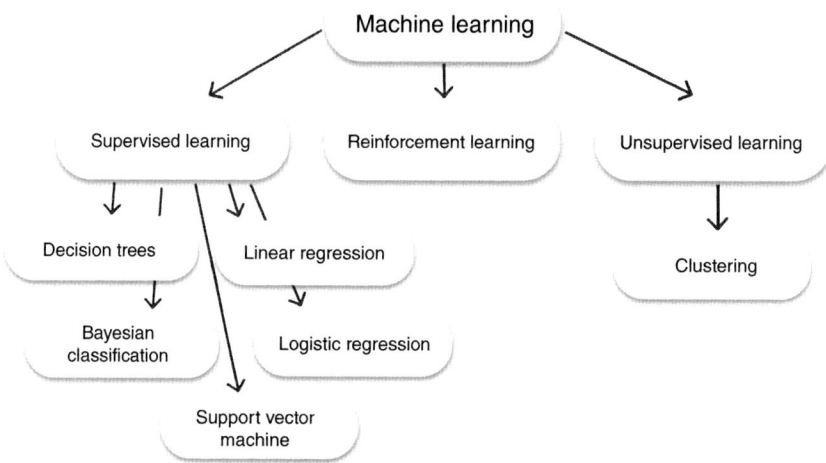

Figure 8.6 Different types of supervised and unsupervised learning methods. Machine learning comprises supervised, unsupervised, and reinforcement learning. Within supervised learning, there are decision trees, ordinary least squares regression, logistic regression, Bayesian classifiers, and support vector machines. Within unsupervised learning, there are clustering and associative algorithms. Table 8.1 provides a summary of the different supervised learning algorithms. In this chapter, the different types of supervised learning methods include regression (both linear and logistic), Bayesian classifiers, SVM, and decision trees. For unsupervised learning the chapter introduces clustering.

Table 8.1 A summary of the different supervised learning algorithms

Algorithm	Description	Applications
Linear regression	Finds the line of best fit for data that has a linear trend	Describing trends in linear data Predicting future continuous data with linear relationships
Logistic regression	Finds a sigmoidal function that fits data along a range between 0 and 1	Separating two classes of data using a single type of input
Bayesian classifier	Uses conditional probabilities to predict whether or not an event will occur based on the occurrence of other events	Classifying data into classes when the prior probability of events is well understood
Support vector machine	Creates a hyperplane that maximizes the separation between two or more classes	Classifying data with a larger number of features
Decision tree	Uses yes/no questions in sequence to separate data into distinct classes	Classifying data when a sequence of yes/no questions can be answered

of reinforcement learning? It helps determine which situation requires an action. It has a reward function and it determines which action has the highest reward over a certain period of time.

Supervised learning can have varying degrees of complexity. The type of response variable typically indicates the type of predictive modeling problem being performed. For example, a **numerical output** or continuous output indicates a regression predictive model, and a **discrete output** variable indicates a predictive modeling problem. Predictive linear regression models the linear relationship between the independent variable *x* and dependent variable *y* using numerical values, as opposed to class labels, and the output is continuous data. An **independent variable** does not change as other variables change. A **dependent variable** changes as the independent variable changes. Unlike linear regression, **logistic regression** falls into the category of predictive modeling. Logistic regression does not assume a linear relationship between the dependent and independent variables and the outcome is discrete (not continuous) – for example, positive or negative disease. In other words, linear regression handles continuous data, whereas logistic regression provides a discrete output.

Detailed explanation of linear, multiple linear, and logistic regression: Equation 8.1 shows the equation for a line, where *y* is the dependent variable, *x* is the independent variable, *b* is the slope, and *c* is the value of the *y*-intercept. For **linear regression**, all points can be modeled as points on a single straight line. Ordinary least squares, also known as least squares, is a method of estimation of the goodness of fit of a linear regression model. The **ordinary least squares** equation minimizes the **sum of squared errors** (SSE) or **mean squared error** (MSE) between the observed value (y_i) and the predicted value $(\hat{y}_i)$, where the **residual error**, *e*, is the observed value minus the model prediction value shown in Equation 8.2. For SSE, the error is squared and then summed for all points. For MSE the error is squared and then averaged across all points. The line that has the smallest SSE or MSE is chosen as the optimal regression line and can be used to make predictions about the values of future data:

$$\hat{y}_i = bx + c, \tag{8.1}$$
$$e = y_i - \hat{y}_i. \tag{8.2}$$

Figure 8.7 illustrates the use SSE to obtain a line of best fit for a linear regression. The plus signs represent the actual data points, y_i, while the corresponding points on the line, $\hat{y}_i$, represent the calculated or fit values. In this case, SSE is used for fitting by adding all of the squared errors together and selecting the line that results in the lowest SSE. Linear regression has only one *y* and one *x* variable.

Multiple linear regression has the same underlying concept as a simple linear regression. The formula for multiple linear regression is shown in Equation 8.3. In multiple linear regression equation, *y* is the predicted or expected value of the dependent variable, $x_1, x_2, \ldots$ are the independents of predictor variables. b_0 is the value of *y* when all the independent variables

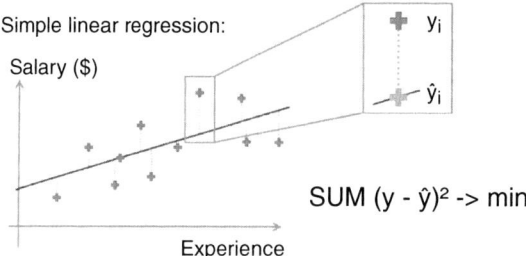

Figure 8.7 Illustration of using SSE to obtain a line of best fit for a linear regression. The plus signs represent the actual data points, y_i, while the corresponding points on the line, $\hat{y}_i$, represent the calculated or fit values. In this case, SSE is used for fitting by adding all of the squared errors together and selecting the line that results in the lowest SSE.

are set to zero and b_1, b_2, and b_3 are the estimated regression coefficients. Each of these coefficients represents the change in y relative to a change in the respective independent variable:

$$y = b_0 + b_1 x_1 + b_2 x_2 + \cdots + b_n x_n. \tag{8.3}$$

Example: Linear Regression

Question: A biomedical engineer performed a linear regression analysis on data showing changes in T cell levels following treatment with a novel immunotherapy. The results of the regression analysis are shown in the table below. Calculate the SSE and the MSE.

y_i	5	8	11	14	17	20	23	26
$\hat{y}_i$	6	7	9	15	18	19	22	28

Answer: First we need to calculate the error using Equation 8.2. Subtracting the second row from the first row gives:

y_i	5	8	11	14	17	20	23	26
$\hat{y}_i$	6	7	9	15	18	19	22	28
e	−1	1	2	−1	−1	1	1	−2

To calculate the squared error, we square each value for e:

y_i	5	8	11	14	17	20	23	26
$\hat{y}_i$	6	7	9	15	18	19	22	28
e	−1	1	2	−1	−1	1	1	−2
e^2	1	1	4	1	1	1	1	4

To calculate the SSE, we add all of the values in the bottom row:

$$SSE = 1 + 1 + 4 + 1 + 1 + 1 + 1 + 4 = 14.$$

To calculate the MSE, we divide the SSE by the number of data points, in this case 8:

$$MSE = 14 / 8 = 1.75.$$

Logistic regression models fit a wide, S-shaped curve to the data set that is positioned between the binary classification values of 0 and 1. How close the data point is to the top or bottom of the curve reveals the probability that it belonging to that particular class. A classification threshold is used to establish which class a point belongs to. A linear relationship is not assumed between the independent and dependent variables.

In order to understand the equation for logistic regression, it is instructive to understand a few important concepts. The **probability (P)** that an event will occur is the fraction of times you expect to see that event. If the probability of an event occurring is P, then the probability of the event not occurring is $1 - P$. **Probabilities** always range between 0 and 1. The **odds** are defined as the probability that the event will occur divided by the probability that the event will not occur. The logistic regression function is defined as the probability of an event occurring, P. It is related to the linear regression model as shown below and describes a sigmoid function. Linear regression needs a linear relationship between the dependent and independent variables, whereas logistic regression does not. Figure 8.8 shows a comparison of linear and logistic regression. Linear regression attempts to fit a straight line to the input data using a linear equation. A logistic model fits a sigmoidal curve (s-curve) to the data and therefore does not require linear data. If the data is bound (i.e., has finite lower and upper limits),

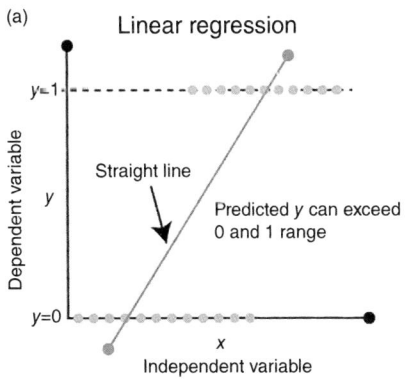
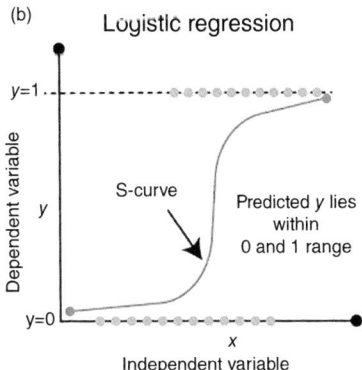

Figure 8.8 Comparison of linear and logistic regression. Linear regression attempts to fit a straight line to the input data using a linear equation. A logistic model fits a sigmoidal curve (s-curve) to the data and therefore does not require linear data.

linear regression can predict values outside of that range. As shown in the example, if the lower limit is 0 and the upper limit is 1, linear regression could result in values below 0 or above 1. Conversely, logistic regression can keep all predicted values within the 0–1 range.

Example: Logistic Regression

Question: Given the data below relating systolic blood pressure with the lifetime likelihood of having a heart attack, decide whether linear regression or logistic regression is a more appropriate model. Explain your rationale using the equations for linear and logistic regression.

Systolic (mmHg)	120	110	150	145	115	125	170	165	118
Lifetime heart attack probability (%)	5	2	20	18	4	6	25	22	4

Answer: Given that the model input is systolic blood pressure, and the model output is a probability with fixed bounds between 0 and 1, a logistic regression model would be best for this type of data. A linear regression model of the form $y = bx + c$ would allow for values outside the 0–1 range, which are not possible given the nature of a probability output. A logistic regression in the form of a sigmoidal function guarantees that the outputs will be contained within the range of 0–1.

Detailed explanation of Bayes' theorem: Bayes' theorem is based on the probability of an event occurring given the occurrence of another related event. For example, Bayes' theorem could be used to provide the probability of having a heart attack given that a person has high blood pressure. Bayes' theorem is shown in Equation 8.4, where $P(A|B)$ is the probability of event A occurring given that event B occurred, $P(B|A)$ is the probability of event B occurring given that event A occurred, $P(A)$ is the probability of event A occurring, and $P(B)$ is the probability of event B occurring. Note that in Equation 8.4 $P(B) \neq 0$. The basic principle behind Bayes' theorem can be expanded to the case where multiple features are present. To construct a classifier, a cutoff point can be set – for example, $P(B) > 0.5$ – to assign the set of features to a given positive or negative class:

$$P(A|B) = \frac{P(B|A) \times P(A)}{P(B)}. \tag{8.4}$$

Example: Calculating Probabilities Using Bayes' Theorem

Question: Patients with cervical cancer often experience abdominal cramps as one of their symptoms; however, not all people experiencing abdominal cramps have cervical cancer. Assuming 80 percent of patients with cervical cancer experience abdominal cramps, the prevalence of disease is 1/100,000, and 100/100,000 healthy people experience abdominal cramps, what is the probability that a person with abdominal cramps has cervical cancer?

Answer: We can use Equation 8.4 to answer this question if we rewrite it as below:

$$P(Cancer \mid Symptoms) = \frac{P(Symptoms \mid Cancer) \times P(Cancer)}{P(Symptoms)}.$$

We have two of these variables already from the assumptions given in the question prompt:

$$P(Symptoms \mid Cancer) = 0.8,$$
$$P(Cancer) = 0.000001.$$

The only variable that we do not have at present is $P(Symptoms)$; however, we can use logic to determine this probability given the information in the question. The probability of having symptoms would be the sum of two different probabilities: (1) the probability of having symptoms for a person with cancer multiplied by the probability of having cancer, plus (2) the probability of having symptoms for a person without cancer multiplied by the probability of not having cancer:

$$P(Symptoms) = P(Symptoms \mid Cancer) \times P(Cancer) + P(Symptoms \mid Healthy)$$
$$\times P(Healthy)$$
$$= 0.8 \times 0.000001 + 0.0001 \times 0.999999$$
$$= 0.000108.$$

Plugging everything into the original equation gives

$$P(Cancer \mid Symptoms) = \frac{0.8 \times 0.000001}{0.000108} = 0.0074.$$

Therefore, the probability that a person with abdominal cramps has cervical cancer is 0.74 percent.

Detailed explanation for support vector machine: **SVM classifiers** find a hyperplane (the number of dimensions that can be more than two dimensions) that maximizes the distance between data points from two or more classes, such that future data points can be classified with reliable confidence into one of these classes. SVMs are typically applied to unstructured and semi-structured data. SVMs operate by creating a dividing boundary, or hyperplane, between different classes of data in n-dimensional space (with n being

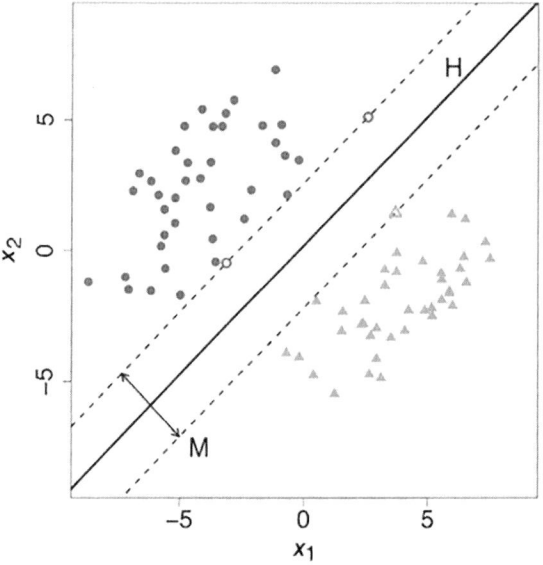

Figure 8.9 Illustrative example of a hyperplane for the 2D SVM. The data set consists of two variables, x_1 and x_2 for each data point and the circles correspond to one class and the triangle symbols correspond to the other. The hyperplane is represented by the solid black line labeled H. The dashed lines separated by the arrow M represent the boundaries of the hyperplane that separate x_1 and x_2.

equal to the number of features used for classification). Figure 8.9 shows an illustrative example of a hyperplane for the 2D SVM. The data set consists of two variables, x_1 and x_2, for each data point and the circles correspond to one class and the triangle symbols correspond to the other. The hyperplane is represented by the solid black line labeled H. The dashed lines separated by the arrow M represent the boundaries of the hyperplane that separate x_1 and x_2. The SVM will calculate the best line or hyperplane that separates the two classes of data, aiming to maximize the margin (distance) between the hyperplane and class data points.

How does SVM find the optimal hyperplane? First, let us consider a two-dimensional case. Two-dimensional linearly separable data can be separated by a line, as shown in Equation 8.1. For the purposes of rewriting the equation for a hyperplane, we can rename x with x_1 to represent the first feature and y with x_2 to represent the second feature, shown in Figure 8.8. Substituting into the equation for a line, we get Equation 8.5, the equation for a hyperplane:

$$bx_1 - x_2 + c = 0. \tag{8.5}$$

Given that both x_1 and x_2 each represent a vector, we can use matrix notation to define vector $\boldsymbol{x} = (x_1, x_2)$ and $\boldsymbol{w} = (b, -1)$. Equation 8.6 is derived from the **dot product** of two-dimensional vectors, $\boldsymbol{w}$ and $\boldsymbol{x}$, and represents the equation

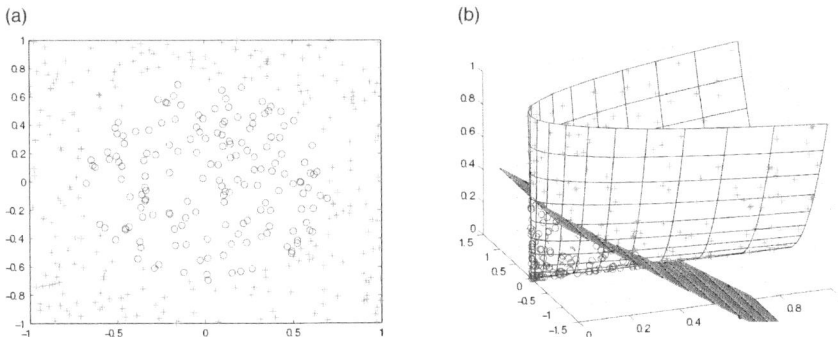

Figure 8.10 Example of a nonlinear SVM. (a) One class designated by small circles is encompassed by the second class designated by pluses. In this case, a circular plane (b), would better separate the two classes.
Source: Author "Machine Learner" under a CC-BY-SA-4.0 license.

of the hyperplane. In Equation 8.6 $|w|$ is the magnitude (length) of **w**, $|x|$ is the magnitude of **x**, and θ is the angle between **w** and **x**:

$$w \cdot x = |w| \times |x| \times \cos(\theta) + c = 0. \tag{8.6}$$

We now can define a hypothesis function $h(x_i)$ that will be used to predict to which class (i) a data point belongs, as shown in Equation 8.7:

$$h(x_i) = +1 \text{ if } w \cdot x + c \geq 0; \text{ and } -1 \text{ if } w \cdot x + c < 0. \tag{8.7}$$

Any points above or on the hyperplane (in this case, the line) will be classified as class +1, and points below the hyperplane will be classified as class −1.

The equations and example above represent the case for a linear hyperplane that separates two classes; however, it is possible that a linear hyperplane is not the optimal solution for separating two or more classes. In this case, a nonlinear SVM can be developed using a different type of hyperplane. Figure 8.10 shows an example of a nonlinear SVM. As seen in (a), one class designated by small circles is encompassed by the second class designated by pluses. In this case, a circular plane (b), would better separate the two classes. The development of a nonlinear SVM is beyond the scope of this book.

Example: Support Vector Machines

Question: Suppose the below equation defines the hyperplane separating two classes of patients with breast cancer, where class 1 responds to a novel treatment and class 2 does not respond to a novel treatment. Two features, x_1 and x_2, are available for each patient.

$$h(x_i) = +1 \text{ if } w \cdot x + c \geq 0; \text{ and } -1 \text{ if } w \cdot x + c < 0,$$
$$w = (3,-1); x = (x_1, x_2); c = 4.$$

(a) Given the new data below, determine which class each patient falls into if $h = 1$ corresponds to responds to treatment and $h = -1$ corresponds to does not respond to treatment.
(b) Suppose the patients are treated based on the recommendation from the SVM classifier and you follow them for response. Clinically, patients 1, 2, 4, 6, 7, and 8 responded to treatment. Calculate the sensitivity and specificity for the SVM.

Patient	1	2	3	4	5	6	7	8
x_1	1	−1	−2	3	−3	0	−2	2
x_2	2	2	1	4	−2	2	0	2

Answer:
(a) We can use the data points and plug each one into the equation shown. If the result is less than 0, the patient is not responsive to treatment; otherwise, the patient responds to treatment.
Using the dot product gives the following equation:

$$3x_1 - x_2 + 4 = ?.$$

Plugging in patient 1 gives:

$$3(1) - 2 + 4 = 5.$$

Using the same method gives the below results for all patients:

Patient	1	2	3	4	5	6	7	8
x_1	1	−1	−2	3	−3	0	−2	2
x_2	2	2	1	1	−2	2	0	2
h	5	−1	−3	9	−3	2	−2	6

Staying with patient 1 as an example, since h is 5, which is larger than 0, the prediction would be that patient 1 will respond to treatment. The only other patients with h greater than or equal to 0 are 4, 6, and 8. Therefore, it is predicted that patients 1, 4, 6, and 8 would respond to treatment.
(b) To calculate the sensitivity and specificity, we need to know the number of true positives (TP), true negatives (TN), false positives (FP), and false negatives (FN).
The number of TPs is the number of patients who were responsive to therapy that the algorithm correctly determined; these are patients 1, 4, 6, and 8, so TP = 4.
The number of TNs is the number of patients who were not responsive to therapy that the algorithm correctly determined; these are patients 3 and 5, so TN = 2.

The number of FPs is the number of patients who were not responsive to therapy that the algorithm incorrectly determined; there were no patients in this category.

The number of FNs is the number of patients who were responsive to therapy that the algorithm incorrectly determined; there are a total of two patients.

$$\text{Sensitivity} = \frac{TP}{TP + FN}$$
$$= \frac{4}{4+2} = 67\%,$$

$$\text{Specificity} = \frac{TN}{TN + FP}$$
$$= \frac{2}{2+0} = 100\%.$$

Detailed explanation of decision trees: A **decision tree** is made up of a minimum number of yes/no questions that one has to ask to make a correct decision. Decision trees run data through a series of nodes, with each node representing a condition statement and splitting into a "true" or "false" branch. The branches parse the data set out into smaller and smaller sections with the goal of dividing the data into groups corresponding to their labels. Decision trees are one of the most easily interpretable models for classification and regression.

When designing a decision tree, there are three main parameters that can be set. First, there is the number of nodes within the tree. The top of a decision tree is the root *and the first split from the root* occurs at the **internal node**, creating branches or **edges**. Each branch can end either in another node, which would split into more branches, or a leaf, which indicates a decision has been reached. The second parameter is the depth of the tree, which is the maximum number of nodes that are allowed before reaching a leaf. The third is a cost function, which is used to penalize incorrect decisions. The algorithm designing the decision tree will iterate through different numbers of nodes and tree depths to try to minimize the cost function (i.e., reduce the number of incorrect decisions) based on the training data provided. The performance of a tree can be further increased by *pruning*, or removing paths along the tree. Figure 8.11 shows an example of a decision tree for breast cancer diagnosis and treatment. The root of the tree is the box with *lump detected by self-exam*. There are two nodes in this tree: mammogram suspicious and biopsy shows malignancy. There are four leaves: the self-exam, no biopsy, nonmalignant cyst, and lumpectomy + chemo.

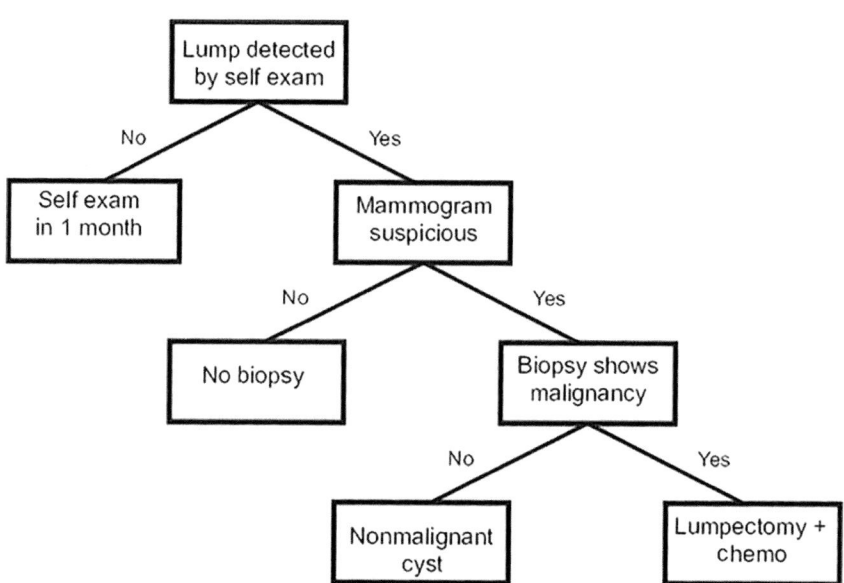

Figure 8.11

Example of a decision tree for breast cancer diagnosis and treatment. The root of the tree is the box with lump detected by self-exam. There are two nodes in this tree: mammogram suspicious and biopsy shows malignancy. There are four leaves: the self-exam, no biopsy, nonmalignant cyst, and lumpectomy + chemo.

Example: Decision Trees

Question: Determining whether or not a patient has cancer as well as the cancer stage is a complex process that involves multiple rounds of test results. Take the basic tree from

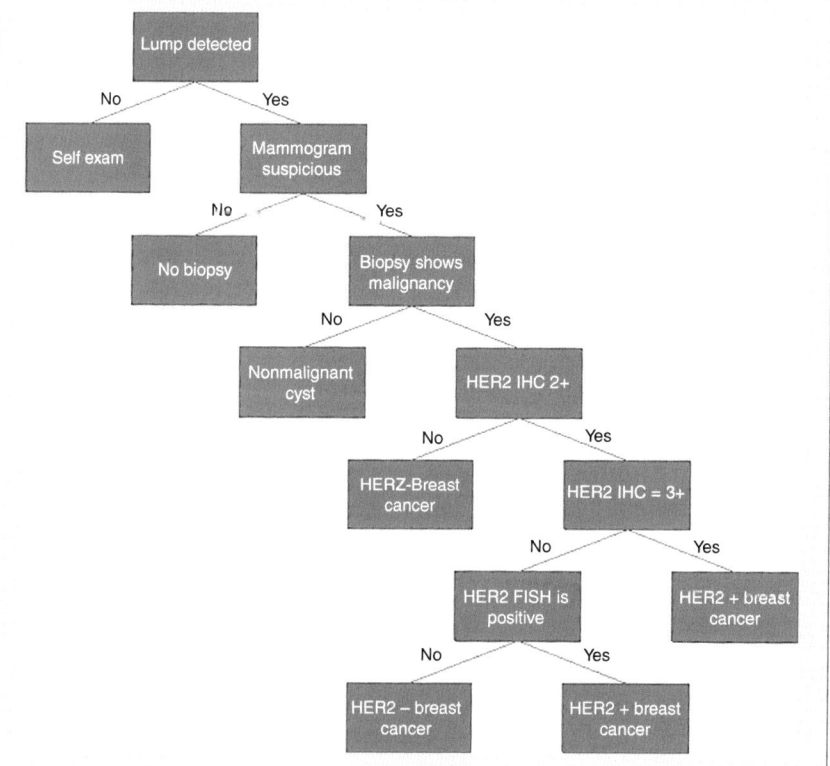

Figure 8.12

The updated decision tree for breast cancer diagnosis.

Figure 8.11, showing breast cancer diagnosis, and expand it to make it specific for HER2-positive breast cancer. Consider that there are two tests for HER2: immunohistochemistry (IHC) and fluorescence in situ hybridization (FISH). How does this change the number of nodes in the tree? How does it change the depth of the tree?

Answer: The updated tree is shown in Figure 8.12. Because up to two tests can be required to determine whether a breast cancer is HER2+ (IHC and FISH), at least two more nodes would be required, one for IHC and one for FISH. However, FISH is only required in the event that the IHC result is 2+. Since decision trees require yes/no questions, two nodes are required for IHC testing, one to check if the IHC result is 0 or 1 (i.e., <2+), and one to check if the IHC result is 2+ or 3+ (i.e., = 3+). The tree shown in Figure 8.11 had two nodes. The new tree has five nodes. The previous tree had a maximum depth of two, the new tree has a maximum depth of five.

Detailed explanation of clustering: Thus far we have focused on supervised learning. In the case of unsupervised learning, the most common approach is to perform clustering. **Clustering** is an unsupervised learning technique that segments the data into groups according to patterns within the data. It aims to maximize intergroup differences and minimize intragroup differences. There are two main goals in clustering: first, identification of similarities between two data points; and second, finding similarities/differences between similar data points. Figure 8.13 shows the difference between supervised learning (classification) and unsupervised learning (clustering). The same data points can be used for supervised learning for classification or unsupervised learning for clustering. In (a) the data is labeled (circles for class 1 and crosses for

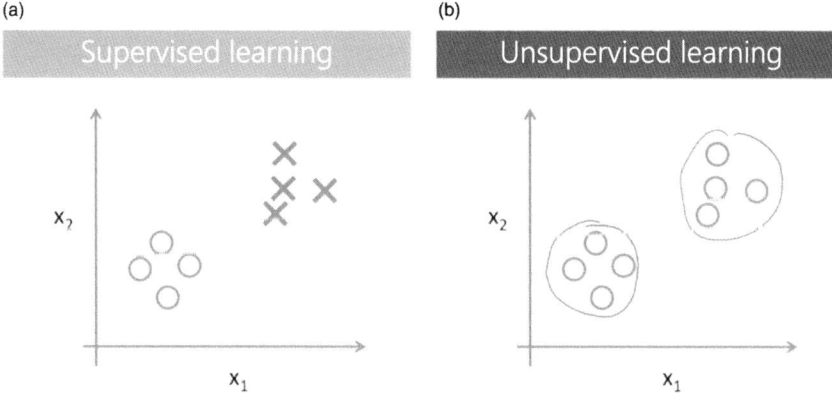

Figure 8.13 The difference between supervised learning (classification) and unsupervised learning (clustering). The same data points can be used for supervised learning for classification or unsupervised learning for clustering. In (a) the data is labeled (circles for class 1 and crosses for class 2), whereas in (b) the data is unlabeled (all points are considered as the same class). The goal of the clustering algorithm is to group points that are similar to each other, as shown by the circles surrounding the two clusters.
Source: Author "Pouya Tahmasbpour" under a CC-BY-SA-4.0 license.

class 2), whereas in (b) the data is unlabeled (all points are considered as the same class). The goal of the clustering algorithm is to group points that are similar to each other, as shown by the circles surrounding the two clusters.

Centroid-based clustering is considered one of the simplest clustering algorithms, yet the most effective way of creating clusters and assigning data points to it. In iterative clustering algorithms, the notion of similarity between points is derived by the closeness of a data point to the centroid (center) of the clusters. K-means clustering algorithms are a popular class of algorithms that falls into the centroid clustering category. In k-means clustering, k clusters are randomly assigned or selected based on prior knowledge of the data set. K is chosen based on the number of classes desired. Next, the cluster centroids are calculated, and this step is iterated until the assignment of data points to the clusters no longer changes. After clustering has been performed, silhouette scores can be calculated to quantify how effective the clustering algorithm was at separating the data into clusters.

Silhouette scores are a metric of how similar points in a cluster are to each other and how different they are from points in different clusters. Equation 8.9 describes how to calculate a silhouette score, s_i. In this equation, a_i is the average distance between point i in a cluster and all points within the same cluster, b_i is the average distance between point i in a cluster and all points within a different cluster, and $\max(a_i,b_i)$ is the maximum of a_i and b_i. In general, a positive silhouette score indicates that the specific point is more similar to the other points within its cluster than points within a different cluster, whereas a negative silhouette score indicates that the specific point is more similar to the points within the other cluster than points within the same cluster:

$$s_i = \frac{b_i - a_i}{\max(a_i, b_i)} \tag{8.9}$$

Example: Clustering

Question: A researcher interested in predicting risk of stroke based on blood pressure and platelet count has collected data from 10 patients and performed k-means clustering with k = 2 to see if there might be any clusters within the data. The algorithm divides the patients into two clusters, with four patients in cluster 1 and six patients in cluster 2. The researcher wants to determine how well the clustering algorithm performed. Calculate the silhouette score for patient 8 in the table below.

Patient	1	2	3	4	5	6	7	8	9	10
Blood pressure	155	127	119	143	172	147	133	135	117	126
Platelet count	507	367	457	463	428	306	374	512	324	408
Cluster	1	2	2	1	1	2	2	1	2	2

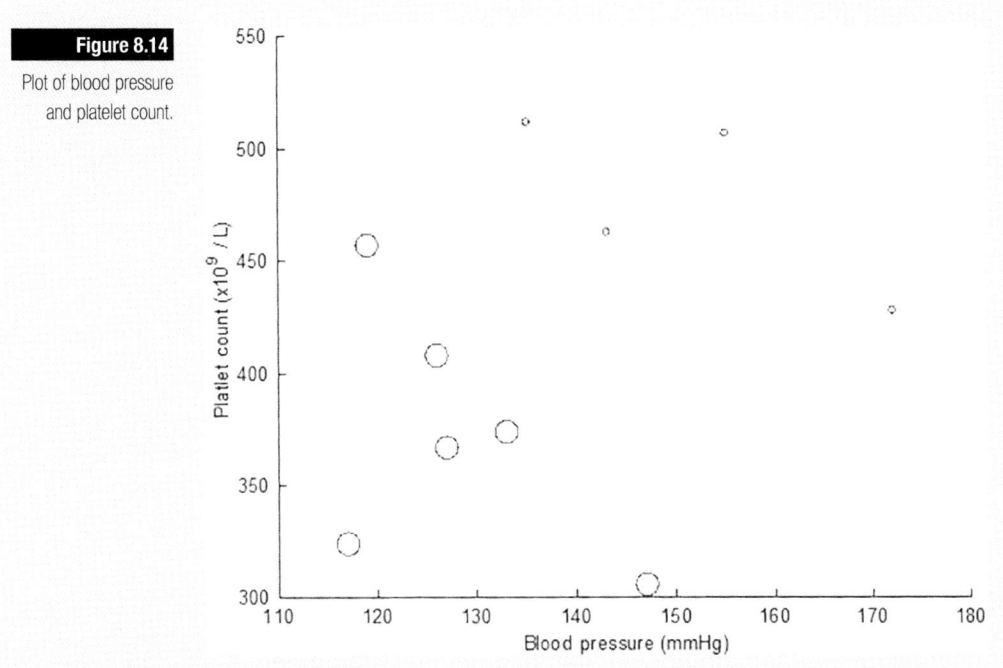

Figure 8.14
Plot of blood pressure and platelet count.

Answer: It may first be helpful to plot the data so that it can be easily visualized, as shown in Figure 8.14. Small circles represent points assigned to cluster 1. Large circles represent points assigned to cluster 2.

The first step for calculating the silhouette scores for patient 8 is to calculate the distances from patient 8 to all other patients. The Pythagorean theorem can be used to calculate the distance between two points as the hypotenuse between the x and y distances. We will show the calculation for this distance between patient 8 and patient 1, $D_{8,1}$:

$$D_{8,1}^2 = (135-155)^2 + (512-507)^2$$
$$= 400 + 25$$
$$= 20.62.$$

This same method can be applied to calculate the remaining distances:

$$D_{8,1} = 20.62,$$
$$D_{8,2} = 145.22,$$
$$D_{8,3} = 57.28,$$
$$D_{8,4} = 49.65,$$
$$D_{8,5} = 91.79,$$
$$D_{8,6} = 206.35,$$
$$D_{8,7} = 138.01,$$

$$D_{8,9} = 188.86,$$
$$D_{8,10} = 104.39.$$

Next, we need to calculate a and b from Equation 8.9, which are the mean distances within and between clusters:

$$a = \frac{D_{8,1} + D_{8,4} + D_{8,5}}{3}$$
$$= 54.02,$$
$$b = \frac{D_{8,2} + D_{8,3} + D_{8,6} + D_{8,7} + D_{8,9} + D_{8,10}}{6}$$
$$= 140.02.$$

The max of a and b is b; therefore, b will be used as the denominator of Equation 8.9:

$$s = \frac{140.02 - 54.02}{140.02}$$
$$= 0.61.$$

Since the silhouette score is positive, the point is more similar to the other points within the same cluster than it is to the points in the other cluster, suggesting the clustering algorithm did a good job of choosing to include patient 8 in cluster 1.

Deeper Look: The Perils of Missing Data

Advances in diagnostic technologies, coupled with data analytics, is poised to address global health inequities. However, several factors may make it difficult to conduct research for hard-to-reach populations, such as language, cultural, and educational barriers. This problem is compounded by missing data. Data can be lost due to a variety of factors, including human error, data sourcing, collection, and processing, not to mention intentional suppression of data. Missing data can be incomplete, inconclusive, inconsistent, or outdated. The problem of missing data is relatively common in almost all research and can have a significant effect on the conclusions that can be drawn from the data. First, the absence of data reduces statistical power. Second, the lost data can cause bias in the estimation of parameters. Third, it may complicate the analysis of the study. Missing data can potentially call into question the validity of the clinical studies.

A common assumption about missing data is that it can be addressed through post hoc methods. However, these methods can artificially inflate correlation among scores, introduce trends not supported by data, bias the results, and result in incorrect inferences (Lee et al., 2019). What is missing data? Figure 8.15 shows a conceptual illustration of the two main types of missing data. **Missing at random** (MAR) corresponds to data points that are a random subset of the original data. **Missing not at random** (MNAR) means there is missing data within a particular group. For example, people with the lowest education are most likely to drop out of the study. The cases of MNAR data are more realistic but highly susceptible to bias.

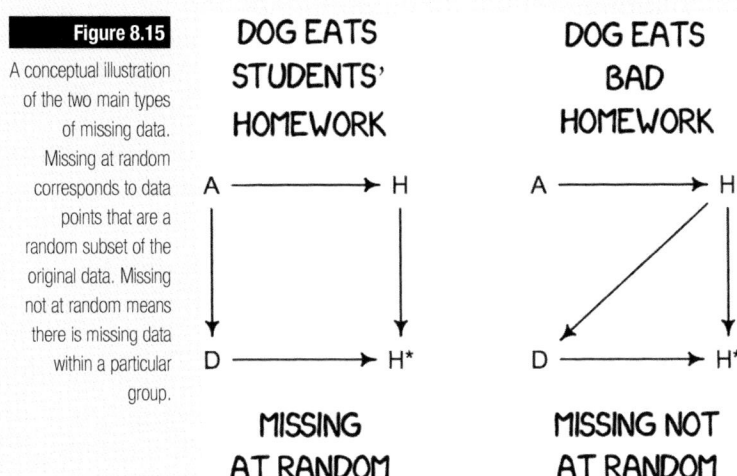

Figure 8.15 A conceptual illustration of the two main types of missing data. Missing at random corresponds to data points that are a random subset of the original data. Missing not at random means there is missing data within a particular group.

There are several available missing data techniques, including (a) listwise deletion, (b) pairwise deletion, (c) maximum likelihood (ML), (d) single imputation, and (e) multiple imputation. The robust methods are *maximum likelihood* (ML: e.g., EM algorithm or full information maximum likelihood/FIML) or multiple imputation. The least robust are likewise and pairwise deletion.

Listwise deletion omits cases with missing data and analyzes the remaining data. **Pairwise deletion** of missing data means that cases relating to each pair of variables with missing data involved in an analysis is deleted. In the **maximum likelihood method**, missing data may be estimated by using the conditional distribution of the other variables. **Imputation** preserves all cases by replacing the missing data with a probable value estimated using other available information. In **multiple imputation** the missing values are replaced with a set of plausible values which contain the natural variability and uncertainty of the right values. Multiple imputation has been shown to produce valid statistical inference that reflects the uncertainty associated with the estimation of the missing data.

The best solution to the missing data problem is to maximize data collection for the study being implemented. Application of post hoc statistical analysis should only be used after maximal efforts have been employed to reduce missing data in the design and prevention techniques. By focusing on the research objectives of the study and only collecting data that is absolutely necessary to fulfill the objectives, the likelihood of missing data will be reduced. It can also reduce the burden on research staff who are more likely to miss data owing to large amounts of data collection.

Dimension Reduction and Generalizability

Now that we have described the different types of machine learning algorithms that can be used for data analytics, how are the inputs selected for the algorithm? Feature selection and extraction approaches are core elements in diagnosis, classification, clustering, recognition, and detection. **Feature selection**, a supervised learning approach, is used if the requirement is to maintain the original features or there are only a small number of features. Feature selection techniques are used when explanation of a model is a key requirement. The selection of the original features that are statistically significant between the classes of interest can be carried out using the tests of statistical significance discussed in Chapter 7. For example, if the original features measured to determine response to a cancer drug are white blood cell count, tumor size, and the cancer antigens CA 125, a test of statistical significance may be used to identify which of the three parameters are significantly different pre- and post-therapy prior to creating a predictive model.

Feature extraction is a common approach to retain the important features of the data in a much smaller dimensional space with minimal loss of relevant information. For example, a classification algorithm that uses the entire human genome is not practical and it will be challenging to perform a test of significance of thousands of variables to select salient features. As mentioned previously, the features extracted from this approach may not be explainable given that this is an unsupervised learning method.

Feature extraction is also important when the input feature size is comparable to or greater than the data sample size, which may lead to overtraining the algorithm. In other words, the algorithm becomes too specific to the training data. While this algorithm may perform well on the training data, it will likely not be generalizable to new data. Two commonly used feature extraction techniques are linear discriminant analysis (LDA) and principal component analysis (PCA). LDA is supervised, whereas PCA is unsupervised; in other words, PCA ignores class labels (e.g., whether a sample is cancer or not cancer). Figure 8.16 shows differences between PCA and LDA. In (a), PCA finds the directions of maximal variance, as shown in the graph where PCA consolidates three variables into two dimensions.

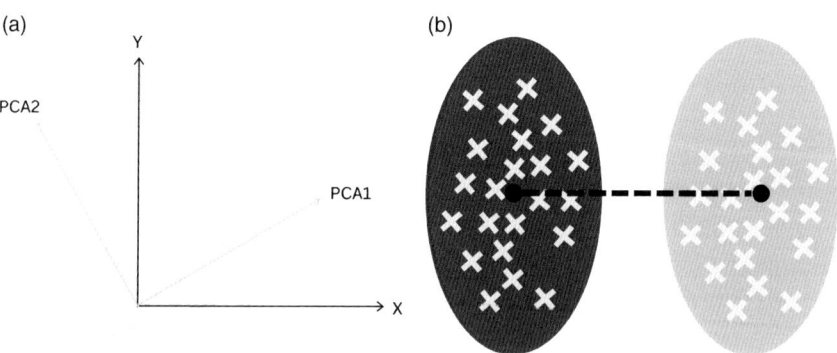

Figure 8.16 Differences between principal component analysis and linear discriminant analysis. (a) PCA finds the directions of maximal variance, as shown in the graph where PCA consolidates three variables into two dimensions. (b) LDA attempts to find a feature subspace that maximizes class separability. Both are linear transformation methods.

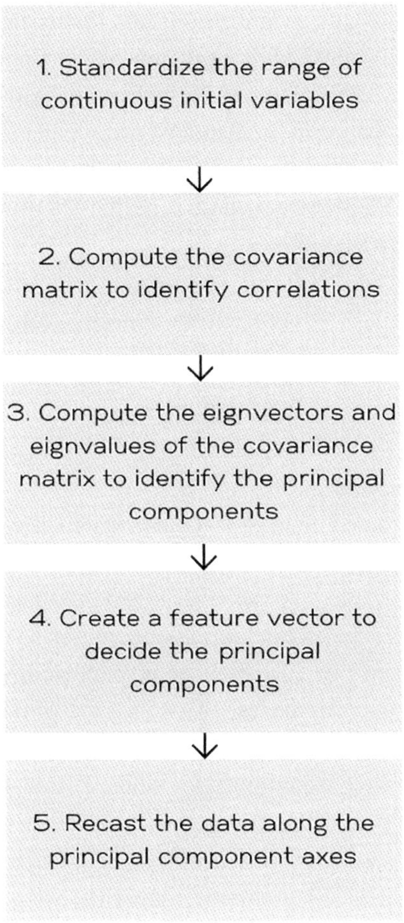

Figure 8.17

Five key steps of PCA. Step 1 standardizes the input data and step 5 recasts the input data onto the new principal component space. The steps in between can be considered the linear transformation steps.

1. Standardize the range of continuous initial variables

↓

2. Compute the covariance matrix to identify correlations

↓

3. Compute the eignvectors and eignvalues of the covariance matrix to identify the principal components

↓

4. Create a feature vector to decide the principal components

↓

5. Recast the data along the principal component axes

In (b), LDA attempts to find a feature subspace that maximizes class separability. Both are linear transformation methods.

Detailed explanation of PCA: The goal of PCA is to reduce the number of variables into principal components (PCs), where the number of PCs is significantly smaller than the number of variables in the original data set. Figure 8.17 shows the five key steps of PCA. Step 1 standardizes the input data and step 5 recasts the input data onto the new PC space. The steps in between can be considered the linear transformation steps.

For the sake of simplicity, we can start with a data matrix that has two variables, x_1 and x_2. Each row corresponds to an individual sample, for a total of 100 samples:

$$X = \begin{bmatrix} x_1^1 & x_2^1 \\ x_1^2 & x_2^2 \\ \vdots & \vdots \\ x_1^{100} & x_2^{100} \end{bmatrix}.$$

Step 1: The next step is to standardize the data matrix in order to put all of the variables on the same scale. This is important as the ranges can be different for each variable, thereby weighting one variable more than others. In order to standardize the variable, the mean is calculated using Equation 8.10, where x is each sample and N is the number of samples; the standard deviation is calculated using Equation 8.11 and the standardization is performed using Equation 8.12:

$$\mu = \sum_{i=1}^{N} \frac{x_i}{N}, \tag{8.10}$$

$$\sigma = \sqrt{\frac{\sum_{i=1}^{N}(x_i - \mu)^2}{N}}, \tag{8.11}$$

$$z_i = \frac{x_i - \mu}{\sigma}. \tag{8.12}$$

Step 2: The standardized matrix is converted to a covariance matrix, which will inform whether there is a positive, negative, or no relationship between each of the variables. A positive covariance means two variables are positively correlated (i.e., as one variable increases so does the other). A negative covariance means two variables are inversely correlated (i.e., as one variable increases the other decreases). A covariance of 0 means there is no correlation between two variables. The covariance between two variables x and y can be calculated using Equation 8.13, where $\underline{x}$ is the sample mean of x, $\underline{y}$ is the sample mean of y, and N is the total number of samples. An example of a covariance matrix is shown below. It should be noted that the covariance between the same variables (diagonals) is simply the variance:

$$\text{cov}_{x,y} = \frac{\sum_{i=1}^{N}(x_i - \underline{x})(y_i - \underline{y})}{N-1} \\ \begin{bmatrix} \text{cov}_{x,x} & \text{cov}_{x,y} \\ \text{cov}_{y,x} & \text{cov}_{y,y} \end{bmatrix}. \tag{8.13}$$

The covariance matrix can be simplified into matrix A, where variables a and d correspond to the covariance (variance) of x_1 and x_1, and x_2 and x_2, respectively. The variables b and d are the covariances between x_1 and x_2, and x_2 and x_1, respectively:

$$A = \begin{bmatrix} a & b \\ c & d \end{bmatrix}.$$

Step 3: The eigenvectors and eigenvalues will be computed from the covariance matrix. An **eigenvector** is a vector whose direction remains unchanged when a linear transformation is applied to it. The **eigenvalue** can be thought of as a scaling factor. All eigenvectors of a matrix are orthogonal to one another, which is one of the requirements for PCA. The eigenvectors and eigenvalues for any matrix are defined by Equation 8.14, where A is the original matrix, $\underline{v}$ is an eigenvector, and λ is an eigenvalue:

Dimension Reduction and Generalizability

$$Av_- = \lambda v_-. \tag{8.14}$$

Linear algebra can be used to demonstrate how to calculate the eigenvalues and eigenvectors for a matrix. First, Equation 8.14 can be rearranged as follows, where I is the **identity matrix** (1s along the diagonal and 0s everywhere else) and is the same size as A:

$$Av_- - \lambda v_- = 0,$$
$$v_-(A - \lambda I) = 0.$$

For the above equation to be true, the **determinant** of $A - \lambda I$ must be zero, as defined by Equation 8.15:

$$\det(A - \lambda I) = 0. \tag{8.15}$$

The determinant of matrix A can be used to generate Equation 8.16 to solve for the eigenvalue, λ:

$$
\begin{aligned}
A &= \begin{bmatrix} a & b \\ c & d \end{bmatrix} \\
A - \lambda I &= \begin{bmatrix} a & b \\ c & d \end{bmatrix} - \lambda \begin{bmatrix} 1 & 0 \\ 0 & 1 \end{bmatrix} \\
A - \lambda I &= \begin{bmatrix} a-\lambda & b \\ c & d-\lambda \end{bmatrix} \\
\det(A - \lambda I) &= (a-\lambda)(d-\lambda) - bc = 0 \\
\lambda^2 &- (a+d)\lambda + ad - bc = 0.
\end{aligned}
\tag{8.16}
$$

The above equation can be written as a quadratic equation, Equation 8.17, which will provide two eigenvalues, λ_1 and λ_2.

$$A\lambda^2 + B\lambda + C = 0, \tag{8.17}$$

$$\lambda_1 = \frac{-B + \sqrt{B^2 - 4AC}}{2A}$$

$$\lambda_2 = \frac{-B - \sqrt{B^2 - 4AC}}{2A}.$$

The eigenvector corresponding to each eigenvalue can be determined by plugging the eigenvalues back into Equation 8.14, as shown below. This system of equations can be used to solve the first eigenvectors (v_{11}, v_{12}). The same process can be used to determine the second eigenvector (v_{21} and v_{22}):

$$\begin{bmatrix} a & b \\ c & d \end{bmatrix} \begin{bmatrix} v_{11} \\ v_{12} \end{bmatrix} = \lambda_1 \begin{bmatrix} v_{11} \\ v_{12} \end{bmatrix},$$

$$\begin{bmatrix} av_{11} + bv_{12} \\ cv_{11} + dv_{12} \end{bmatrix} = \begin{bmatrix} \lambda_1 v_{11} \\ \lambda_1 v_{12} \end{bmatrix}.$$

Step 4: The fourth step is to rank the eigenvalues and corresponding eigenvectors from first to last, beginning with the largest eigenvalue and finishing with the smallest eigenvalue. The reason the eigenvalues are ranked highest to lowest is that the larger the eigenvalue, the more variance (Var) of the original data it accounts for. The amount of variance for each eigenvalue, λ_i, can be calculated as shown in Equation 8.18. In this particular case there are only two eigenvalues and corresponding eigenvectors. It should be noted that if there are a large number of eigenvectors, the goal will be to keep the number of PCs manageable. In most cases, two or three PCs should describe most of the variance in the data:

$$\text{Var}_i = \frac{\lambda_i}{\sum_{k=1}^{n} \lambda_k} \times 100. \tag{8.18}$$

Step 5: The fifth step is to project the original data set onto the principal component axes. This is a fairly straightforward process. The transpose of the eigenvector vector is multiplied by the transpose of the original data set to project the data onto the PCs, as shown in Equation 8.19, where $v_{1\_}$ is the eigenvector and $X\_$ is the original matrix of features or variables:

$$PC1 = v_1^T \times X^T$$
$$PC1 = \begin{bmatrix} v_{11} & v_{12} \end{bmatrix} \begin{bmatrix} x_1^1 & x_1^2 & \cdots & x_1^{100} \\ x_2^1 & x_2^2 & \cdots & x_2^{100} \end{bmatrix}. \tag{8.19}$$

Example: Principal Component Analysis

Question: A researcher is performing a study using two variables to classify patients as responsive or nonresponsive to a particular therapy. The researcher wishes to reduce the dimensionality to simplify the inputs into their algorithm. Suppose they found the covariance matrix below. Calculate the eigenvalues and eigenvectors corresponding to the two PCs. What percentage of the variance in the data is described by the first principal component?

$$A = \begin{bmatrix} 1 & 2 \\ 2 & 5 \end{bmatrix}.$$

Answer: To find the eigenvalues and corresponding eigenvectors of A, we first need to use Equation 8.10:

$$\det(A - \lambda I) = 0.$$

For a 2×2 matrix, this equation turns into the below, where $a = 1$, $b = 2$, $c = 2$, and $d = 5$:

$$\lambda^2 - (a+d)\lambda + ad - bc = 0,$$
$$\lambda^2 - 6\lambda + 1 = 0.$$

Using the quadratic formula to solve for λ gives:

$$\lambda_1 = 3 + 2\sqrt{2} \approx 5.83,$$

$$\lambda_2 = 3 - 2\sqrt{2} \approx 0.17.$$

Now that we have found the eigenvalues, we can use Equation 8.14 to solve for the two eigenvectors using two systems of equations. The system for the first eigenvector is shown below; the same methodology can be used for the second eigenvector by substituting in the second eigenvalue:

$$A\vec{v} = \lambda \vec{v},$$

$$\begin{bmatrix} 1 & 2 \\ 2 & 5 \end{bmatrix} \begin{bmatrix} x_{11} \\ x_{21} \end{bmatrix} = (3 + 2\sqrt{2}) \begin{bmatrix} x_{11} \\ x_{21} \end{bmatrix}$$

$$x_{11} + 2x_{21} = 3x_{11} + 2\sqrt{2}x_{21},$$
$$2x_{11} + 5x_{21} = 3x_{11} + 2\sqrt{2}x_{21}.$$

The system of equations can be solved to find:

$$\vec{v}_1 = \begin{bmatrix} x_{11} \\ x_{21} \end{bmatrix} = \begin{bmatrix} -1 + \sqrt{2} \\ 1 \end{bmatrix} \approx \begin{bmatrix} 0.41 \\ 1 \end{bmatrix}.$$

Using the same methodology to get the second eigenvector gives:

$$\vec{v}_2 = \begin{bmatrix} x_{12} \\ x_{22} \end{bmatrix} = \begin{bmatrix} -1 - \sqrt{2} \\ 1 \end{bmatrix} \approx \begin{bmatrix} -2.41 \\ 1 \end{bmatrix}.$$

Equation 8.18 can be used to calculate the percentage of the variance contained within the first principal component:

$$\text{Var}_{\text{PC1}} = \frac{3 + 2\sqrt{2}}{3 + 2\sqrt{2} + 3 - 2\sqrt{2}} \times 100 \approx 97.14 \text{ percent.}$$

Therefore, 97.14 percent of the variance is explained by the first principal component and the remaining variance is accounted for by the second principal component.

We have already discussed the fact that having more variables than the actual sample size can lead to overfitting. Having an appropriate training and validation set can also help prevent overfitting. During training, the algorithm adapts particular parameters to better recognize patterns to classify the data. The **training set** is the portion of the data that is used to optimize the machine learning approach, and then to optimize the selected algorithm. The training set should be representative of the entire data set – for example, it has the same class balance. Training sets are used to develop the model, and the model *sees* and *learns* from this data. The **validation set** is a subset of the training set that is used to spot-check the model's performance before continuing to tune its parameters. Validation sets are a segment of the data used during training that the algorithm has not yet seen.

One of the first considerations when developing a machine learning algorithm is deciding how to split the data into training and validation sets. Overfitting occurs when an algorithm learns the details and noise associated with the training data to the extent that it negatively impacts the performance of the model on a validation set. The noise or random fluctuations in the training data may not apply to the validation data and impacts the algorithm's ability to be adept as a predictor in new populations. If left uncorrected, overtraining can reduce classification accuracy, which is the number of correctly classified samples divided by the total number of samples to be classified. A classification of 90 percent, for example, means that 9 out of 10 instances are classified correctly by the algorithm. Ideally, an infinite amount of data would be available; however, in a real-world scenario this will not be the case. There are quite a few factors to consider when deciding how to split the data to train the algorithm: How many samples are available for analysis, how many variables are available for each sample, how many groups the algorithm will need to be able to distinguish, and how many samples fall into each of these groups.

Imbalanced data sets occur when the number of samples within each group in the training data set are not equal. For example, classifying an image as positive or negative for cervical cancer would likely be unbalanced because most images are going to be negative. The classification accuracy of the entire data set is not the best output to determine the training size, but rather the classification accuracy of samples that are positive or negative for disease, particularly prediction of positive disease. The reason is intuitive: Let us assume that the true negative is the dominant input. Then we can achieve high accuracy by predicting true negatives as negative (specificity) most of the time at the expense of predicting the true positives as positive (sensitivity). In a real-world setting, the consequences could be dire. This could lead to a low false positive rate but high false negative rate, in which case the cancers would be missed.

Once the algorithm has been developed on a training set, it is then tested on a validation set. The validation set contains data that can be used to provide an evaluation of a model fit on the training data set and for tuning the algorithm through a back-and-forth between the training and validation set. However, the evaluation on the validation set is not sufficient as the results on the validation set can be used as feedback to refine the algorithm. This is why a separate **test set**, also referred to as a holdout set, is required. It is used to calculate the final performance metrics after all the optimizations have been made. It is only used once a model is completely trained and validated (using the training and validation sets). The test set is generally well curated and contains carefully sampled data that spans the various classes that the model would face when used in the real world.

Dimension Reduction and Generalizability

> **Example: Imbalanced Data Sets**
>
> Question: In Malawi, HIV has a prevalence rate of 9 percent among people aged 15–49, according to the WHO. The same prevalence is reflected in a data set of 100 patients. If the algorithm correctly classifies only three of the nine patients as positive for HIV, and correctly classifies all 91 patients that are negative for HIV, what is the accuracy, sensitivity, and specificity of that algorithm? Why may the accuracy not be the best indication of the algorithm's performance?
>
> Answer: The algorithm's accuracy is 94 percent (94 patients out of 100 were correctly classified). The sensitivity of the algorithm is 33 percent (three of the nine positive patients were correctly classified) and the specificity of the algorithm is 100 percent (all 91 negative patients were correctly classified.) Because of the low prevalence, the high accuracy masks the poor sensitivity of the algorithm.

Figure 8.18 summarizes of the process for training and evaluating a machine learning algorithm. The model is initially trained on the training set, which changes different parameters of the algorithm to minimize the classification error. Once the algorithm has gone through one iteration of training to minimize the classification error on the training set, the algorithm is applied to the validation set to check for the level of classification error. This process is repeated until the error on the validation set reaches a minimum. The algorithm is then applied to the test set to demonstrate the algorithm is generalizable to new data.

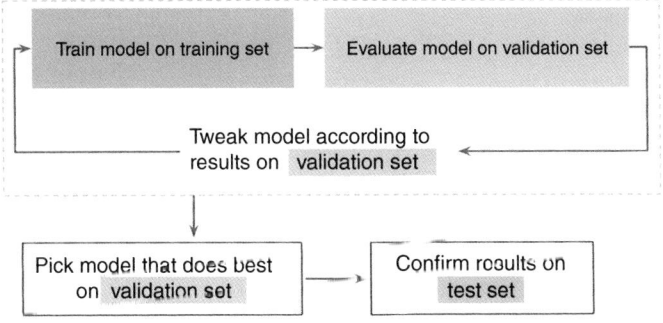

Figure 8.18 Summary of the process for training and evaluating a machine learning algorithm. The model is initially trained on the training set, which changes different parameters of the algorithm to minimize the classification error. Once the algorithm has gone through one iteration of training to minimize the classification error on the training set, the algorithm is applied to the validation set to check for the level of classification error. This process is repeated until the error on the validation set reaches a minimum. The algorithm is then applied to the test set to demonstrate the algorithm is generalizable to new data.

An alternative to a test set is the process of **cross validation**. Cross validation is a method in which, through multiple iterations, random samples of the training set are divided into either training or validation portions. The method is used to prevent overfitting on smaller data sets, where having a traditional test set would reduce the size of the training set to a point where it was too small to adequately train the algorithm. Cross validation is typically performed if the sample size is not sufficiently large to have independent training and validation sets. In this case, a randomly chosen X percentage of the training data is used to actually train the algorithm and the remaining ($100 - X$ percent) is used for validation, where X is a fixed number (e.g., 80). The model is then iteratively trained and validated using the same process by repeating this with another randomly chosen training and validation set. This process can be repeated multiple times to determine the performance difference between different training and validation sets.

Cross validation avoids overfitting and is gaining popularity, with **k-fold cross validation** being the most popular method. K-fold cross validation is one of the best approaches for limited input data. K corresponds to the number of times cross validation is performed. K-fold ensures that every instance from the original training data set has the chance of appearing in both the training and validation sets. The first step is to split the entire data randomly into k folds, for example 5–10, depending on the data size. The next step is to fit the model using the $k - 1$ folds and validate the model using the remaining fold. The next step is to repeat this process until every k serves as the test set and the average of the recorded scores from every remaining k serves as the performance metric for the model. Figure 8.19 shows an example of

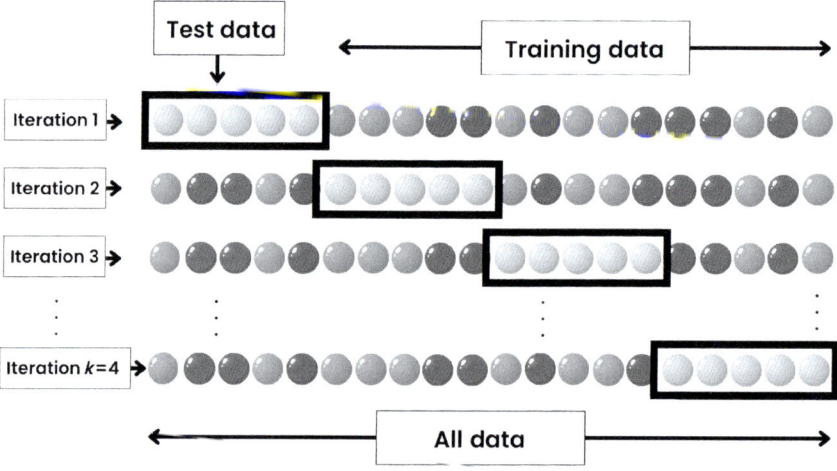

Figure 8.19 Example of K-fold cross validation with $K = 4$. In the case shown here, four iterations are performed. With four iterations, the data is randomly split into four equal-sized partitions, with 25 percent of the data in each partition. The first round through, three of the partitions are combined into the training set and the fourth is used for testing. This process repeats, cycling through all of the partitions being used for testing.

Dimension Reduction and Generalizability

k-fold cross validation with $k = 4$. In the case shown here, four iterations are performed. With four iterations the data is randomly split into four equal-sized partitions, with 25 percent of the data in each partition. The first round through, three of the partitions are combined into the training set and the fourth is used for testing. This process repeats, cycling through all of the partitions being used for testing.

A common value for k is 10. How do we actually know this is the right value to use? One approach to addressing this question is to compare the performance for a given value of k to an ideal scenario. When the amount of data available is not a constraint, then the methodology shown in Figure 8.15 can be used. If not, the ideal scenario can be simulated with a computationally more intensive version of k-fold validation, referred to as leave-one-out cross validation (LOOCV), where $k = N$, and N is the total number of samples in the training data set. Figure 8.20 shows an illustration of the variance, bias, and required computational power for LOOCV (ideal scenario) and k-fold cross validation for different values of k. As the value of k decreases, the bias increases (i.e., the error between the predicted and expected value). Increasing k reduces bias; however, it also increases the variance (i.e., the spread of predicted value, relative to the average value). Note that repeated cross validation is shown where the k-fold validation is performed, and the entire process is repeated multiple times.

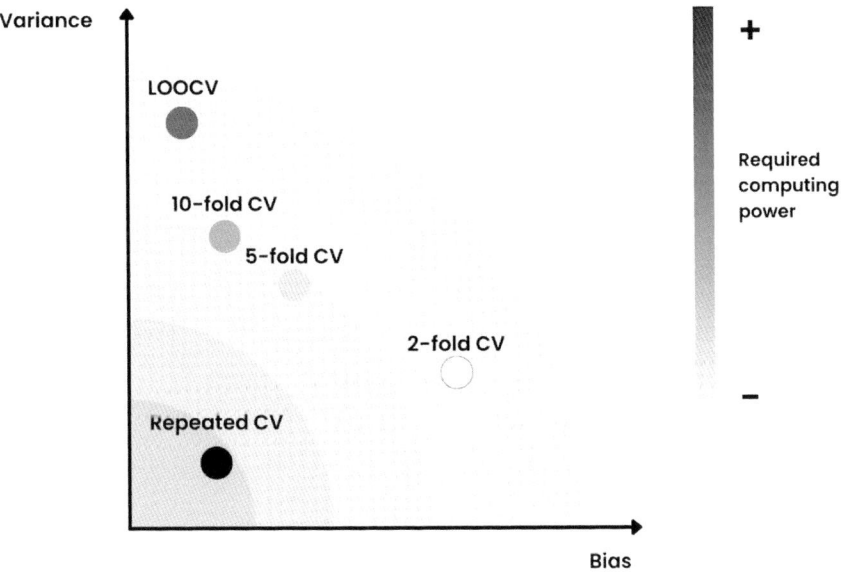

Figure 8.20 Illustration of the variance, bias, and required computational power for LOOCV (ideal scenario) and k-fold cross validation for different values of k. As the value of k decreases, the bias increases (i.e., the error between the predicted and expected value). Increasing k reduces bias; however, it also increases the variance (i.e., the spread of predicted value, relative to the average value). Note that repeated cross validation (CV) is shown where the k-fold validation is performed, and the entire process is repeated multiple times.

Deeper Look: Explainable or Accurate?

A radiologist is a physician who specializes in medical imaging. Radiologists analyze images, such as X-rays, to help diagnose, monitor, and treat various conditions or injuries. Figure 8.18 shows an image of a radiologist looking at a patient's chest X-ray. The interpretation of the images can be affected by a number of factors, such as the quality of the image, the number of images the radiologists looked at prior to the current image, and experience. Let us assume a lab at Duke University is interested in exploring the decisions made by radiologists in reviewing breast mammograms based on their dictation notes. They first identify relevant words to map what types of decisions were made by radiologists in different hospitals. There are two critical steps in the model's decision-making process: first, a topic (decisions) and then a classification – for example, in a binary classification assigning a radiologist to either a good or bad decision category. To start, the researchers use a dozen variables, which they dimensionally reduce to two PCs, which are then used as inputs to an SVM algorithm. They are able to differentiate radiologists who made good decisions from bad decisions using pathology as the gold standard. The algorithm makes excellent predictions in future scenarios. The question, however, is: How does this lead to something actionable? Without knowing the root cause of the problem, a simple decision would be to fire bad radiologists, which would not be good for the morale of the community. As an alternative approach, the researchers now ask expert radiologists to rank the 12 variables in order of which is most likely to distinguish a good from a bad decision. A multiple linear regression model using two or three of the top-ranking variables is used for classification. The classification is now simply the equation of a line. The simplistic model has less accuracy in predicting a future good or bad decision owing to the fact that much less information is used to train the model. However, the radiologists are able to identify image quality and the lighting in the room as key variables. Now they can do something about it.

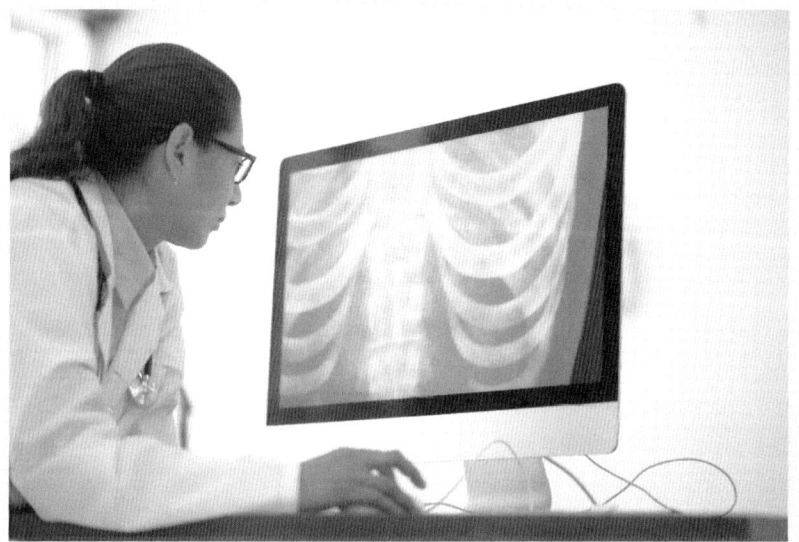

Figure 8.21

A radiologist looking at a patient's chest X-ray. The interpretation of the images can be affected by a number of factors, such as the quality of the image, the number of images the radiologists looked at prior to the current image, and experience. Source: ©FatCamera/ E+/Getty Images.

> Explainability is a very important aspect of machine learning, especially in scenarios where the decisions made by the model affect many people in a potentially negative way (firing radiologists because they are not good). However, there is a big difference between the types of explanations desired by people who produce machine learning models. A decision scientist may want explanations that help them improve the models. A decision-maker wants to understand issues such as data sources and how reliable that output is. A person who received a decision based on a model wants to know what the contributing factors were that led to the answer. Use cases with low criticality require less explainability, and allow for a complex model in order to improve accuracy. On the other hand, use cases with high criticality necessitate greater explainability and therefore may need to use simpler models at the expense of accuracy. The complexity of a model is broadly attributed to the number of variables, nonlinearity of the data, and lack of **monotocity** (always changes in one direction).

Looking Ahead

The impact of machine learning on data analytics continues to grow, reflecting its significance in decision-making. As machine learning becomes increasingly important in healthcare, there will be opportunities to solve progressively more advanced problems. Figure 8.22 shows the number of machine learning publications over a 40-year period. The number of overall publications has been exponentially increasing since

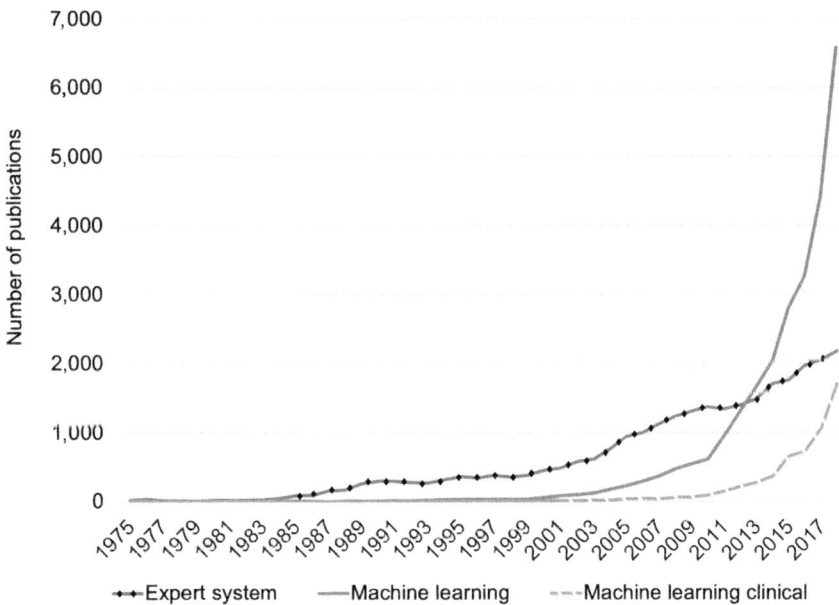

Figure 8.22 Number of machine learning publications over a 40-year period. The number of overall publications has been exponentially increasing since the early 2000s. Clinical applications related to machine learning began increasing exponentially the following decade (Peiffer-Smadja et al., 2020).
Source: Peiffer-Smadja et al. (2020). © 2019 European Society of Clinical Microbiology and Infectious Diseases. Published by Elsevier Ltd.

the early 2000s. Clinical applications related to machine learning began increasing exponentially in the following decade (Peiffer-Smadja et al., 2020).

Many of the machine learning techniques presented provide the basic framework for the process of data analytics. These methods work best on relatively small data sets, which can be classified with simple and straightforward algorithms. As the size and complexity of the data increases, more advanced types of machine learning frameworks must be developed to keep pace with the intricacies of healthcare. Chapter 9 will focus on more advanced machine learning methods, particularly ANNs and CNNs, which more closely mimic the decisions that would be made by the human brain. These more sophisticated algorithms can be used to solve some of the most pressing issues in healthcare globally.

Even though many of the techniques described in this chapter are restricted to small data sets, these approaches are foundational to developing the more complex algorithms described in the next chapter. For example, these methods can be used to look for patterns in the data that can aid with interpretation, and/or inform decision-making. An additional important aspect of these methodologies is that they can be tailored for numerical outputs, discrete outcomes, or categories or classes. With more sophisticated algorithms, the outputs are largely restricted to assignment of outputs into classes (for example, normal or abnormal). Also significant is the much lower computational burden of these approaches compared to ANNs and CNNs. This is precisely why this chapter precedes the next chapter on deep learning – to provide an appreciation of relatively simpler techniques that can reveal information that would otherwise be masked in black-box algorithms.

SUMMARY

Data analytics attempts to take past data to help make predictions about what may happen with future data. The data analytics model can be divided into four parts: What is happening (descriptive analytics); why it is happening (diagnostic analytics); what is likely to happen (predictive analytics); and what should be done (prescriptive analytics). Machine learning is one method of data analytics that can be used to look for patterns within data or classify new data based on patterns observed from existing data. The key features of machine learning models are inputs, a method of simplifying the number of variables into their salient features, and a classification technique used to analyze the extracted features.

There are three different types of learning that can be used in machine learning: supervised, unsupervised, and reinforced. Supervised learning is used to train an algorithm on past data to make predictions on future data. Unsupervised learning is used to look for patterns within the data that could be used to develop a supervised learning model. Reinforcement learning iterates through scenarios that either reward or punish the decisions made by the algorithm based on whether or not the desired outcome in achieved. There are five major methods used for supervised machine learning: linear regression, logistic regression, Bayesian classifiers, SVMs, and decision trees.

Linear regression models the linear relationship between the independent variable x and dependent variable y using numerical values, as opposed to class labels. Logistic regression models fit a wide, S-shaped curve to the data set that is positioned between the binary classification values of 0 and 1. How close the data point is to the top or bottom of the curve reveals the probability of it belonging to that particular class. Linear regression is designed for continuous outputs and logistic regression algorithms are specific to discrete outputs.

Bayesian theorem and decision tree networks leverage *a priori* information to strengthen decision-making. Bayesian classifiers provide the probability of an event based on the prior probability of that event occurring. The output is the likelihood of a particular class of a new instance based on the feature distributions within each class in the data set. A decision tree is made up of a minimum number of yes/no questions that one has to ask to make a correct decision. Decision trees run data through a series of nodes, with each node representing a condition statement and splitting into a "true" or "false" branch. The branches parse the data set into smaller and smaller sections with the goal of dividing the data into groups corresponding to their labels.

Support vector machine and clustering algorithms categorize objects into one or more classes based on the features. SVM classifiers find a hyperplane (there can be more than two dimensions) that maximizes the distance between data points from two or more classes, such that future data points can be classified with reliable confidence into one of these classes. Clustering is an unsupervised learning technique that segments the data into groups according to patterns within the data. It aims to maximize intergroup differences and minimize intragroup differences. Silhouette scores, which measure how similar points within a cluster are to each other and how different they are from points in other clusters, can be used to assess how well a clustering algorithm performed.

Another application of unsupervised learning is dimension reduction. One of the most common uses of dimensionality reduction is to reduce the complexity of a problem by projecting the feature space to a lower-dimensional space so that less correlated variables are considered in a machine learning system. LDA and PCA are two examples of dimension reduction. PCA finds the directions of maximal variance, whereas LDA attempts to find a feature subspace that maximizes class separability. A key feature of PCA is linear transformation, where a total of k variables, each representing a specific feature, is combined to form a single principal component, such that: $PC_1 = w_1 v_1 + w_2 v_2 + \cdots + w_k v_k$, where w is a weighted value and v corresponds to a specific variable. The goal is to reduce the number of variables into principal components (PCs), where the number of PCs is significantly smaller than k or can be plotted on two or at most three axes.

Another important consideration to reduce overfitting is the process of training and validation as a way to optimize a classification model. The model is initially optimized on a training set, which changes different parameters of the algorithm to minimize the classification error. Once the algorithm has gone through one iteration of training to minimize the classification error on the training set, the algorithm is applied to the validation set to check for the error. This process is repeated until the error on the validation set reaches a minimum. The algorithm is then applied to the test set to demonstrate the algorithm is generalizable to new data. Cross validation is a method in which, through multiple iterations, random samples of the training set are divided into either training or validation portions. The method is used to prevent overfitting on smaller data sets, where having a traditional test set would reduce the size of the training set to a point where it was too small to adequately train the algorithm. Cross validation is typically performed if the sample size is not sufficiently large to have independent training and validation sets.

PROBLEMS

Data Analytics for Classification

1. What is the difference between predictive and prescriptive analytics? How is each relevant in healthcare?
2. A scientist is designing a model that will cluster data based on similarities and differences among the features describing the data set. Which type of machine learning model (supervised, unsupervised, or reinforcement) should they use, and why?
3. Three biomarkers are collected for a patient population that has breast cancer, and the goal is to predict which cancers are going to respond to therapy and which ones are not. A retrospective study is performed on the patients who are already labeled as responders or nonresponders. The goal is to identify which population each of the biomarkers fall into. From clustering analysis, the responders cluster in the first biomarker category, and the nonresponders cluster in the second biomarker category and both responders and nonresponders are equally represented in the third biomarker category. Which biomarker(s) are expected to separate the two groups? Why?

4. In the above example, to further understand the data, additional variables are included, specifically pre-menopausal, post-menopausal, and peri-menopausal status. How many classes or categories are there in the patient group being analyzed?
5. A researcher shows that the amount of sugar, or glucose, in the blood changes the behavior of blood vessels, making them contract more than normal. What type of learning model would you use, supervised or unsupervised?
6. A physician observes that blood pressure by itself is not able to provide any diagnostic information to act upon. In order to make a decision on what action to take, what steps does the physician need to take, or in other words, what is the key information needed to translate observation to action.

Supervised and Unsupervised Learning

7. What method would you use to determine if there is a relationship between blood pressure and blood glucose level? Based on this data, are you able to determine the independent or dependent variable? Why or why not?
8. Using the table below, calculate the SSE and MSE for the data in the case where

$$\hat{y} = 6x + 7,$$
$$\hat{y} = 5.9x + 7.$$

x	1	8	5	3	9	7	4	2	6
y	14	56	36	24	60	48	32	18	42

Which regression line better fits the data in the table? Why?

9. A biomedical engineer is trying to decide whether to use linear or logistic regression to model data on treatment response for patients with pancreatic cancer. They end up performing both linear and logistic regression on the data and find that the SSE is lower for linear than logistic regression. The data provided was of the form 1 if the patient responded and 0 if the patient did not respond. Should the engineer proceed with the linear model because it had a lower error? Explain your reasoning.
10. Patients with cardiovascular disease often experience abnormal heartbeat as one of their symptoms; however, not all people experiencing an abnormal heartbeat have cardiovascular disease. Assume 100 percent of patients with cardiovascular disease have abnormal heartbeat, the prevalence of cardiovascular disease is 1/1,000, and 1/100,000 healthy people experience abnormal heartbeat. What is the probability that a person with an abnormal heartbeat has heart disease?
11. Suppose the below equation defines the hyperplane separating two classes of patients with cervical cancer, where class 1 responds to a novel treatment and class 2 does not respond to a novel treatment. Two features, x_1 and x_2,

are available for each patient. Given the new data below, determine which class each patient falls into if $h = 1$ corresponds to responds to treatment and $h = -1$ corresponds to does not respond to treatment. Suppose the patients are treated based on the recommendation from the SVM classifier and you follow them for response. Clinically, patients 1, 2, 4, 6, 7, and 8 responded to treatment. Calculate the positive predictive value and negative predictive value for the SVM.

$$h(x_i) = +1 \text{ if } w \cdot x + b \geq 0; \text{ and } -1 \text{ if } w \cdot x + b < 0,$$
$$w = (2, -1); x = (x_1, x_2); b = 1.$$

Patient	1	2	3	4	5	6	7	8
x_1	1	-1	-2	3	-3	0	-2	2
x_2	2	2	1	4	-2	2	0	2

12. Could Bayes' theorem be used to cluster data in an unsupervised manner? Why or why not?
13. Tamoxifen is a commonly used hormonal therapy for patients with ER+/PR+ breast cancer. Update the decision tree for diagnosing and treating breast cancer to include treatment with tamoxifen. What is the new maximum depth of the decision tree with the additional nodes?
14. A researcher interested in predicting risk of stroke based on blood pressure and platelet count has collected data from 10 patients and performed k-means clustering with $k = 2$ to see if there might be any clusters within the data. The algorithm divided the patients into two clusters with four patients in cluster 1 and six patients in cluster 2. The researcher wants to determine how well the clustering algorithm performed. Calculate the silhouette scores for patients 3 and 9 in the table below. What do these silhouette scores tell you about how well the clustering algorithm did at assigning each patient to cluster 2?

Patient	1	2	3	4	5	6	7	8	9	10
Blood pressure	155	127	119	143	172	147	133	135	117	126
Platelet count	507	367	457	463	428	306	374	512	324	408
Cluster	1	2	2	1	1	2	2	1	2	2

Dimension Reduction and Generalization

15. A biomedical engineer is performing an analysis on treatment response in patients with cervical cancer. The available data includes tumor volume

following treatment, which ranges from 0.5 to 2 cm diameter; change in white blood cell count in the blood (range: 1,000–13,000 cells per microliter); and age (range: 42–71 years). Suppose the researcher wants to see if the data can be clustered into three groups: responders, nonresponders, and partial responders. How might the different magnitudes of the data for each variable affect a clustering algorithm? How could this be mitigated?

16. A subset of the data from question 15 is shown below. Assuming it is representative of the rest of the data set (i.e., the sample mean and standard deviation are the same as the population mean and standard deviation), perform z-standardization for each data set.

Patient	1	2	3	4	5	6	7	8	9
Tumor volume (cm)	0.5	1.8	1.2	0.7	0.8	1.9	1.3	1.2	1.1
White blood cell count (cells per microliter)	5,000	2,200	12,000	3,300	9,900	11,100	6,700	4,200	8,900
Age	49	58	47	70	64	53	68	52	67

17. A researcher is performing a study using three variables to classify patients as responsive or nonresponsive to a particular therapy. The researcher wishes to reduce the dimensionality to simplify the inputs into their algorithm. Suppose they performed PCA, and found the covariance matrix below. Calculate the eigenvalues and eigenvectors corresponding to the three PCs. What percentage of the variance in the data is described by the first eigenvector? What about the second? Does it seem appropriate to reduce the dimensionality of the data?

$$A = \begin{bmatrix} 2 & 0 & 3 \\ 0 & 1 & 2 \\ 3 & 2 & 3 \end{bmatrix}.$$

18. Using the data from question 16, project the first two PCs using the eigenvectors you found in question 17.

19. What is the purpose of a validation set? What is the purpose of a test? Why is it important to have both?

20. An engineer is designing a machine learning algorithm to classify whether or not a patient with diabetes is at increased risk of heart attack based on clinical characteristics. There are 500 patients available for analysis, so the engineer decides that a cross validation approach is the best way to test their algorithm. The engineer does 5-, 10-, and 15-fold cross validation. The engineer finds that 10-fold had a lower error rate than 5-fold cross validation. Explain why the error rate may be higher for 5-fold than for 10-fold? The same engineer finds that 15-fold validation results in high variability in the validation set. Explain why this occurs?

REFERENCES

GBD. 2019. Human resources for health collaborators. *The Lancet* 399(10341), P2129–2154. https://doi.org/10.1016/S0140-6736(22)00532-3.

Lee, N. T., Resnick, P., & Barton, G. 2019. Algorithmic bias detection and mitigation: best practices and policies to reduce consumer harms [Online]. Available: www.brookings.edu/articles/algorithmic-bias-detection-and-mitigation-best-practices-and-policies-to-reduce-consumer-harms (accessed April 16, 2024).

Martignon, L., Vitouch, O., Takezawa, M., & Forster, M. R., 2003. Naive and yet enlightened: From natural frequencies to fast and frugal decision trees. In Hardman, D., & Macchi, L., (eds), *Thinking: Psychological Perspectives on Reasoning, Judgment and Decision Making*. Wiley, Chichester.

Myszczynska, M. A., Ojamies, P. N., Lacoste, A. M., et al. 2020. Applications of machine learning to diagnosis and treatment of neurodegenerative diseases. *Nature Reviews Neurology*, 16, 440–456. https://doi.org/10.1038/s41582-020-0377-8.

Peiffer-Smadja, N., Rawson, T. M., Ahmad, R., et al. 2020. Machine learning for clinical decision support in infectious diseases: a narrative review of current applications. *Clinical Microbiology and Infection*, 26, 584–595.

Qayyum, R. 2020. A roadmap towards big data opportunities, emerging issues and Hadoop as a solution. *International Journal of Education and Management Engineering*, 10, 8–17.

Toh, T. S., Dondelinger, F., & Wang, D. 2019. Looking beyond the hype: applied AI and machine learning in translational medicine. *EBioMedicine*, 47, 607–615.

Yu, C., Liu, J., & Nemati, S. 2019. Reinforcement learning in healthcare: a survey. *arXiv preprint arXiv:1908.08796*.

9 Deep Learning

The last chapter focused on the use of analytical methods that rely on feature extraction or selection. These techniques provide a variety of ways in which to analyze and interpret data, whether it be continuous or discrete. These models are particularly useful when attempting to see important patterns in the data and/or classify data from a small sample size. Other attributes of these approaches are that the results are mostly explainable, and these algorithms can be trained relatively quickly. These classification methods, specifically machine learning algorithms such as support vector machine (SVM), fall under the broader umbrella of machine learning. This family of algorithms also encompasses artificial neural networks (ANNs) and convolution neural networks (CNNs), both of which belong to the family of **deep learning**.

Why is deep learning important? The analytical methods described in the previous chapter are appropriate when the sample size is manageable (hundreds of samples). However, as the sample size increases to tens of thousands, alternative classification techniques – such as ANNs and CNNs – can provide advantages over traditional machine learning algorithms. An ANN is a digital web of processing nodes that receive and pass signals to each other, much like neurons in the biological brain. The nodes and signals are optimized during the training process to obtain the desired output from the network. A CNN is a type of ANN that excels in processing images because it preserves spatial features within the image inputs. Deep learning algorithms learn by examples; therefore, the availability of very large data sets opens the door for development of image interpretation, personalized diagnostic and prognostic tools, and advanced clinical support.

Figure 9.1 shows the growth in machine learning use since 2010 and the different data types being used for information (Alloghani et al., 2019). Applications of deep learning to diagnostic imaging and genetic data far exceed those in other areas. Deep learning benefits from a large amount of data to learn from. Therefore, leveraging existing data rather than waiting to amass new information can lead to "ready to use" algorithms. There is a tremendous amount of imaging and genetic databases that already exist. Therefore, predictive and diagnostic analysis can immediately benefit from these data analytics methods.

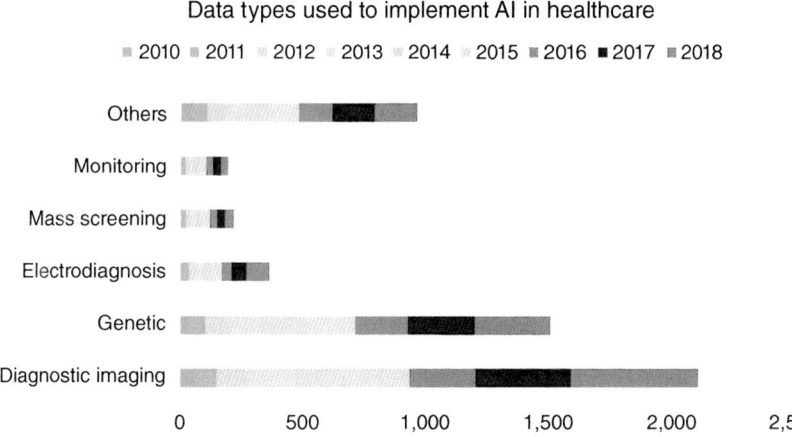

Figure 9.1
The growth in machine learning use since 2010 and the different data types that are being used for information (Alloghani et al., 2019). Applications of deep learning to diagnostic imaging and genetic data far exceed those in other areas.
Source: Alloghani et al. (2020)

Large data sets of breast mammograms exist owing to the fact that this is a widely used screening tool and has been used for decades. In a recent breast cancer screening study, more than one million breast mammograms were each read by 14 radiologists and a deep learning algorithm. The results showed that a hybrid model combining the diagnosis averaged across the 14 radiologists *and* the algorithm was superior to that of either approach alone. In this particular example, information content generated by the radiologists and the algorithm was synergistic.

Another area where vast amounts of data can be mined for diagnostics is genomics. A deep algorithm called the DeepVariant (Poplin et al., 2018) has been created by Google. DeepVariant reconstructs the true genome sequence from high throughput sequencing data with significantly greater accuracy than previously used methods. The idea behind DeepVariant is to identify anomalies in genetic data that can be used for a variety of applications, including diagnosis and treatment. DeepVariant provides deep learning-based genomics tools to the community with the broader goal of making this technology accessible for solving both healthcare and scientific problems (Poplin et al., 2018).

Deep learning can also be used to continuously collect and analyze data about an individual, such as the amount of physical activity and heart rate. An FDA-cleared electro-diagnosis sensor can measure electrical waves in real time from an individual, and can then indicate conditions such as atrial fibrillation. The sensor can then alert the need for an intervention for health conditions that need immediate attention. Another example is population health screening. For example, a smartphone app that collected activity tracker data, as well as self-reported symptoms, can differentiate COVID-19 positive versus negative cases in symptomatic individuals, where the actual diagnosis was used as the gold standard (Quer et al., 2021).

LEARNING OBJECTIVES

Artificial Neural Networks
- Key components of an ANN;
- the function of a neuron and the relationship between neurons and layers;
- the process by which gradient descent algorithms work for optimizing ANN error.

Convolutional Neural Networks
- Differences between a CNN and conventional machine learning algorithms;
- the architecture of a CNN;
- the understanding and calculation of convolution, pooling, and flattening.

Algorithm Bias
- The effect of bias and variance errors on the performance and generalizability of a CNN;
- the components of the network that can be modified for reducing bias and variance error;
- different technologies to generalize a model that is overtrained.

Artificial Neural Networks

Artificial neural networks are computer models of human neural network structures that can learn and render intelligent decisions on their own. Figure 9.2 shows the key components of an ANN. They consist of five components: an **input layer**, **hidden layers**, an **output layer**, and two propagation functions – forward and backward – to optimize the network. A **layer** is a collection of nodes that perform parallel processing on the data. **Forward propagation** delivers the "predicted value" and **backward propagation** delivers the "error value" to optimize the network.

The input layer, as the name suggests, receives the inputs for the algorithm; the inputs are typically all of the variables in the original data set. The output layer provides the classification result. The hidden layer(s) are termed as such because they do not directly "see" the inputs or outputs. There can be more than one hidden layer. The more layers in the network, the deeper and more complex the network is. During forward propagation, the ANN is trained by mapping the relationship between the input data and the output. Once the model has produced an output, back propagation is used to compare the predicted output against the given target output and a loss function is computed. The **loss function** is the main driver of a neural network, which works to minimize the loss, or error. During training,

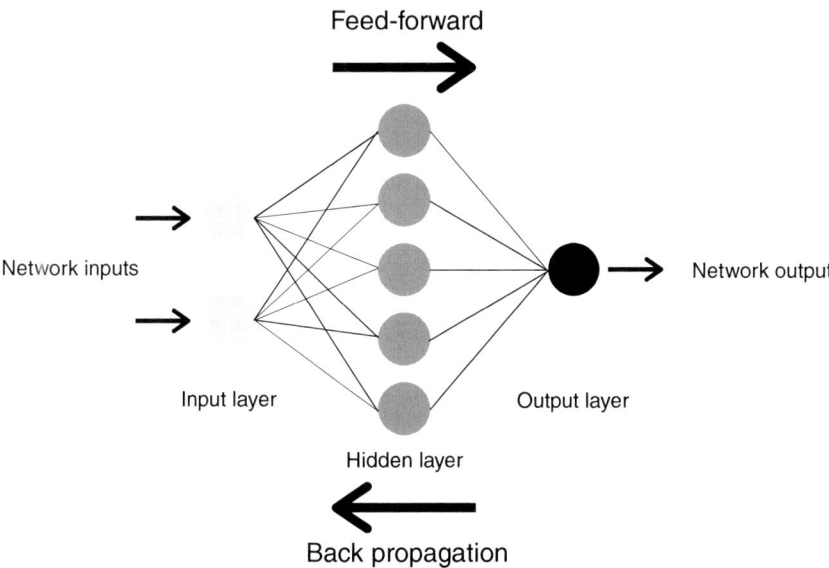

Figure 9.2 Key components of an artificial neural network. ANNs consist of three components: an input **layer**, hidden **layers**, an output **layer**, and two propagation functions to optimize the network. A **layer** is a collection of nodes that perform parallel processing on the data. **Forward propagation** delivers the "predicted value" and **backward propagation** delivers the "error value" to optimize the network.
Source: Based on Santhana Krishnan and Palanisamy (2021).

the ANN will adjust the weights for each connection within the network based on the results of the loss function to generate an updated output through an iterative process so that it now outputs a result closer to the target output.

Figure 9.3 shows the process through which the value of each node is calculated. A node is the sum of the product of each input (X_1 to X_m ...) multiplied by the corresponding weight (w_1 to w_m ...). In addition, a bias term is added $(1 \times w_o)$, where w_o has the effect of shifting the activation function by a constant amount. The sum is then passed into an activation function to determine the output of the neuron. An activation function takes the sum of the node's inputs and converts the sum into an output value for the node. An activation function is the mathematical function that adds nonlinearity to the network. The most basic activation function is the identify function, shown in Equation 9.1, which simply sets the output, $f(x)$, equal to the input, x. With an identify function, the equation of the line has a slope of 1 and goes through the origin. The output could be binary (e.g., 0 or 1) or continuous. If the output is continuous, it can be bounded (e.g., continuous along the interval 0 to 1) or unbounded (e.g., from negative infinity to infinity):

Artificial Neural Networks

$f(x) = x$
(see illustration on right).

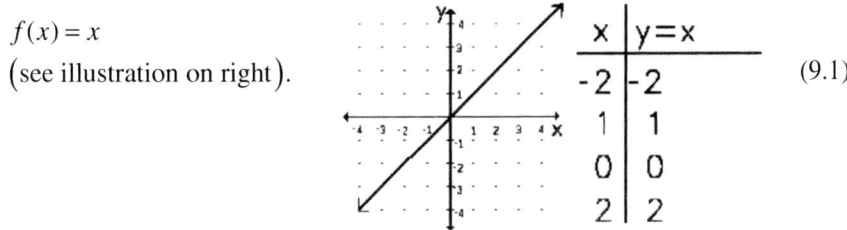

(9.1)

Figure 9.4 shows an example of a network with six nodes and three layers. Nodes 1 and 2 are in the input layer and receive the inputs to the network. Nodes 3–5 are in the hidden layer and receive inputs from N1 and N2 after they have been manipulated by weighting factors (labeled W) W1–W6. Node 6 is the output layer and receives inputs from N3–N5 after they have been manipulated by weighting factors W7–W9. Using the identity activation function (i.e., output = input), the inputs to N3, N4, and N5 can be represented as:

$$N3 = W1 \times N1 + W2 \times N2,$$
$$N4 = W3 \times N1 + W4 \times N2,$$
$$N5 = W5 \times N1 + W6 \times N2.$$

The same process can be applied to N6 to calculate the overall output of the network in terms of the nodes in the hidden layer:

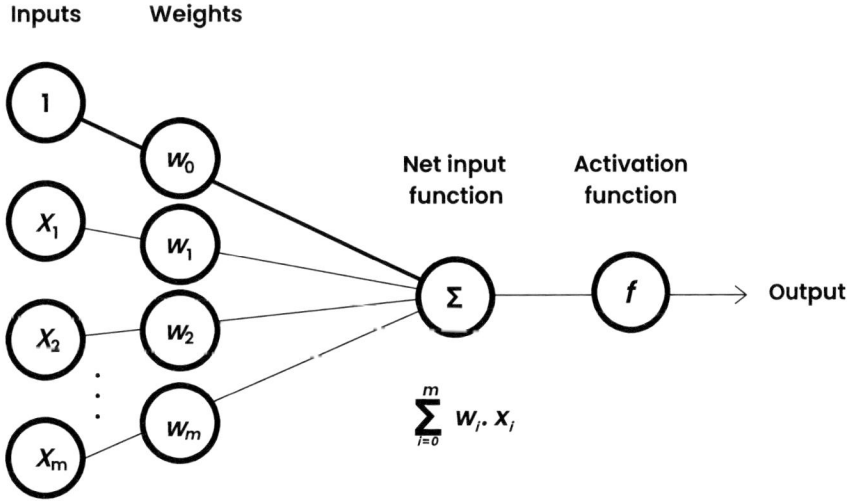

Figure 9.3 The process through which the value of each node is calculated. A node is the sum of the product of each input (X_1 to X_m ...) multiplied by the corresponding weight (w_1 to w_m ...). In addition, a bias term is added ($1 \times w_0$), where w_0 has the effect of shifting the activation function by a constant amount. The sum is then passed into an activation function to determine the output of the neuron. An activation function takes the sum of the node's inputs and converts the sum into an output value for the node.

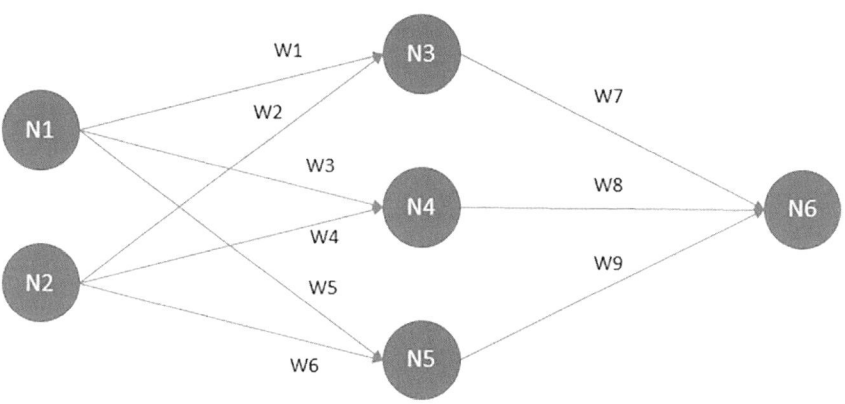

Figure 9.4 Example of a network with six nodes and three layers. Nodes 1 and 2 are in the input layer and receive the inputs to the network. Nodes 3–5 are in the hidden layer and receive inputs from N1 and N2 after they have been manipulated by weighting factors (labeled W) W1–W6. Node 6 is the output layer and receives inputs from N3–N5 after they have been manipulated by weighting factors W7–W9.

$$N6 = W7 \times N3 + W8 \times N4 + W9 \times N5.$$

Substituting in for the equations representing N3–N5 gives the final equation for the entire network, relating the inputs to the outputs as Equation 9.2:

$$N6 = W7 \times (W1 \times N1 + W2 \times N2) + W8 \\ \times (W3 \times N1 + W4 \times N2) + W9 \times (W5 \times N1 + W6 \times N2). \quad (9.2)$$

Example: Calculating the Output for an Eight-Node, Four-Layer Network

Question: A researcher is developing an ANN that receives three inputs (age, systolic blood pressure, and diastolic blood pressure) to determine whether blood pressure medication should be administered to lower the risk of heart disease. Based on the diagram of the network in Figure 9.5), determine the equation that calculates the output of the network based on the inputs. Assume an identity activation function is used.

Answer: In order to calculate the output value, in this case N8, we first need to determine the equations for the nodes within the hidden layers (N4–N5 and N6–N7). Beginning with the first hidden layer, we can determine the equations for N4 and N5 as the sum of the inputs multiplied by their respective weights:

$$N4 = W1 \times N1 + W2 \times N2, \\ N5 = W3 \times N2 + W4 \times N3.$$

Next, we can determine the equations for N6 and N7 as the sum of the outputs from N4 and N5 multiplied by their respective weights:

Artificial Neural Networks

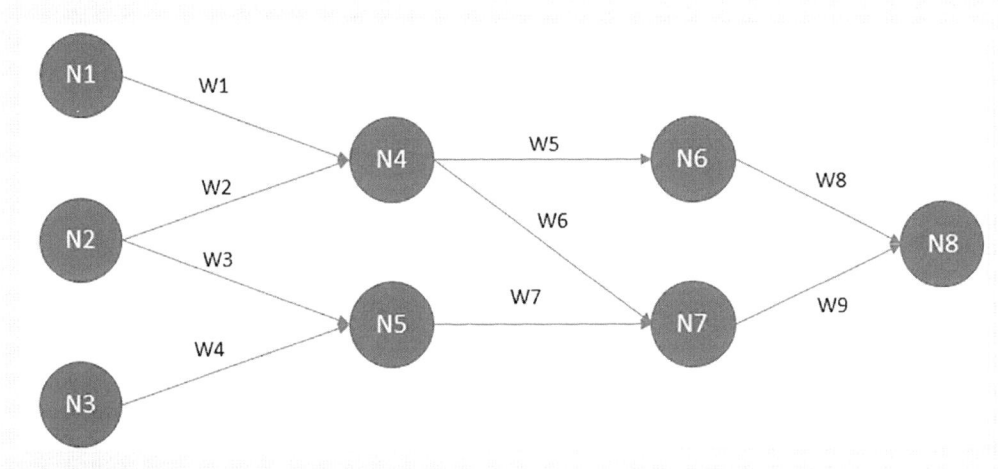

Figure 9.5 Example ANN with inputs age, systolic blood pressure, and diastolic blood pressure.

$$N6 = W5 \times N4,$$
$$N7 = W6 \times N4 + W7 \times N5.$$

Plugging in the equations for N4 and N5 will give N6 and N7 in terms of the input:

$$N6 = W5 \times (W1 \times N1 + W2 \times N2),$$
$$N7 = W6 \times (W1 \times N1 + W2 \times N2) + W7 \times (W3 \times N2 + W4 \times N3).$$

Now we are ready to determine the equation for the output in terms of the second hidden layer nodes (N6–N7):

$$N8 = W8 \times N6 + W9 \times N7.$$

Plugging in for N6 and N7 gives the final equation relating inputs to output:

$$N8 = W8 \times \left[W5 \times (W1 \times N1 + W2 \times N2)\right] + W9$$
$$\times \left[W6 \times (W1 \times N1 + W2 \times N2) + W7 \times (W3 \times N2 + W4 \times N3)\right].$$

As you can see, when the **identity activation function** is used the relationship between the input and output variables is a simple linear transformation (Equation 9.2). While a linear transformation is still a useful implementation of an ANN, more complex activation functions can help solve nonlinear problems. A second activation function is the **Heaviside step function**, which is similar to a biological neuron firing, as shown in Equation 9.3. It is a simple classification function where the class is either 1 or 0, determined by $f(x)$, which is 0 if $x < 0$ and 1 otherwise. The final activation function we will cover is a **logistic function**, which offers a continuous range of outputs between 0 and 1, and is defined by Equation 9.4. While there are numerous other activation functions, the three provided here give a flavor of the main types: (1) identity function that has a continuous output that spans $(-\infty, \infty)$; (2) the Heaviside step function with a binary output of $\{0,1\}$; and (3) a logistic function with a continuous output that spans $(0,1)$. If the ANN is developed to solve a regression problem, the output may be continuous, in which case an output from a single node along a continuum might make the most sense. If the goal of the network is to perform classification, then one or more output nodes could be used. In the case of a single node, a function would be needed to determine the class.

$$f(x) = \begin{cases} 1, & x \geq 0 \\ 0, & x < 0 \end{cases}, \tag{9.3}$$

$$f(x) = \frac{1}{1 + e^{-x}}. \tag{9.4}$$

Example: Determining the Type of Output (Continuous or Binary) and the Activation Function Needed

Question: A researcher is interested in predicting the price of future cancer drugs based on historical data. The data available to them for training includes the type of drug (e.g., chemotherapy, hormone therapy, etc.), the year, and the price. Given this information, how many inputs would they use in their ANN? How many outputs? What type of problem are they solving?

Answer: The researcher has three pieces of data available for training: (1) drug type, (2) year, and (3) price. The ANN would have two inputs, drug type and year, since the goal is to predict the price. The ANN would have one output, the predicted price. Because the output is continuous, the ANN is solving a regression problem and would use an identity activation function.

Now that we have examined how the outputs of an ANN can be used for linear regression, logistic regression, or classification, we will cover how training is performed. There are two important components to training an ANN, as mentioned previously: (1) a method for updating the weights within the network, which aims to reduce the network error; and (2) the loss function, which determines the network error. We will cover methods for updating the algorithm weights first.

An ANN can be thought of as an optimization problem, where the ANN seeks to optimize a set of weights so that the error in output from the algorithm is minimized. It is important to understand the loss function before understanding how the network error is introduced. In Figures 9.3 and 9.4, the weights of the nodes in a given layer are important in determining the values of the nodes in the next layer. If all of the training data are run through the ANN algorithm – say, the first time – an error needs to be determined to inform the network that further optimization of the weights is needed. An ANN uses a loss function to determine the error.

The most frequently used loss functions for ANNs fall under the umbrella of maximum likelihood estimation. The goal of **maximum likelihood estimation** is to determine how similar two distributions are to one another. The two distributions being compared are (1) the distribution of outputs (classes, for example) from the ANN based on the training data; and (2) the ground truth distribution of outputs of the training data. The exact method for comparing the two distributions is the **loss function**, which is also referred to as the cost function. For classification applications the most commonly used loss function is cross entropy, also referred to as logarithmic loss. The details of calculating cross entropy are beyond the scope of this book. For regression applications, the most commonly used loss function is **root mean squared error** (RMSE). It is shown here in Equation 9.5, where $\hat{y}$ is the predicted values, y is the observed values, and n is the number of observations; this can also be referred to as **mean square error** (MSE), where the square root sign is removed:

$$\text{RMSE} = \sqrt{\sum_{i=1}^{n} \frac{(\hat{y}_i - y_i)^2}{n}}. \quad (9.5)$$

Referring back to Figure 9.3, we will walk through how to identify the weights that minimize the error between the predicted and expected output. Figure 9.6 shows an example of a 3D plot of an ANN output error as a function of the ANN weights. Consider the case where there are two weights, W1 and W2, that are used in an ANN. The error (e.g., RMSE) can be plotted as a function of the two weights and may resemble the 3D plot shown in Figure 9.6. The goal of the ANN is to find the global minimum, where the error is the lowest; however, as you can see, there are multiple local minima that the algorithm could falsely identify as the global minimum. As a result, ANNs typically use a gradient descent algorithm to find the global minimum.

Detailed explanation of stochastic gradient descent: First, it is instructive to discuss the **gradient descent algorithm**. There are two basic values that a gradient descent algorithm uses while finding the minimum – the error for the two weights, W1 and W2, and the corresponding slope (gradient). For Figure 9.6 this means that the entire training data would be run through the ANN algorithm, for all possible weight combinations, W1 and W2, and the resulting error and gradient would be calculated. Beginning with the weight combination with the steepest gradient, the weights can be iteratively updated in small increments to reach the global minimum. Equation 9.6 shows how the weights are updated in a gradient descent algorithm (a visual representation of the gradient descent path is shown in Figure 9.6):

$$W_x' = W_x - a \frac{\partial Error}{\partial W_x}. \quad (9.6)$$

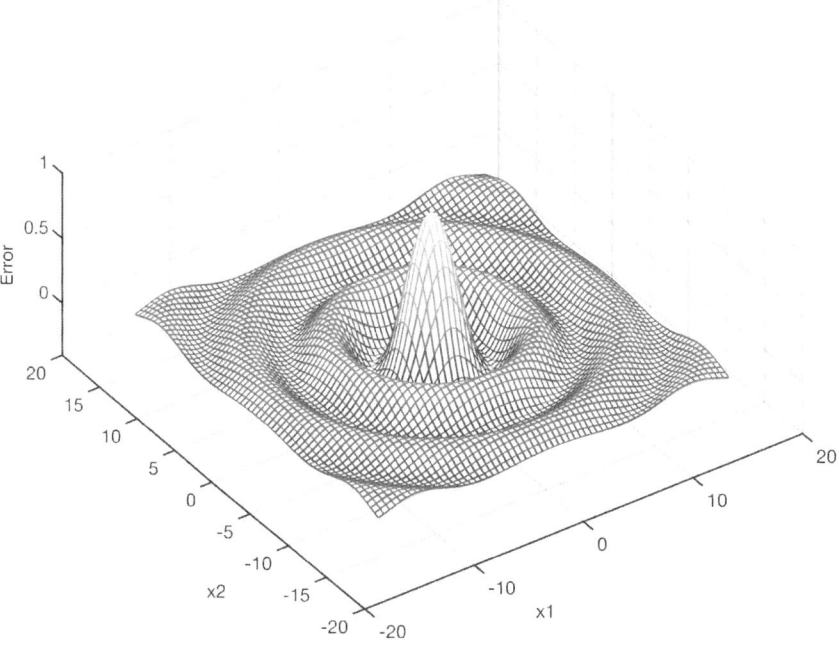

Figure 9.6 Example of a 3D plot of an ANN output error as a function of the ANN weights. Consider the case where there are two weights, W1 and W2, that are used in an ANN. The error can be plotted as a function of the two weights and may look something like the 3D plot shown here. The goal of the ANN is to find the global minimum, where the error is the lowest; however, as you can see, there are multiple local minima that the algorithm could falsely identify as the global minimum. As a result, ANNs typically use a gradient descent algorithm to find the global minimum.

where $W_{1,2}$ are the initial weights, $W'_{1,2}$ are the new weights, and a is the learning rate, or the step size for each iteration of the descent. The third component is the derivative of error or loss with respect to the old weight

While gradient descent might be feasible for a small number of weights, ANNs can contain hundreds of layers and nodes, which would make it impractical to calculate the values and gradients for all possible combinations of weight values. Stochastic gradient descent reduces this computational burden. Figure 9.7 shows a conceptual representation of both the gradient descent and stochastic gradient descent error minimization approach. For a given weight combination, both approaches calculate the error output from the algorithm and the "steepest" downward direction (akin to walking down a mountain and always moving in the steepest direction). The process begins with an arbitrary weight and repeatedly modifies it in small steps (learning rate) to reach the minimum. The gradient descent updates the weight after summing over errors of all of the training samples. Stochastic gradient updates the weight incrementally, after calculating the error for each individual training sample.

A frequently used alternative approach is to break the training data into smaller batches. In the case of batches, the algorithm would shift the weights

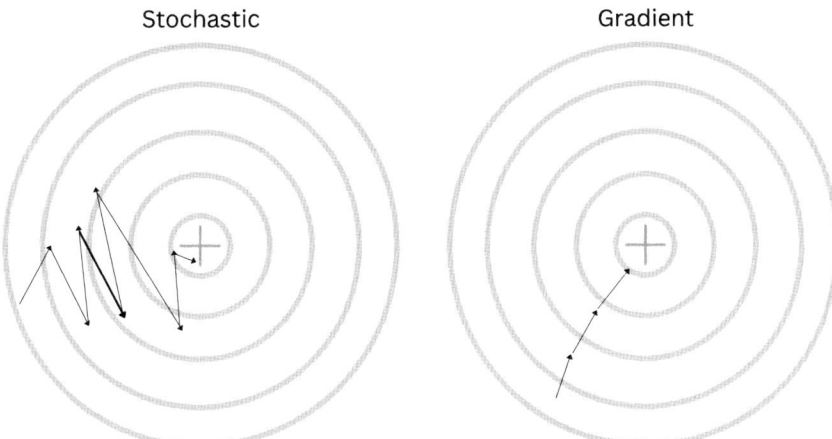

Figure 9.7 Conceptual representation of both the gradient descent and stochastic gradient descent error minimization approach. For a given weight combination, both approaches calculate the error output from the algorithm and the "steepest" downward direction (akin to walking down a mountain and always moving in the steepest direction).

after calculating the error on the first batch, calculate the error on the second batch, and move forward to the third batch with either the first or second set of weights, depending on which resulted in a lower error. Using the batch approach may help the algorithm find the minimum faster and with fewer iterations through the training data. The efficiency of this approach is intermediate between gradient and stochastic gradient descent.

Example: Determining which Optimization Algorithm to Use

Question: When developing an ANN to predict tumor volume following therapy, the engineer is trying to decide whether to use a stochastic or maximum gradient descent algorithm. They decide to train the algorithm on a small number of samples first to see which method seems to be performing better before training on all samples. They get the following outputs compared to ground truth:

Ground truth	Stochastic output	Maximum output
35 mm	37 mm	36 mm
18 mm	15 mm	17 mm
54 mm	49 mm	59 mm
23 mm	24 mm	19 mm
42 mm	44 mm	40 mm

Calculate the RMSE for each method. Which one should the engineer continue with?

Answer: The RMSE can be calculated by plugging the results into Equation 9.5 for each method:

$$\text{RMSE}_{\text{Stochastic}} = \sqrt{\frac{(35-37)^2 + (18-15)^2 + (54-49)^2 + (23-24)^2 + (42-44)^2}{5}}$$
$$= 2.9,$$

$$\text{RMSE}_{\text{Maximum}} = \sqrt{\frac{(35-36)^2 + (18-17)^2 + (54-59)^2 + (23-19)^2 + (42-40)^2}{5}}$$
$$= 3.1.$$

Because the RMSE is lower for stochastic gradient descent, the engineer should proceed with that algorithm.

In summary, ANNs use a branching structure of nodes and weights to convert inputs into a desired output, whether that be for classification or regression. The output of each node is determined based on an activation function, which is chosen by the algorithm designer. Activation functions can have continuous or binary outputs. ANNs are trained using stochastic gradient descent algorithms to reduce computational burden when updating weights. The error of the algorithm is typically calculated using a maximum likelihood estimation with a cross entropy loss function for classification applications or MSE for regression applications.

Deeper Look: Perceptron – It Is Not a Perception

The neural network is composed of multiple neurons connected via synapses (which are basically weighted inputs). Figure 9.8 shows an actual neuron and a neuron from a neural network. There is a striking similarity between the structure of each. In fact, the birth of the neural network was inspired by the neuron in the brain. In a real neuron, the dendrites serve as the portion of the neuron that accepts multiple "input" signals; through the cell body and the axon it outputs through the terminal axon. In a single layer of a neural network, multiple inputs are processed through a function to output a value or set of values. The involvement of synapses in both cases is very similar. This basic structure of a neuron in a network is called the perceptron. The idea was conceived by two psychologists – McCulloch and Pitts – in 1943, and was first implemented as a mathematical model in 1958 by Frank Rosenblatt, funded by the United States Office of Naval Research.

Convolutional Neural Networks

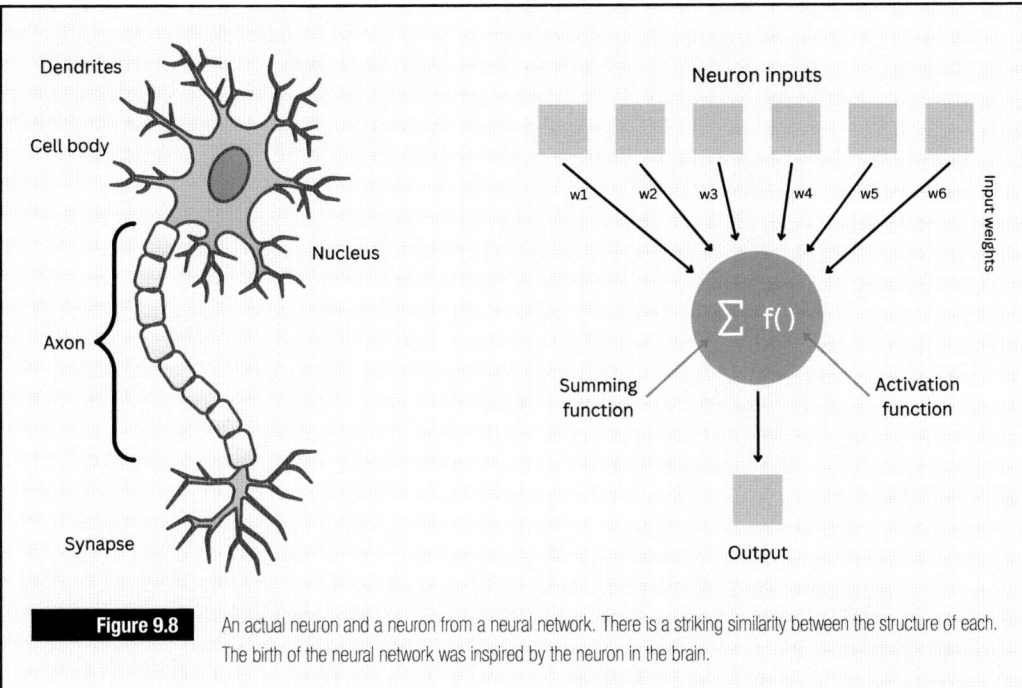

Figure 9.8 An actual neuron and a neuron from a neural network. There is a striking similarity between the structure of each. The birth of the neural network was inspired by the neuron in the brain.

The perceptron takes a set of binary inputs (nearby neurons), multiplies each input by a continuous valued weight (the synapse strength to each nearby neuron), and thresholds the sum of these weighted inputs to assign the output as 1 if the sum exceeds a certain threshold; otherwise it assigns it 0, in the same way that neurons either fire or do not fire. Perceptrons also have a "bias" input, which has a value of 1 and basically ensures that more functions are computable with the same input by being able to offset the summed value.

Skeptics insisted that the perceptron was incapable of reshaping the relationship between human and machine. Specifically, another renowned researcher, Marvin Minsky, argued that the perceptron is a function and therefore far too simple to do the equivalent to the task of a neuron. The problem was not that it was too simple; Rosenblatt's perceptron had only one layer, while modern neural networks have millions. Today, perceptrons can be viewed as the building blocks of a single layer of a neural network.

Convolutional Neural Networks

Artificial neural networks are useful for classifying data with defined features that can be input into a node, such as blood pressure, heart rate, and age. But what if the features for classification are contained within an image instead? Neural networks can still be used in this case; however, this requires a special type of network, referred to as a **convolutional neural network**. A CNN is a deep learning algorithm that exploits the local connectivity between spatial locations in an input image to greatly reduce the number of learnable parameters, enabling the network to use upwards of hundreds of thousands of input pixels.

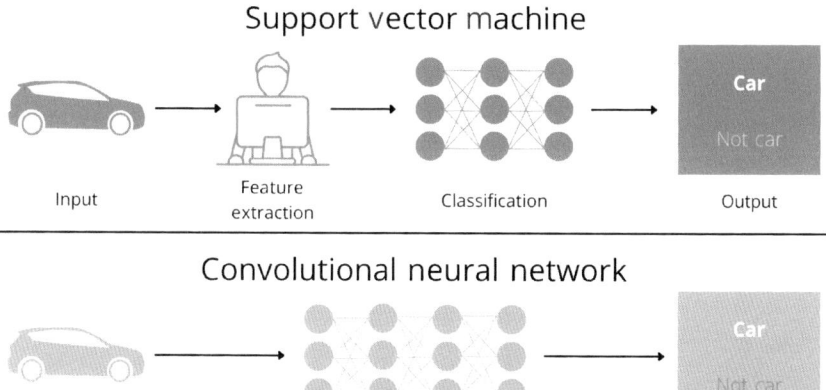

Figure 9.9 Comparison between an SVM and a CNN for identifying a car. Traditional machine learning techniques, such as an SVM, require a step between image acquisition and input into the classifier to extract features that can be used for classification. On the other hand, the CNN will correctly classify an image of a car based on a large number of examples of images of cars.

Figure 9.9 shows a comparison between an SVM and a CNN for identifying a car. Traditional machine learning techniques, such as an SVM, require a step between image acquisition and input into the classifier to extract features that can be used for classification. On the other hand, the CNN will correctly classify an image of a car based on a large number of examples of images of cars. Traditional machine learning is similar to the case where an individual looks at an image of a car to identify its defining features. The person has a general idea of the shape and sizes of different features, such as the windows, headlights, and wheels. The individual uses prior knowledge based on these features to discern a car from a tree, for example. CNNs, on the other hand, do not require this *a priori* feature identification. In an ideal scenario, the CNN operates as the person, looking at an image of the car. However, this requires that CNNs are trained with large amounts of data.

The basic architecture of a CNN consists of three main layers, as listed below. A detailed explanation will follow this summary.

- **Convolutional layer:** This layer consists of filters and feature maps. Filters carry the input weights according to that output value and the feature map is the output according to the weight applied on the filter.
- **Pooling layers:** The basic work of the pooling layer is to downsample the feature map.
- **Fully connected layer:** This is a conventional feed-forward neural network, which consists of an activation function in order to make predictions.

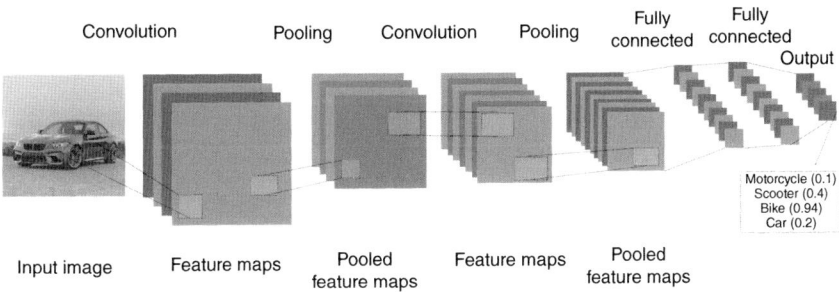

Figure 9.10 Example of the basic architecture of a CNN. The CNN uses the steps of convolution and pooling to generate feature maps from which the general features can be recognized in future unknown images, which is achieved with a standard ANN, represented by fully connected layers.

Figure 9.10 shows an example of the basic architecture of a CNN. The CNN uses the steps of convolution and pooling to generate feature maps from which the general features can be recognized in future unknown images, which is achieved with a standard ANN, represented by fully connected layers. The first step in the CNN is a series of transformations to the image using convolution. Convolution is the simple application of a filter to an input. Repeated application of the same filter to an input results in a feature map, indicating the location and strength of a detected feature in an input, such as an image. To limit the computational burden, a process called pooling is performed after convolution to reduce the size of the output image. **Pooling** is a technique for generalizing features extracted by convolutional filters and helping the network recognize features independent of their location in the image. The process of performing convolution and pooling can be performed multiple times to convert the original image into a finite number of distinct features, which can then be input into a more traditional ANN for classification. The ANN step is represented by the fully connected layers leading to an output. Each of these steps will be described in greater detail below.

The first several layers of the network are responsible for extracting primitive features, such as edges or big color blocks of the car. The deeper layers resolve more complex features such as the person driving the car. To reduce extraneous information in the input image, the image can be cropped to provide the network with only the relevant information. For example, if there is both a tree and a car in the image, the cropping step can remove the tree from the image before running it through a car classification CNN. There are **object detection** networks that can automatically create a box around the object of interest. Training a CNN to create the bounding box requires training on a large number of images containing the bounding box coordinates of the car as labels, similar to the images and ground truth labels that are required when training a network to classify an image of a car. As more layers are added to the CNN, more and more complex features can be discerned. For example, with enough layers, all of the characteristics to replicate the original image can be accounted for. The more data that can be incorporated into a CNN, the more accurate the output will be, akin to the case where a less experienced healthcare provider can learn from the experts and over time can become a surrogate expert.

Detailed explanation of convolution: In a CNN, the convolution uses a filter or **kernel**, a matrix that is used in a convolution to extract features or information from an input image. The output image can be referred to as a **feature map**. Figure 9.11 shows an example of a 2D convolution. In the case shown here, an input image with five rows and five columns (i.e., a 5 × 5 image) is being convolved with a 3 × 3 kernel. The convolution is performed by superimposing the kernel on top of the image and multiplying each pixel in the image by the superimposed pixel from the kernel. For a 3 × 3 kernel, this would mean nine multiplications. The resulting multiplications are then summed to determine the output value. The kernel is then moved one pixel to the right and the process is repeated until the kernel has been shifted through every pixel in the image. Because the output at each step in the convolution is a single value, the resulting image or feature map is the same size as the input image. The **stride** is the size of the step that the convolution filter moves each time. A stride size is usually 1, meaning the filter slides pixel by pixel. By increasing the stride size, the filter slides over the input image in larger intervals and thus has less overlap between the cells in the image matrix. This entire process is repeated for each kernel (if there is more than one) and the number of output images is equivalent to the number of kernels. This entire convolution process can be represented mathematically as shown in Equation 9.7, where $f[n]$ is the input image and $g[n]$ is the kernel:

$$f[n] \times g[n] = \sum_{m=-\infty}^{\infty} f[n]g[m-n] \qquad (9.7)$$

In Figure 9.11, when the 3×3 kernel matrix is centered on the pixel (pixel value of 75) located at the intersection of the second row and column, all pixels of the kernel are within the input image. What would happen, however, when the kernel is placed so the center pixel in the kernel aligns with the top left-most pixel in the input image (pixel value of 0)? In this case, only four of the pixels in the kernel would overlap with pixels in the input image. To accommodate this, the input image can be padded by adding rows and columns to the ends of the image. Frequently the padded rows and columns consist of zeros (called zero padding).

Convolutional Neural Networks

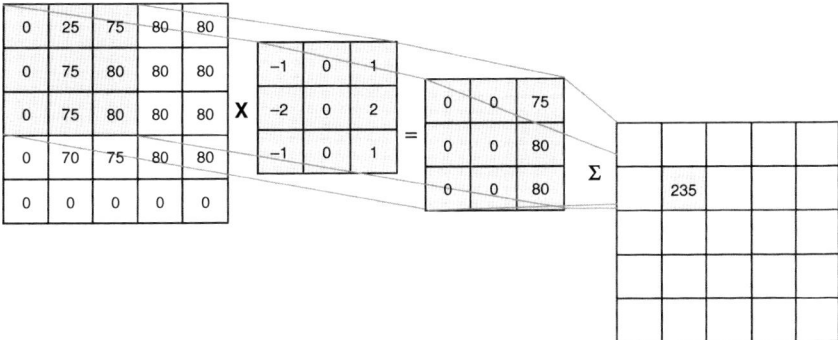

Figure 9.11 An example of a 2D convolution. In the case shown here, an image with five rows and five columns (i.e., a 5 × 5 image) is being convolved with a 3 × 3 kernel. The convolution is performed by superimposing the kernel on top of the image and multiplying each pixel in the image by the superimposed pixel from the kernel. For a 3 × 3 kernel, this would mean nine multiplications. The resulting multiplications are then summed to determine the output value. The kernel is then moved one pixel to the right and the process is repeated until the kernel has been shifted through every pixel in the image. Because the output at each step in the convolution is a single value, the resulting image or feature map is the same size as the input image.

Example: Calculation of Convolution

Question: A biomedical researcher is developing a CNN that will look at lung X-rays to determine whether or not a tumor is present. A representative 5 × 5 sample of the image is shown below. One of the convolutional layers is designed to extract vertical edges within the image using the 3 × 3 Prewitt kernel below. Calculate the resulting output values after applying the Prewitt kernel centered over pixel locations (1,1) and (3,3) of the input image, using zero padding where needed:

$$\text{Image} = \begin{bmatrix} 10 & 11 & 18 & 14 & 20 \\ 17 & 21 & 20 & 25 & 23 \\ 85 & 110 & 120 & 90 & 113 \\ 131 & 87 & 108 & 124 & 79 \\ 111 & 133 & 93 & 103 & 127 \end{bmatrix},$$

$$\text{Kernel} = \begin{bmatrix} -1 & 0 & 1 \\ -1 & 0 & 1 \\ -1 & 0 & 1 \end{bmatrix}.$$

Answer: Begin by creating the appropriate sub-image with zero padding:

$$\text{Sub-image} = \begin{bmatrix} 0 & 0 & 0 \\ 0 & 10 & 17 \\ 0 & 11 & 21 \end{bmatrix}.$$

Next, multiply the kernel by the sub-image pixel by pixel:

$$\text{Kernel} \times \text{sub-image} = \begin{bmatrix} -1\times 0 & 0\times 0 & 1\times 0 \\ -1\times 0 & 0\times 10 & 1\times 17 \\ -1\times 0 & 0\times 11 & 1\times 21 \end{bmatrix}$$

$$= \begin{bmatrix} 0 & 0 & 0 \\ 0 & 0 & 17 \\ 0 & 0 & 21 \end{bmatrix},$$

Finally, sum all of the resulting values to get the output:
$$\text{Output} = 17 + 21$$
$$= 38.$$

Now we will repeat the process for (3, 3), beginning by creating the appropriate sub-image. No zero padding is required in this case:

$$\text{Sub-image} = \begin{bmatrix} 21 & 90 & 113 \\ 20 & 87 & 108 \\ 25 & 79 & 111 \end{bmatrix}.$$

Next, multiply the kernel by the sub-image pixel by pixel:

$$\text{Kernel} \times \text{sub-image} = \begin{bmatrix} -1\times 21 & 0\times 90 & 1\times 113 \\ -1\times 20 & 0\times 87 & 1\times 108 \\ -1\times 25 & 0\times 79 & 1\times 111 \end{bmatrix}$$

$$= \begin{bmatrix} -21 & 0 & 113 \\ -20 & 0 & 108 \\ -25 & 0 & 111 \end{bmatrix}.$$

Finally, sum all of the resulting values to get the output:
$$\text{Output} = -21 - 20 - 25 + 113 + 108 + 111$$
$$= 26$$

The final output value is 26. In general, the higher the output value, the more likely it is that there is an edge. Since tumors would have sharp border edges, anywhere that there are strong responses to the kernel could indicate the presence of a tumor.

Detailed explanation of pooling: Now that we have discussed convolution, we will talk about pooling. The pooling step compresses the size of each feature map to accomplish two goals: (1) reduce the size of the feature map to improve computational efficiency; and (2) distill each feature map down to the most critical information. There are typically two different types of pooling methods: average pooling and maximum pooling. Figure 9.12 illustrates the difference between average and maximum pooling. A 4×4 image is divided into four 2×2 sub-images as represented by the grid. Maximum pooling condenses the 4×4 image into a 2×2 image by selecting the maximum value within each of the sub-images. Average pooling accomplishes the same reduction in size by taking the average of all pixels of each sub-image as a single value. As you can see, the two pooling methods result in different outputs with different trends. For example,

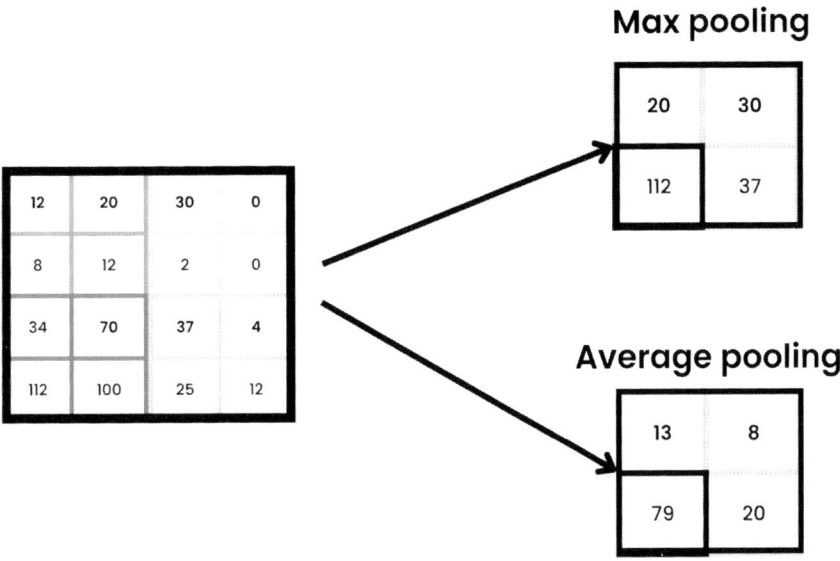

Figure 9.12 The difference between average and maximum pooling. A 4×4 image is divided into four 2 × 2 sub-images as represented by the grid. Maximum pooling condenses the 4×4 image into a 2×2 image by selecting the maximum value within each of the sub-images. Average pooling accomplishes the same reduction in size by taking the average of all pixels of each sub-image as a single value.

with maximum pooling position (1,1) is smaller than position (1,2) (20 vs. 30), whereas in the case of average pooling (1,1) is larger than (1,2) (13 vs. 8).

Average pooling can be performed using convolution. The 2×2 kernel shown here could be used to take the average value of four pixels within an image when it is convolved with the image:

$$\text{Average kernel} = \begin{bmatrix} \frac{1}{4} & \frac{1}{4} \\ \frac{1}{4} & \frac{1}{4} \end{bmatrix}.$$

The reason this kernel takes the average value is somewhat intuitive: each pixel in the 2×2 grid is multiplied by ¼ and then added together, which is the same as adding all four pixel values together and then dividing by four to calculate the average. However, if we perform convolution as we described in the previous detailed explanation where the kernel is moved one pixel at a time, we will not actually reduce the size of the image. In order to reduce the size, we have to increase the **stride size** for the convolution from 1 to 2. What this means in practice is that after each convolution is performed, the kernel is moved over two pixels instead of one pixel. When the kernel reaches the end of a row, it will then start over two rows below instead of one row. By increasing the stride size to 2, the size of the image is reduced by a factor of four (half as many rows and half as many columns).

The convolution and pooling steps are designed by the user to gradually extract information from the input image and distill the input image down to

Deep Learning

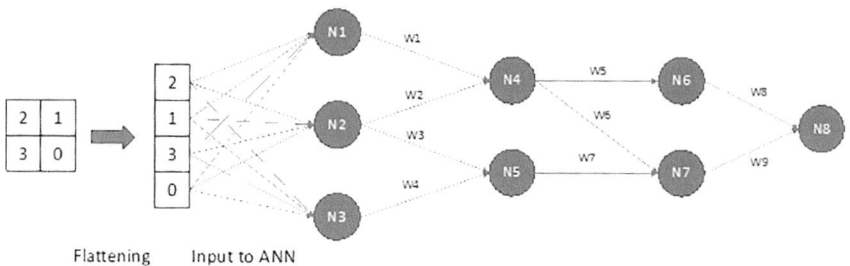

Figure 9.13 Example of flattening for input into an ANN. A 2×2 matrix is flattened into a 1×4 vector and then input into an ANN for classification. Flattening is performed by taking the top row of the 2×2 matrix and transposing it into a 1×2 column vector. The bottom row of the 2×2 matrix is then transposed and concatenated to the end of the first 1×2 column vector, forming the final 1×4 column vector that serves as inputs into an ANN.

a smaller subset of salient features that can be used for classification. How are the pooled features maps actually converted into a classification? The first step is a process called **flattening**, which converts the image into a vector from which a classification score can be determined. It needs to be in the form of a one-dimensional linear vector so that it can be input into the fully connected layer, which is simply an ANN as described in the previous section. Figure 9.13 shows an example of flattening for input into an ANN. A 2×2 matrix is flattened into a 1×4 vector and then input into an ANN for classification. Flattening is performed by taking the top row of the 2×2 matrix and transposing it into a 1×2 column vector. The bottom row of the 2×2 matrix is then transposed and concatenated to the end of the first 1×2 column vector, forming the final 1×4 column vector that serves as inputs into an ANN.

In summary, a CNN uses similar methods to an ANN for classification, with the added advantage that it uses spatial information within the input. The spatial information is extracted by performing a sequence of convolutions with pooling to reduce the size of the input image to a vector that can be input into a more traditional ANN architecture for classification. During training, the algorithm updates not only the weights associated with the ANN, but also the convolution and pooling steps in an attempt to improve classification performance.

Deeper Look: The Regulatory Challenges Associated with Deep Learning

Just as the FDA reviews safety and efficacy of devices and drugs, it also plays an important role in regulating machine learning algorithms. These algorithms have different levels of sophistication, in that they can be "locked" or "adaptive," also referred to as "continuous learning." In a locked algorithm, the same input will always produce the same result. Locked algorithms can degrade as new treatments and clinical practices arise or as populations alter over time. In contrast, an adaptive algorithm has the potential to update itself based on new data. In other words, the same input could generate different decisions over time. To date, the FDA has cleared or approved several medical devices using "locked" algorithms. However, the FDA presently does not have regulatory frameworks designed for adaptive algorithms that change and can adapt over time.

While locked algorithms are relatively straightforward from a regulatory standpoint, they may be hard to generalize to new populations. One major issue is the makeup of the database that was used to train the algorithm in the first place. Companies do not always publicly report detailed information on the data sets they use to develop or validate algorithms, limiting the ability of healthcare providers to evaluate how well the AI algorithm will perform for their patients. For example, a report examining companies' public summaries about their FDA-approved AI tools found that, of the 10 products approved for breast imaging, only 1 included a breakdown of the racial demographics in the data set used to validate the algorithm. Breast cancer is more likely to be fatal in Black women, who may be diagnosed at later stages of the disease and who experience greater barriers to care. Therefore, lack of public disclosure means that healthcare providers and patients might not have all the information they need to make informed decisions about the use of these products.

Even though this might be true for adaptive algorithms, they have the opportunity to redeem themselves, so to speak. For example, Google researchers developed an algorithm to detect diabetic retinopathy with 90 percent accuracy in a controlled setting. However, when put into use it was far less accurate due to problems presented in realistic scenarios, such as lack of high-quality images, among other issues. In this case, an adaptive algorithm could continue to improve results by retraining with the new observations. Because of regulatory challenges, many adaptive AI algorithms are marketed for nonmedical applications – for example, for lifestyle purposes.

The FDA recognizes this as an issue. It has a workflow to regulate machine learning algorithms that include an adaptive component. In addition, the FDA has announced the names of companies selected to participate in a first-of-its kind pilot pre-certification program. Figure 9.14 shows the pre-certification model. It is intended to inform a tailored approach toward

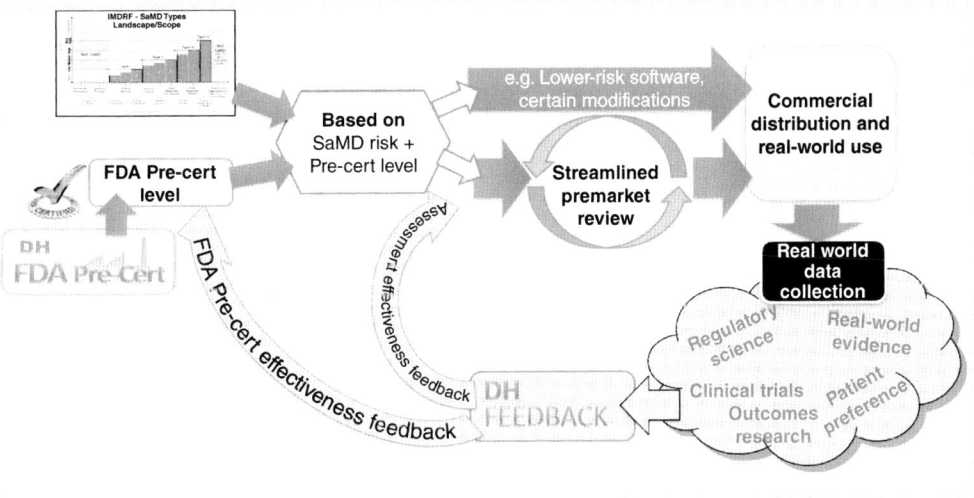

Figure 9.14 FDA pre-certification model. It is intended to inform a tailored approach toward digital health technology by looking at the software developer or digital health technology developer, rather than primarily at the product. Source: U.S. Food and Drug Administration. "Developing a Software Precertification Program: A Working Model," 2017.

digital health technology by looking at the software developer or digital health technology developer, rather than primarily at the product. The pilot participants represent a wide range of companies, including small startups and large companies, medical product manufacturers, and software developers. Participants selected include Apple, Fitbit, Johnson & Johnson, Pear Therapeutics, Phosphorus, Roche, Samsung, Tidepool, and Verily.

Algorithm Bias

In machine learning, an error is a measure of how accurately an algorithm can make predictions on a validation data set. Recall that in the first section, a loss function was defined based on RMSE to compare the difference between the predicted and actual value and gradient descent algorithms were used to minimize the error. That discussion did not discuss the types of errors that need to be considered, which are reflected by the complexity of the model and the amount of training data available to optimize it. There are two main types of error that are present. **Irreducible errors** will always be present in the model regardless of which algorithm has been used. The cause of these errors is unknown variables whose value cannot be reduced. **Reducible errors** are errors that can be reduced to improve the model accuracy. Such errors can further be classified into bias and variance.

Bias and variance errors were discussed in the context of cross validation in the previous chapter. Here they will be elaborated on in greater detail. Figure 9.15 illustrates the impact of bias error and variance error on the performance of a machine learning algorithm. Bias error leads to **underfitting** (a), variance error results to **overfitting** (c), and a trade-off between bias and variance is required to create an optimal balance (b). In the case of high **bias** the model is not of sufficient complexity to capture the structure in the data. In the case of high variance, the model is too complex and it learns parts of the noise as well as the true problem structure. This is called overfitting or model **variance**.

Figure 9.16 illustrates the effect of different combinations of bias and variance with a bullseye graphic. These combinations include low and high

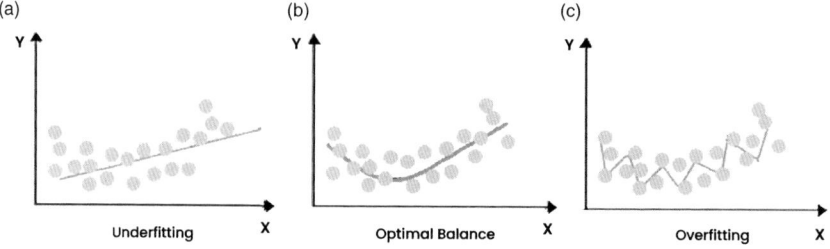

Figure 9.15 The impact of bias and variance error on the performance of a machine learning algorithm. Bias error leads to underfitting (a), variance error results in overfitting (c), and a trade-off between bias and variance is required to create an optimal balance (b).

Algorithm Bias

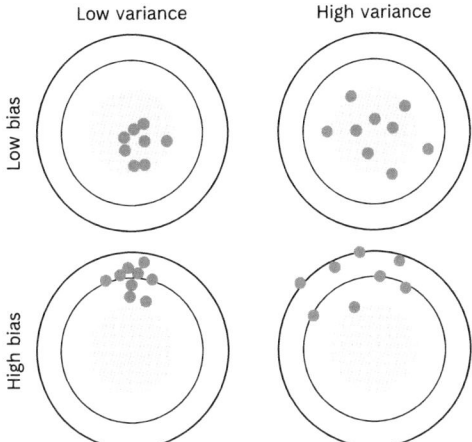

Figure 9.16 The effect of different combinations of bias and variance with a bullseye graphic. These combinations include low and high bias, variance pairs, high variance and low bias, and high bias and low variance. The combination of low bias and low variance shows an ideal machine learning model.

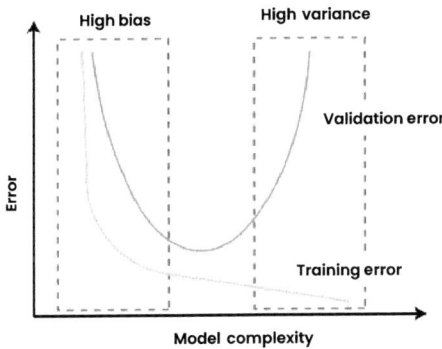

Figure 9.17 The effect of high bias and high variance on the training and validation data. Both high bias and high variance increase error on the validation set, as shown by the U-shaped curve. There are several ways to reduce bias and variance errors. Bias error can be decreased by increasing the number of tunable parameters in the training set and/or increasing the complexity of the model. Variance error can be reduced by increasing the training data and/or reducing the input features or number of parameters as a model is overfitted.

bias, variance pairs, high variance and low bias, and high bias and low variance. The combination of low bias and low variance shows an ideal machine learning model. However, it is not realistic. With low bias and high variance, model predictions are inconsistent, but accurate on average in that the data is centered on the bullseye. With high bias and low variance, predictions are consistent but deviate from the bullseye. With high bias and high variance, predictions are inconsistent and also inaccurate (worst case scenario).

Figure 9.17 shows the effect of high bias and high variance on the training and validation data. Both high bias and high variance increase error in the validation set as shown by the U-shaped curve. When there is high bias, the algorithm can perform similarly on both the training and testing sets, but this is at the expense of a large difference between the prediction values and the expected values, thereby leading to increased error. In the case of high variance, the algorithm has excellent performance on the training set, but leads to high error on the validation set. Another way to think about this error is variation in the prediction if different training data was used. Picking the minimum point in the U-shaped error curve strikes a balance between bias and variance errors.

Example: Assessing Fit, Bias, and Variance

Question: A biomedical engineer is designing a deep learning algorithm to predict the probability of survival for breast cancer following different treatment regimens. As they train their model, they notice the following:

- The initial training and validation errors begin at around 30 percent and the residuals are almost all negative.
- After 100 rounds of training, the training error is around 3 percent, the validation error is around 6 percent, and the residuals are uniformly distributed around zero.
- After 200 rounds of training, the training error is 1 percent (residuals are uniformly distributed around zero) and the validation error is 16 percent (residuals are almost all positive).

At each stage of training, is the algorithm overtrained, undertrained, or adequately trained? Is there variance or bias error? Why?

Answer: During the initial training, the model is undertrained as both the training and validation error are high (30 percent). The algorithm has both high variance and bias because the error is high and the residuals all fall in one direction. After 100 rounds of training, the algorithm is adequately trained as the training error is low and the trade-off between training and validation error is low (6 − 3 = 3 percent). The bias and variance are both low due to low training and validation errors and a random distribution of residuals. After 200 rounds of training, the algorithm is overtrained because the difference between the validation and training error is high (16 − 1 = 15 percent) compared to the training error (1 percent). The variance is high because the residuals are not uniformly distributed around zero.

The **dropout method** can reduce overfitting by randomly dropping neurons from the network during training. We can use a Bernoulli distribution to decide which neurons should be dropped. A Bernoulli distribution applies to events that have one trial and two possible outcomes (for example, drop or do not drop neuron). Recomputing dropout during training allows us to build multiple unique models to learn from the data. Dropout can be performed on any hidden or visible layer. **Early stopping** is another approach to decreasing overfitting. As discussed before, we can assess the performance

Algorithm Bias

Figure 9.18

An illustration the (a) drop out and (b) early stopping methods. In the dropout method, the neural network on the left represents a typical neural network where all units are activated. On the right, some units have dropped out of the model. The values of their weights and biases are not considered during the training phase. In early stopping the error for the validation set plateaus at approximately five epochs even though the error for the training set continues to decrease. Source: Adapted from Srivastava et al. (2014).

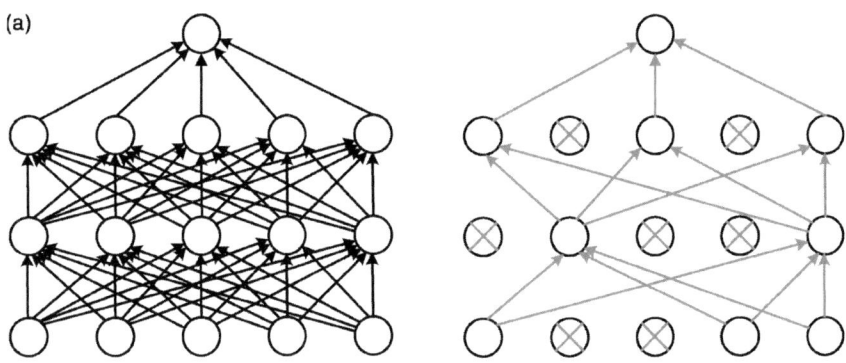

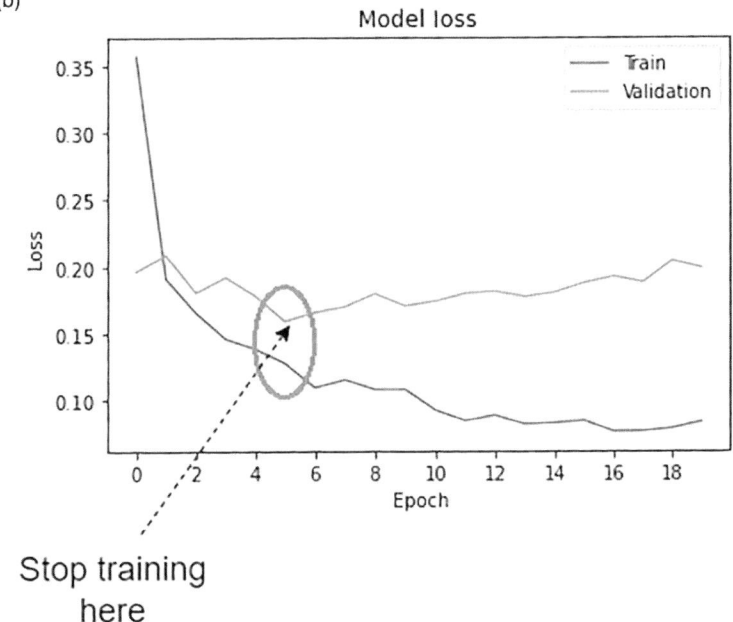

Stop training here

Right fit region

of a neural network algorithm using a loss function and continue iterating until the error is minimized. With early stopping, the number of iterations is terminated when there is no improvement on the validation set. Figure 9.18 illustrates the drop out and early stopping methods. In the dropout method (a), the neural network on the left represents a typical neural network where all units are activated. On the right, many units have dropped out of the model. The values of their weights and biases are not considered during the training phase. In early stopping (b), the error for the validation set plateaus at approximately five epochs even though the error for the training set continues to decrease.

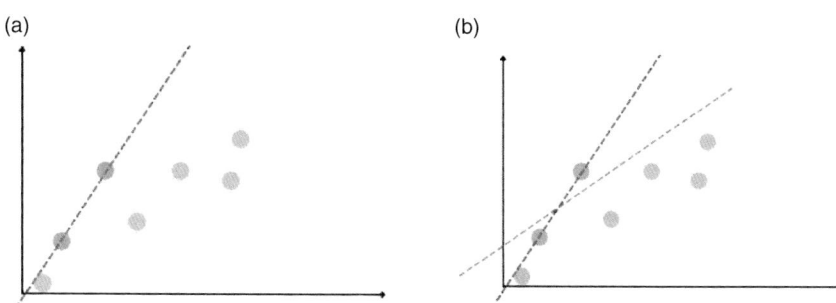

Figure 9.19 The goal of the regularization methods is to generalize a model that is overtrained. The graphic illustrates two sets of data, training data (dark gray) and validation data (light gray). It can be seen that the best fit to the training is overtrained and therefore not generalizable to the validation set as shown in (a). The **regularization** method introduces a small amount of bias for the new fitted line on the training data set to get a low variance for the testing data (b).

The longer a network is trained, the larger the weights will grow and the more specific they will become to the training data; this leads to overfitting. In other words, small changes in the input can lead to large changes in the output. Regularization is a method that constrains or regularizes the weights. There are two ways to penalize the model to restrict the size of the weights. The first is the restriction of the actual size of the weights (lasso or L1), and the second is to add a penalty (ridge or L2). **Lasso** results in more sparse weights (weights with more zero values). **Ridge** penalizes larger weights more severely, but does not necessarily lead to sparse weights. Ridge regression is also referred to as weight decay.

Figure 9.19 illustrates the goal of the regularization methods, which is to generalize a model that is overtrained. The graphic illustrates two sets of data, the training data (dark gray) and validation data (light gray). It can be seen that the best fit to the training data is overtrained and therefore not generalizable to the validation set as shown in Figure 9.19(a). The **regularization** method introduces a small amount of bias for the new fitted line on the training data set to get a low variance for the testing data (Figure 9.19(b)). It is important to point out that the models described here are linear regression models. In the case of the neural networks model, the output in the applications that this chapter pertains to are characterized as classes of data and therefore use an extension of these regularization models – for example, logistic lasso, akin to logistic vs. linear regression.

Linear **lasso regression** and **ridge regression** are mathematically shown in Equations 9.8 and 9.9. The MSE is the sum of the square of residuals, as previously shown in the first section, with additional terms, reflecting the lasso (Equation 9.8) and ridge (Equation 9.9). The lasso regression works very similarly to the ridge regression with a slight change in the training equation.

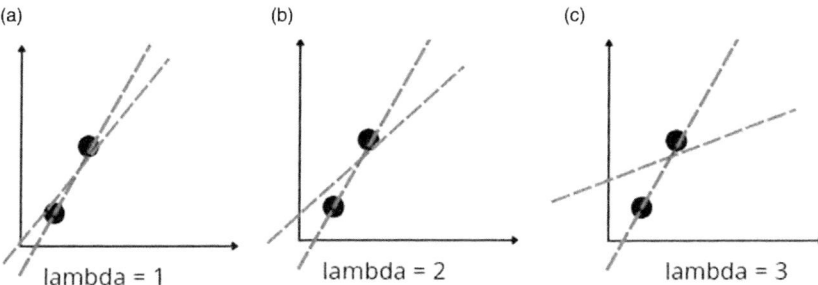

Figure 9.20 The effect of varying the value of λ on the slope of the fit. Notice that as we increase the value of λ, the slope decreases, which means the best-fitted line becomes less sensitive to the input values. λ can be any value from 0 to infinity.

Note that instead of squaring the slope for the penalty term, the lasso regression takes the absolute value of the slope (the absolute value will return all positive values). That means that for the same value of λ, the lasso regression will produce less bias than the ridge regression, as shown in Equations 9.8 and 9.9:

$$\text{MSE}_{\text{Lasso}} = \text{MSE} + \lambda \sum_{i=1}^{n} |m_i|, \qquad (9.8)$$

$$\text{MSE}_{\text{Ridge}} = \text{MSE} + \lambda \sum_{i=1}^{n} m_i^2. \qquad (9.9)$$

where m is the slope of a regression line and λ is the amount of shrinkage.

What do different values of λ mean? Figure 9.20 shows the effect of varying the value of λ on the slope of the fit. Notice that as we increase the value of λ, the slope decreases, which means the best-fitted line becomes less sensitive to the input values. λ can be any value from 0 to infinity. $\lambda = 0$ implies all features are considered and it is equivalent to the linear regression, where only the residual sum of squares is considered to build a predictive model. $\lambda = \infty$ implies no feature is considered; as λ closes to infinity it eliminates more and more features. The bias increases with increase in λ. Variance increases with decrease in λ.

If the bias introduced with lasso and ridge are similar, why choose one over the other? Evaluating Equations 9.8 and 9.9 more closely shows that with the ridge model, the slope will approach zero but will never be zero. However, with the lasso model the slope can be zero. Why is this important? Generally, lasso will perform better where some of the predictors have large coefficients and the remaining predictors have very small coefficients in the linear regression fit. This is due to the fact that predictors with low coefficients will be removed when the slope is zero.

Ridge regression will perform better when the outcome is a function of many predictors, all with coefficients of roughly equal size.

Example: Lasso vs. Ridge

Question: Mathematically explain why lasso and ridge will result in the same regression line if the slope of the regression line is 1 or −1. Why is it highly unlikely that a regression line would have a slope of 1 or −1? What does this tell you about lasso and ridge?

Answer: Lasso takes the magnitude of the slope of the line, whereas ridge takes the square of the slope of the line. Let us first rewrite magnitude according to its mathematical definition:

$$|m| = \sqrt{m^2}.$$

If we equate the lasso and ridge terms to each other, we get:

$$\sqrt{m^2} = m^2.$$

This equation is only true for two values of m: 1 and −1.

It is highly unlikely that a regression line would have a slope of 1 or −1 because it is rarely the case that the input and output have a 1:1 ratio or 1 : −1 ratio. If such a relationship were known, there would be little reason to perform regression. At the same time, this tells us that lasso and ridge are unlikely to ever provide the same change to a regression line, making them complementary techniques.

Deeper Look: Bias in AI in Criminal Profiling and Medical Diagnostics

The idea of overfitting and underfitting has big implications in real life. In 2018, Amazon released a facial recognition algorithm to identify persons who have a criminal record. Figure 9.21 shows the bar chart of the Rekognition algorithm developed by Amazon. The algorithm was tested on members of the US Congress against a database of 25,000 criminal mugshots. Although only 20 percent of members of Congress were people of color, they accounted for 40 percent of the algorithm's false matches to mugshots in the database. This reflects the bias of the training database on which the algorithm was trained, which likely comprised mugshots of mostly people of color. This bias has important and negative implications in real-world scenarios – for example, racial biases in policing.

In another example involving diagnostic imaging, an AI algorithm was developed to identify a collapsed lung from chest X-ray images. The algorithm was trained on different subsets of data and then applied to a new set of chest X-rays. Figure 9.22 shows a representative image of a collapsed lung (a), and the results of detecting collapsed lungs in male and female patients using an AI algorithm (b,c). The area under the curve of a receiver operator has an ideal value of 1. As seen in the results, when the training set comprised largely of female chest X-rays the performance of the algorithm was low when identifying collapsed lungs in male chest rays and vice versa, again emphasizing the impact of sample bias on AI algorithm prediction.

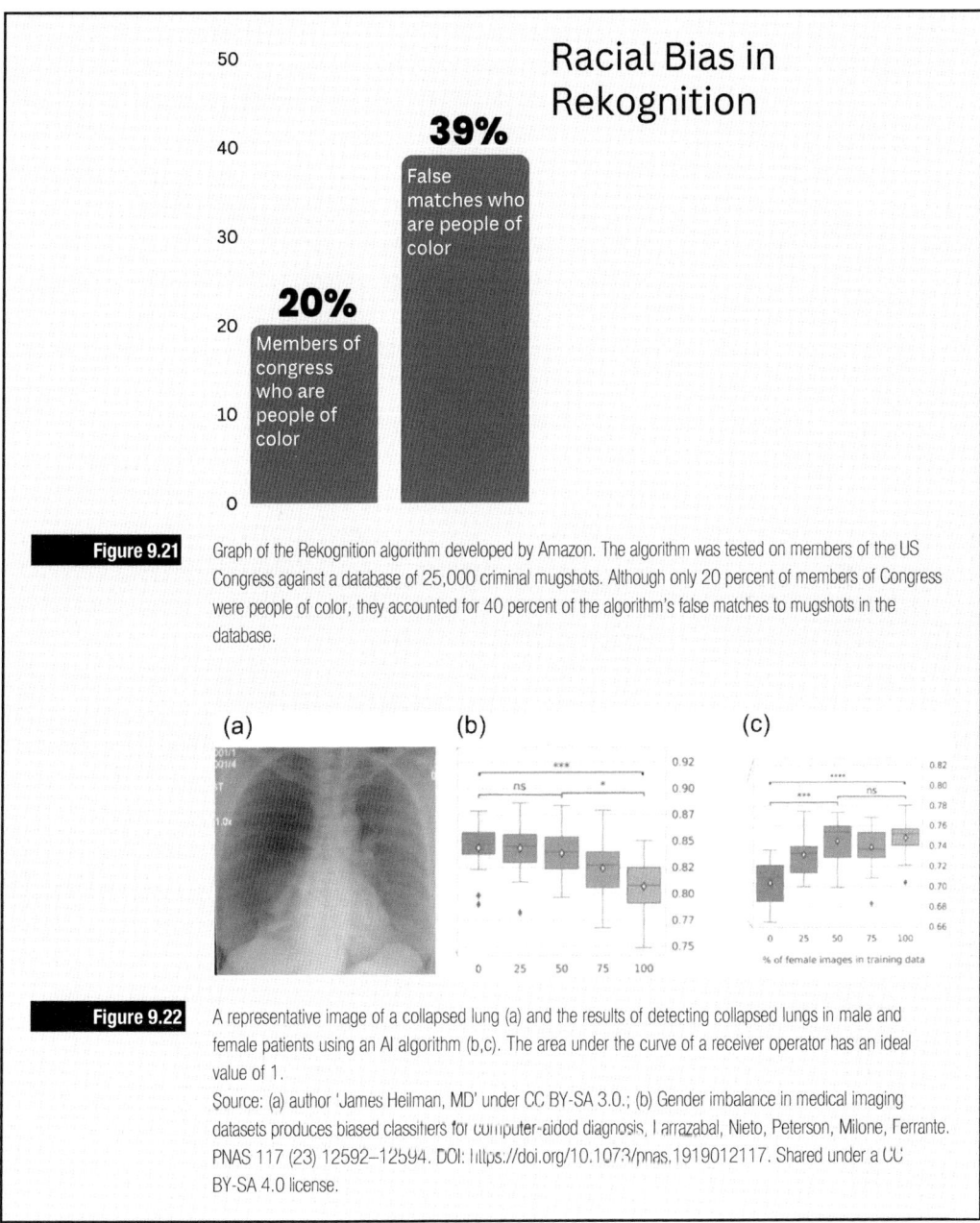

Figure 9.21 Graph of the Rekognition algorithm developed by Amazon. The algorithm was tested on members of the US Congress against a database of 25,000 criminal mugshots. Although only 20 percent of members of Congress were people of color, they accounted for 40 percent of the algorithm's false matches to mugshots in the database.

Figure 9.22 A representative image of a collapsed lung (a) and the results of detecting collapsed lungs in male and female patients using an AI algorithm (b,c). The area under the curve of a receiver operator has an ideal value of 1.
Source: (a) author 'James Heilman, MD' under CC BY-SA 3.0.; (b) Gender imbalance in medical imaging datasets produces biased classifiers for computer-aided diagnosis, Larrazabal, Nieto, Peterson, Milone, Ferrante. PNAS 117 (23) 12592–12594. DOI: https://doi.org/10.1073/pnas.1919012117. Shared under a CC BY-SA 4.0 license.

Looking Ahead

Machine learning algorithms have the potential to revolutionize the way cancer care is delivered. Whether they are used to screen for and diagnose disease or predict outcomes for particular therapies, machine learning can be used in virtually all parts of the cancer care cascade. As computer processors become smaller and less expensive, the potential to implement machine learning tools more widely will continue to increase. For example, if a nurse or midwife performs imaging with a portable colposcope in a mobile clinic or a community clinic, they may not have the expertise to render a decision. Even if these health providers are trained with the appropriate skills, high turnover may make this model challenging to scale. The prospect of having a virtual expert – an AI algorithm that could either serve as an additional expert allowing for both humans and machines to collectively render a decision or, with sufficient validation, as a solo decision-maker – could transform the healthcare landscape.

Before deep learning methods are widely accepted, more work is required. Networks rely on "black-box reasoning" and all knowledge is stored inside the network, making it challenging to provide credible explanations. With respect to the training phase, there are challenges associated with long training times, overfitting or underfitting, and lack of diversity in the training data sets. Further, data acquisition is still a major problem, especially when it is used for medical diagnostics, owing to privacy policies. This is further compounded by the fact that availability of public data is limited. Therefore, there are still multiple issues that need to be addressed before this can be integrated in a practical application. Ultimately, the use of AI, as well as the devices described in Chapters 4–6, will need to undergo rigorous clinical evaluation to ensure that these solutions are safe and effective. In fact, these innovations need to undergo this process in order to be cleared by regulatory agencies to use them in the first place. This is where the significance of training, validation, and testing sets becomes important.

As ANNs and CNNs continue to evolve, there are still effective ways to advance decision-making in scenarios where experts are lacking. One approach, telemedicine, the focus of Chapter 10, is a powerful way to address this gap. Tele-mentoring, which shifts and shares knowledge between an expert and nonspecialist or between nonspecialists, can further expand the workforce to make important decisions at the point of care. All of these approaches will inform deep learning – that is, the processes by which experts operate and the training of nonspecialists to improve their skills over time can serve as exemplars for a new workforce of virtual experts.

SUMMARY

Artificial neural networks consist of three components: an input layer, hidden layers, and an output layer. The input layer, as the name suggests, receives the inputs for the algorithm. The output layer provides the classification result. The layers consist of neurons that are connected by weights. Neurons take inputs multiplied by weights, sum them, and feed that result into an activation function, which determines the output of the neuron. The output can be continuous or discrete, depending on the type of activation function used. The goal of the ANN is to find the global minimum in order to minimize the differences between the measured and expected output. ANNs typically use a stochastic gradient descent algorithm to find the global minimum, which calculates the gradient (slope) at a single randomly chosen point instead of all possible points.

One limitation of traditional ANNs is that they are not adept at image classification, as images contain too many individual pixels for an ANN to adequately learn from. Convolutional neural networks, on the other hand, can take advantage of spatial information within images to distill the images down to a subset of features that can be used for classification. The CNN begins by taking the input image and performing a series of transformations to the image using a process called convolution. The computational burden can become heavy as each convolution step can result in multiple feature maps. Therefore, a process called pooling is performed after convolution to reduce the size of the output image. The process of performing convolution and pooling can be performed multiple times to convert the original image into a finite number of distinct features, which can then be input into a more traditional ANN for classification.

Algorithm optimization is inextricably linked to the training data available and the complexity of the model. Algorithm optimization needs to consider different types of errors. The main types of errors are irreducible (cannot be removed) and reducible errors, which includes bias and variance. High bias can lead to underfitting and poor algorithm performance. On the other hand, high variance can lead to high performance in the optimization process, but will not be generalizable to new observations. Bias error tends to occur when the algorithm is not complex enough (i.e., does not have enough tunable parameters) to adequately learn on the training data. Variance error occurs when the algorithm is too complex (i.e., has too many parameters, some of which may not add any value). There are a number of ways in which bias and variance errors can be reduced, including using multiple CNN models from which to identify relevant parameters (or variables), reducing the number of iterations to optimize the CNN, thereby reducing the complexity of the CNN model itself, and a process called regularization that adds a penalty to prevent the algorithm from being overtrained.

PROBLEMS

Artificial Neural Networks

1. Draw an ANN with the following characteristics:
   a. an input layer with two neurons;
   b. three hidden layers, where the first has two neurons, the second has three neurons, and the third has two neurons;
   c. an output layer with one neuron.
   Assuming that the inputs to the ANN go directly into the input layer without weighting, how many weights are in the network?

2. Determine the equation that would relate inputs to output for the ANN in question 1. Assume there are two inputs that go directly into the input layer, the ANN is fully connected, and an identify activation function is used.
3. A biomedical engineer wants to train the ANN from question 1 to determine whether or not a patient with breast cancer is likely to respond to a novel therapy. Between the identity function and the Heaviside step function, which would be a more appropriate activation function? Explain your reasoning.
4. Based on the diagram of a single neuron in Figure 9.23, determine the number of input patterns the node can receive if each input (x_1, x_2, x_3) can be −1, 0, or 1.

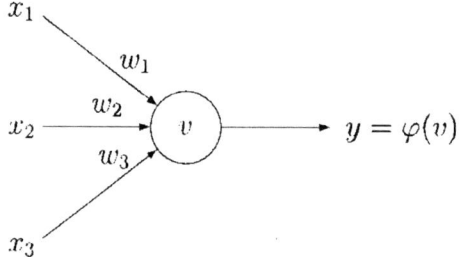

Figure 9.23
A single neuron.

5. Using the neuron from question 4, assume the values of the weights are 2, 1, and −3, respectively. If the activation function (i.e., neuron output) is a 1 if v is ≥0 and 0 otherwise, calculate the output for each input parameter below:
   a. 1, 1, 0
   b. 0, −1, −1
   c. 1, 0, 1
   d. 1, 1, 1
   e. −1, −1, −1.
6. For the same values in question 5, calculate the output value of y when there is no activation function. What is the difference in the relationship between x and y with and without the activation function? Why is the use of the activation function important?
7. Explain one advantage and one limitation of stochastic gradient descent compared to a traditional maximum gradient descent.
8. Suppose you are training an ANN to estimate the likelihood of adverse events occurring when a combination of different drugs is given for cancer treatment. You are trying to decide whether to use a stochastic gradient descent or maximum gradient descent algorithm during training. If you knew *a priori* that the maximum gradient descent would take 75 iterations to converge and each iteration would take 90 minutes, whereas the stochastic gradient descent algorithm would take 140 iterations to converge and each iteration would take 45 minutes, which approach is more computationally efficient?

Convolutional Neural Networks

9. A biomedical engineer is tasked with designing an algorithm based on two variables: CTCs and lesion size. What type of algorithm can be developed with minimal computational burden and why?

10. The biomedical engineer decides to include gene expression and now has thousands of variables as inputs into the algorithm. What type of algorithm should be developed and why?

11. The biomedical engineer observes that there is a relationship between features on the breast MRI images and gene expression and decides to explore the use of images as an alternative to the gene expression data, since it is not always available for all patients. What type of algorithm should be developed?

12. Design a CNN with the following characteristics. Draw a flowchart similar to Figure 9.10 to illustrate your design:
    a. a grayscale image as the input;
    b. three convolutional layers with two kernels in each layer;
    c. one pooling layer after each convolutional layer.

13. How would your design change if the input was a color image (e.g., RGB) instead of grayscale? How would that affect the computational intensity of the CNN?

14. A biomedical engineer is interested in designing a CNN that will use images of a cervix to identify women with cervical precancer. Acetowhite features within images tend to create edges, therefore, an edge-detecting Sobel kernel is one of the convolutional layers, as shown below. What is the output when the Sobel kernel is convolved with the 5×5 image shown here? Use zero padding.

$$\text{Image} = \begin{bmatrix} 10 & 11 & 18 & 14 & 20 \\ 17 & 21 & 20 & 25 & 23 \\ 85 & 110 & 120 & 90 & 113 \\ 131 & 87 & 108 & 124 & 79 \\ 111 & 133 & 93 & 103 & 127 \end{bmatrix},$$

$$\text{Kernel} = \begin{bmatrix} -1 & 0 & 1 \\ -2 & 0 & 2 \\ -1 & 0 & 1 \end{bmatrix}.$$

Repeat with a Sobel kernel that is oriented horizontally:

$$\text{Kernel} = \begin{bmatrix} -1 & -2 & -1 \\ 0 & 0 & 0 \\ 1 & 2 & 1 \end{bmatrix}.$$

15. Based on the results, do you think there is a vertical or horizontal edge present in the image? Explain your reasoning.

16. To reduce the size of the 5×5 feature maps from question 14, the engineer wants to apply average pooling to reduce each feature map to a single

number. Design a kernel that will accomplish this task. What is the result for each feature map from question 14? What stride size would need to be used for the kernel designed in the second part of question 14? By what factor in size would the kernel and stride size reduce a feature map?

Algorithm Bias

17. Explain what you would expect the training and validation error (low vs. high) to be for an algorithm that is adequately trained, undertrained, and overtrained.
18. Label each part of Figure 9.24 with respect to high/low variance and high/low bias or both.

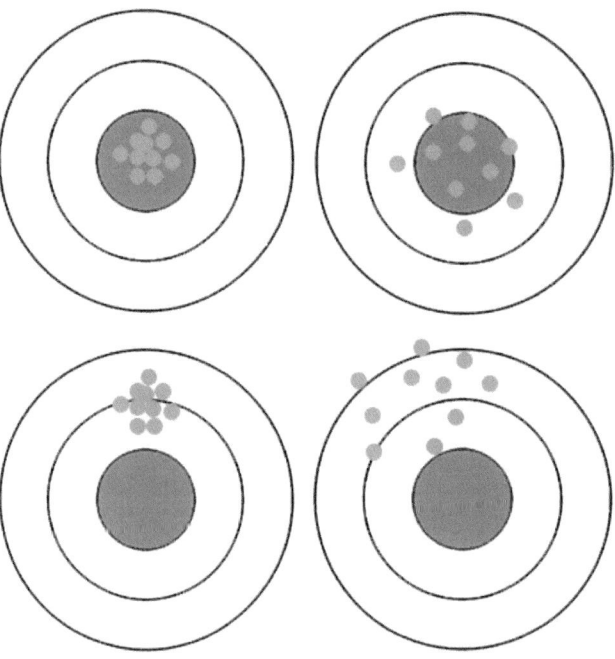

Figure 9.24

Figure for question 18.

19. An algorithm that is used to detect cervical cancer is trained using colposcope images. There is a limited amount of training data available. What type of error (bias or variance) would this introduce during training?
20. If cell phone images are added to the training set from question 19, what type of error (bias or variance) would this introduce assuming equal numbers of colposcope and cell phone images are used?
21. The validation images used for the algorithm in questions 19 and 20 result in a validation error that initially drops but then increases again. What method would be most suitable to prevent the validation error from increasing again and why?
22. Explain two reasons why ridge is more suitable than lasso for resolving bias when the distribution of weights is uniform.

REFERENCES

Alloghani, M., Al-Jumeily, D., Aljaaf, A. J., et al. 2019. The application of artificial intelligence technology in healthcare: a systematic review. In *International Conference on Applied Computing to Support Industry: Innovation and Technology*, Springer, New York.

Alloghani, M., Al-Jumeily, D., Aljaaf, A.J., Khalaf, M., Mustafina, J., Tan, S.Y. 2020. The application of artificial intelligence technology in healthcare: a systematic review. In: Khalaf, M., Al-Jumeily, D., Lisitsa, A. (eds) *Applied Computing to Support Industry: Innovation and Technology. ACRIT 2019.* Communications in Computer and Information Science, vol 1174. Springer, Cham. https://doi.org/10.1007/978-3-030-38752-5_20

Poplin, R., Chang, P.-C., Alexander, D., et al. 2018. A universal SNP and small-indel variant caller using deep neural networks. *Nature Biotechnology*, 36, 983–987.

Quer, G., Radin, J. M., Gadaleta, M., et al. 2021. Wearable sensor data and self-reported symptoms for COVID-19 detection. *Nature Medicine*, 27, 73–77.

Santhana Krishnan, U. S., & Palanisamy, K. 2021. Recycled integrated circuit detection using reliability analysis and machine learning algorithms. *IET Computers & Digital Techniques*, 15, 20–35.

Srivastava, N., Hinton, G., Krizhevsky, A., et al. 2014. Dropout: a simple way to prevent neural networks from overfitting. *Journal of Machine Learning Research*, 15, 1929–1958.

10 The Evolution of Healthcare in the Twenty-First Century

As described in Chapter 1, telemedicine played a significant role during the COVID-19 pandemic. Today, telemedicine is more accessible than ever, owing largely to mobile technologies. Patients now have the ability to interact face to face with providers in real time via live video. Images, lab results, etc., can be communicated efficiently for interpretation synchronously or at a later time. Devices such as digital stethoscopes, ophthalmoscopes, otoscopes, and wearable biosensors can further extend the telemedicine experience for patients and providers through seamless transmission of data. This has made it possible for providers to deliver healthcare to a broader segment of the population than was previously possible.

The impact of COVID-19 was greatest in socioeconomically disadvantaged populations, particularly those in low- and middle-income countries (LMICs). For instance, prior to the pandemic, almost one-third of the population in LMICs lived more than two hours away from essential healthcare services, and the ratio of healthcare workers to population was typically well below the minimum recommended by the WHO. The loss of healthcare workers to COVID-19 and the disruption of transport systems because of lockdowns worsened the impact of these issues. Telemedicine is poised to be the disruptive innovation that can begin to close this gap, particularly physical access to care, a persistent and pervasive obstacle. Additionally, telemedicine could provide access to culturally competent care that may not otherwise be accessible. Coupled with machine learning algorithms, described in Chapters 8 and 9, the impact of telemedicine can stretch even further. Deep learning algorithms can serve as a tool to train nonexpert health providers to help them improve their skills, provide an assistive role when diagnosis of a health condition is not synchronous, and can also serve as a standalone tool when an expert is not available.

The goal of this chapter is to discusses how electronic health (eHealth) can transform the way healthcare reaches patients, particularly when patients are unable to reach health facilities. The term **eHealth** refers to health services and information delivered or enhanced through the internet and related technologies, with the capability to improve healthcare locally, regionally, and globally. The field of eHealth encompasses **telehealth, telemedicine,** and **telecare**. The application of each of the "tele" approaches is distinct and will be described in greater detail in this chapter, along with the ways they can address health inequities.

LEARNING OBJECTIVES

The Growing Shortage of Healthcare Experts in Clinical Deserts
- The challenges associated with healthcare delivery and disease prevention, using the US as the example;
- the distribution of the healthcare workforce across the US;
- the role that technology can play in addressing healthcare provider shortage.

Addressing the Shortage of a Skilled Healthcare Workforce Through eHealth
- The different types of eHealth services;
- the different areas of telemedicine and what impact (direct or indirect) they can have on patients;
- the limitations of telehealth that create racial disparities.

Addressing Healthcare Disparities in Low- and Middle-Income Countries
- Differences in the workforce distribution between high-income countries (HICs) and LMICs;
- the role that telehealth is playing in addressing global health disparities;
- the role of community health providers in telehealth.

The Growing Shortage of Healthcare Experts in Rural and Low-Resource Settings

At the turn of the twentieth century, US healthcare became increasingly reliant on technology. In addition to the use of medical technologies, other tools – such as telephones, automobiles, and paved roads – changed the nature of physician–patient interactions. Hospitals transitioned from serving the poor to the destination for paying patients. The transition from the nineteenth to the twentieth century also brought about a revolution in medical education that extended and intensified the process of becoming a physician. These changes included the increase in the duration of medical school curricula from two to three to four years, along with rising admissions requirements. Teaching hospitals became sites for clinical medical education and medical practice became regulated by licensure laws passed in every state.

While many of the physicians at this time were generalists, a widely publicized national commission in 1932 divided medical care into groups of

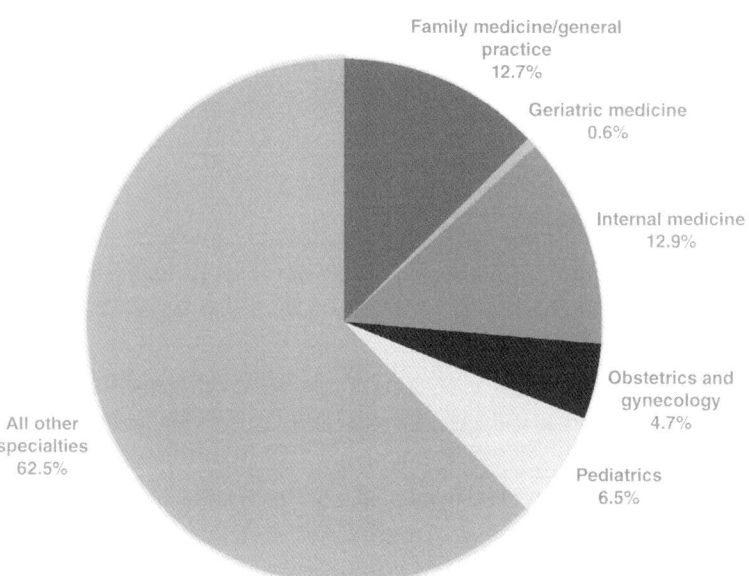

Figure 10.1 Physician characteristics and distribution in the US. Over the last century, generalists have transitioned from comprising 100 percent of all physicians to approximately one-third of the entire physician pool in the US. Data: American Medical Association, 2017.

physicians who specialized in specific organ systems. Ophthalmologists, who focus on the vision system, were the most specialized types of physicians, forming the first specialty board in 1916. Physicians who focused on the use of X-rays created the radiology specialty board in 1934. In the 1960s, Medicare increased the salary differential between primary care physicians and specialists, a trend that has continued to grow. Medical care moved increasingly to specialty clinics and hospitals as specialized care was outside the scope of the primary care physician. While the support for primary care has continued to strengthen within many medical organizations, the appeal of primary care for medical students has not. The shift from primary care to specialized care can be explained in part by the potential for higher incomes as a specialist. Figure 10.1 shows physician characteristics and distribution in the US. Over the last century, generalists have transitioned from comprising 100 percent of physicians to approximately one-third of the entire physician pool in the US.

Primary care is critical to the US healthcare system, given its inextricable link to positive health outcomes and health equity. A greater number of primary care physicians has been linked to longer life spans and better patient outcomes, including lower rates of mortality, according to the United Health Foundation (UHF). The UHF considers primary care physicians' availability as an indication of health when calculating its annual Health Rankings report, which is the longest running annual assessment of the nation's health on a state-by-state basis.

Despite the importance of primary care, the availability of these providers is far from ideal. Figure 10.2 shows the primary care physician shortage in

Shortage of Healthcare Experts in Clinical Deserts

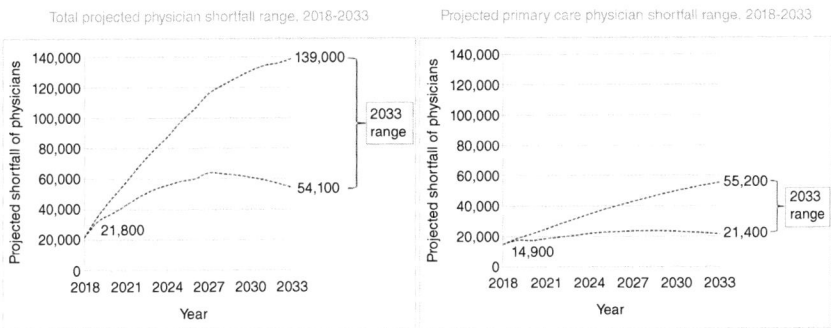

Figure 10.2 Primary care physician shortage in the US. Projections to 2033 show there will be an overall shortfall of physicians, and the shortfall of primary care physicians is expected to grow.
Source: Data according to the AAMC.; AAMC, "The Complexities of Physician Supply and Demand: Projections From 2018 to 2033". Prepared for the AAMC by IHS Markit Ltd.

the US. At least 10 states have primary care physician shortages of greater than 50 percent. The average number of primary care physicians per 1,000 people in the US was 156.7 in 2008. There were 55.1 primary care physicians per 100,000 residents in rural settings compared to 79.3 per 100,000 in urban settings. Unfortunately, the physician to resident ratio continues to decrease. This is not uniformly distributed.

Example: How Many Physicians Do We Need to Address Shortage?

Question: One way to overcome the physician shortage is to incentivize physicians to stay in primary care and to work in rural settings. How many new physicians are needed in the next five years to meet a goal of 100 physicians per 100,000 people if there is an average of 60 per 100,000 currently and a 5 percent retirement rate per year? Assume a US population of 300,000,000.

Answer: If there are currently 60 physicians per 100,000 people and a goal of 100 per 100,000 people, we can multiply by the population size to get the total current and target number of physicians:

$$\frac{60}{100,000} \times 300,000,000 = 18,000 \text{ physicians},$$

$$\frac{100}{100,000} \times 300,000,000 = 30,000 \text{ physicians}.$$

Since 30,000 physicians are needed and there are currently only 18,000, over the next five years 12,000 more physicians are needed. This number, however, does not take into account the physicians who will retire. We can estimate this by taking 5 percent of the current number of physicians and multiplying by 5:

$$0.05 \times 18,000 \times 5 = 4,500.$$

Since 4,500 physicians will retire, the actual number needed in the next five years is $12,000 + 4,500 = 16,500$.

Table 10.1 compares the performance of health systems of 11 HICs. This data was obtained from the Commonwealth Fund Survey, conducted by the SSRS in collaboration with partner organizations in the 10 other countries. Additional data was drawn from the OECD and the WHO. The top-performing countries overall are Norway, the Netherlands, and Australia. The next three countries in the ranking – the UK, Germany, and New Zealand – perform very similarly to one another. The US ranks #11 – the performance of the US falls well below the average of the other countries and far below the two countries ranked directly above it.

Several approaches have been suggested to solve the shortage of primary care providers; for example, incentivizing medical professionals to serve in rural communities through the addition of rural residency programs and the retention of physicians in LMICs, who typically leave to the US and Europe. However, significant resources will be required to build this capacity and, further, this will likely take decades to achieve.

Paradoxically, the most effective way to overcome a worldwide physician shortage may be to rely on physicians less, but how can this be

Table 10.1 Comparison of health systems of 11 HICs

	AUS	CAN	FRA	GER	NETH	NZ	NOR	SWE	SWIZ	UK	US
Overall ranking	3	10	8	5	2	6	1	7	9	4	11
Access to care	8	9	7	3	1	5	2	6	10	4	11
Care process	6	4	10	9	3	1	8	11	7	5	2
Administrative efficiency	2	7	6	9	8	3	1	5	10	4	11
Equity	1	10	7	2	5	9	8	6	3	4	11
Healthcare outcomes	1	10	6	7	4	8	2	5	3	9	11

This data is from the Commonwealth Fund surveys, which were conducted by SSRS in collaboration with partner organizations in the 10 other countries. Additional data were drawn from the Organization for Economic Co-operation and Development (OECD) and the World Health Organization (WHO).

accomplished? One way is to provide midwives, nurses, and community health providers with tools to effectively triage patients such that the majority of the population can receive the care they need within their own communities. The advent of high-quality disruptive innovations (Chapters 4–6) that can translate hospital-based technologies into communities makes this an exciting and realistic prospect. In addition, digital health combined with data analytics can extend the reach of specialists across geographical and knowledge barriers.

Telehealth is a gateway to efficient care for 81 million US citizens living in health professional shortage areas, where access to primary, dental, and mental healthcare services is very limited. Residents generally have lower incomes and are more likely to be uninsured. The COVID-19 pandemic has shown that communication technologies can be leveraged to provide more efficient delivery. During the pandemic, telehealth services increased 78-fold from February to April 2020. Despite in-person options becoming more available in many states, telehealth usage continues to stay at 38 times higher than it was pre-pandemic. With access to telehealth during the pandemic, patients with diabetes, hypertension, thyroid diseases, and other chronic conditions had access to remote patient monitoring options and treatment, if needed. For example, diabetic patients benefited from the timely sharing of blood glucose levels using telehealth.

Artificial intelligence (AI) can further amplify the impact of telehealth on patient outcomes. It can be used to address the issues of misdistribution of the demand versus supply of healthcare services, and develop algorithms to match the availability of care providers with appropriate clinical skills for a given community. Moreover, it can provide mechanisms for human or virtual interactions to occur, and thereby mitigate difficulties in timing and availability of clinicians (such as the time taken to understand the patient's problem or taking a history). Table 10.2 shows examples of how AI is being used in healthcare. These examples can be broadly divided into supportive care, prevention and diagnosis of health issues, and capacity building.

What began as a personalized way to care for the wealthy through home visits is making a comeback through a virtual space and is accessible to individuals at different socioeconomic levels. The advantage of the virtual approach is its reach and its ability to serve more than only the wealthy. In fact, it is a fundamental step forward in democratizing healthcare and is important in facilitating the dissemination of point-of-care technologies. In fact, telemedicine symbolizes in many ways the transition from a fee-for-service model introduced during the Johnson presidency in the 1960s to value-based care, where patients, not hospitals, are at the center of care.

Table 10.2 Examples of how AI is being used in healthcare

These examples can be broadly divided into supportive care, prevention and diagnosis of health issues, and capacity building.

Purpose	Representative applications	Companies
Nursing support	Virtual nursing assistants provide responses to patients through natural language processing	Teladoc
Elderly care	Provide at-home assistance with robots	Carepilot
Scheduling appointments	AI-powered chatbots schedule and remind patients of their upcoming in-person visits	My Check In (Myriad Genetics)
Counseling	AI-powered chatbots provide support and guidance for mental health issues	Wysa
Treatment decision	Analysis of automated health records	IBM, Google, and others
Predict future health risks	Predictive analysis for population management	NurseWise
Remote patient monitoring for medical issues	Gather and transmit data such as vital signs, heart rates, sleep patterns, and physical activity levels	Apple, Google Watch, and other wearables
Reduce hospital readmissions	Determine if hospital visits are necessary by providing real-time feedback to physicians	Teladoc
Medical training	Use health information technology to provide immersive and realistic medical training experiences	Medical Realities

Deeper Look: Nurse Practitioners Can Play an Important Role in Addressing the Primary Care Shortage

Nurses (both nurse practitioners [NPs] and registered nurses [RNs]) make up the largest segment of the healthcare profession. Nurses were introduced in the US more than 40 years ago as a response to the shortage of physicians. The number of nurses gradually increased, and they now play a substantial and accepted role in healthcare. These health providers are not only highly skilled, they are capable of providing many of the same services provided by primary care physicians. At the same time, the labor costs for these health providers are significantly lower than those of physicians.

Addressing the Shortage Through eHealth

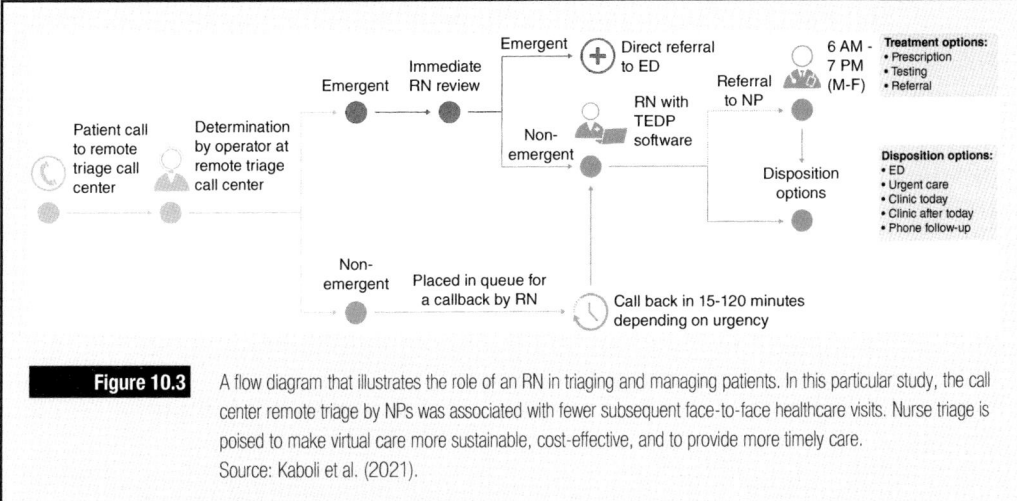

Figure 10.3 A flow diagram that illustrates the role of an RN in triaging and managing patients. In this particular study, the call center remote triage by NPs was associated with fewer subsequent face-to-face healthcare visits. Nurse triage is poised to make virtual care more sustainable, cost-effective, and to provide more timely care.
Source: Kaboli et al. (2021).

Unfortunately, many physician groups may oppose this solution to physician shortage, owing to their belief that this would threaten public safety. Patient skepticism about nurses providing care in lieu of physicians compounds this problem. Further, and understandably so, this model could cut physician wages, as NPs are given greater independence. Only half of the states allow nurses to independently care for patients, but many others have strict scope-of-practice guidelines. This is an ethical dilemma – that is, to not provide care to patients when there is actually a viable solution. The growing number of patients seeking care and increasing physician shortage will only exacerbate this problem.

Telehealth can turn competition between physicians and nurses to a collaboration. One way in which nurses already participate in primary care is patient triage. Nurse advice lines have existed for years. By leveraging experienced nurses prior to a virtual physician visit, organizations can effectively triage care and direct patients to physicians if it is warranted. This alleviates the burden on physicians and at the same time helps patients avoid unnecessary emergencies and urgent care visits. From a cost standpoint, physicians can see patients who need further care rather than those who do not, thereby increasing revenue. Figure 10.3 shows a flowchart that illustrates the role of an RN in triaging and managing patients. In this particular study, call center remote triage by NPs was associated with fewer subsequent face-to-face healthcare visits (Kaboli et al., 2021). Nurse triage is poised to make virtual care more sustainable, cost-effective, and to provide more timely care.

Addressing the Shortage of a Skilled Healthcare Workforce Through eHealth

Figure 10.4 shows the different spheres of eHealth. The field of eHealth encompasses **telehealth**, **telemedicine**, and **telecare**. **mHealth** cuts across all of these different spheres and includes medical services and public health activities enabled by mobile devices. Telehealth corresponds to a wide variety of remote healthcare services beyond the doctor–patient relationship.

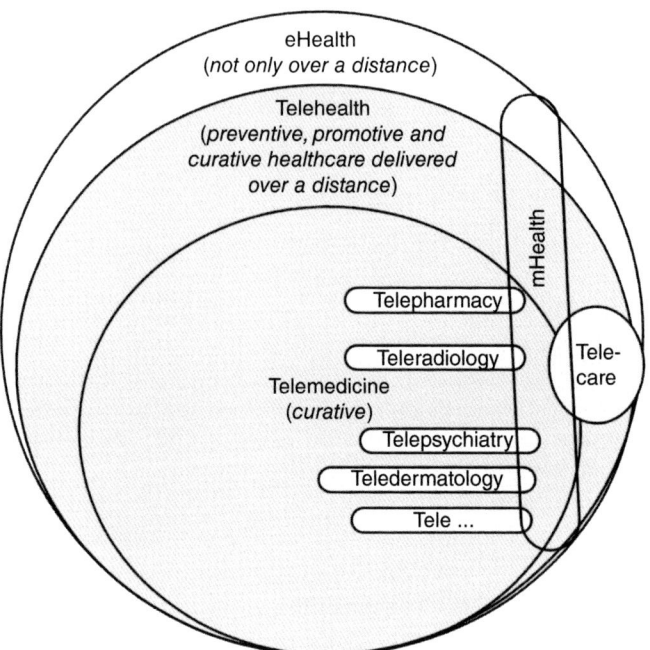

Figure 10.4

Different spheres of eHealth. The field of eHealth encompasses telehealth, telemedicine, and telecare. mHealth, cuts across all of these different spheres and includes medical services and public health activities enabled by mobile devices. Source: Van Dyk (2014). Shared by MDPI under an open access CC BY license.

Telemedicine is the dynamic, real-time, remote interaction between healthcare professionals and patients. Collectively, these three areas are synergistic and provide preventive, curative, and follow-up care that has the potential to improve overall health outcomes by making services more accessible and integrated.

Telehealth or telemedicine often involve services provided by nurses, pharmacists, or social workers, for example, who help with patient health education, social support, and medication adherence. Telecare, on the other hand, generally refers to technology that allows consumers to stay safe and independent in their own homes. For example, telecare may include consumer-oriented health and fitness apps, sensors and tools that connect consumers with family members or other caregivers, exercise-tracking tools, digital medication reminder systems, or early-warning and detection technologies. Table 10.3 shows how telehealth can aid risk stratification by intervention type and patient type.

One example of telemedicine is tele-mentoring, where an expert physician can provide medical guidance to a primary care physician or nurse on managing patients. This includes training on diagnostic tests, closely monitoring a patient's progress after treatment, and facilitating access to specialists. Tele-mentoring may be a more economical method of workforce development than traditional in-person mentoring. Through mentorship it can prevent burnout and improve retention. In rural or remote areas where in-person mentoring

Table 10.3 Telehealth can aid risk stratification by intervention type and patient type.

	Person-specific risk			
Intervention-specific risk	Frail and at-risk	Severe conditions	Chronic and moderated conditions	Healthy living
Monitor and alert	Very high risk	Very high risk	High risk	Medium risk
Diagnose and treat	Very high risk	High risk	Medium risk	Medium risk
Communicate and coordinate	High risk	Medium risk	Low risk	Low risk
Reference and guide	Medium risk	Low risk	Low risk	Very low risk

is more difficult, tele-mentoring can help foster a sense of camaraderie and teach resilience strategies that are valuable to both providers and patients.

Project ECHO is an example of an initiative to provide a novel tele-mentoring strategy to equip primary care physicians in rural areas with the knowledge they need to provide high-quality specialty care. Project ECHO is a nationally and globally recognized model for bringing best-practice healthcare to patients who don't have access to it where they live. In the US alone, 175 ECHO hubs have reached thousands of communities across 46 states. Around the world, ECHO programs operate in 34 countries. By participating in weekly virtual clinics with teams of specialist mentors, primary care practitioners in rural and underserved areas acquire the expertise they need to treat patients with complex health problems – including hepatitis C, HIV, chronic pain, opioid addiction, mental illness, diabetes, and cancer.

Telemedicine can also enable a physician halfway around the world to read scans and images, especially when there is a physician shortage within a particular specialty. One of the earliest examples of telemedicine is teleradiology. Radiologists provide specialized interpretations of medical images in order to improve patient outcomes. Teleradiology expedites this process, and also addresses shortages of radiologists. Digital imaging has provided the opportunity for radiologists to access medical images in a far more proficient manner than the previous technology of film-based radiologic image acquisition. A teleradiologist can be anywhere in the world. Some examples of companies that have established teleradiology are presented below.

Philips has partnered with Digital China Health, the largest provider of cloud-based healthcare services in China, to launch SHINEFLY – a secure, cloud-based platform for teleradiology applications to meet the demands of

China's rapidly expanding healthcare system. Collaboration between radiologists and clinicians at different locations, aided by Philips' image, information, and analysis tools, helps primary and remotely located hospitals in China enhance the quality of – and access to – care. Findings from surveys show that teleradiology currently has the highest rate of established service provision globally (33 percent).

Example: Time for Data Transmission

Question: One of the limiting factors in the adoption of telemedicine is the availability of high-speed internet to transmit data, particularly large images, to clinicians who may be hundreds or thousands of miles away from where a medical exam is being performed. Suppose a remote clinic has brought in a portable mammography machine to take mammograms for women in a clinic. The goal is to send the mammogram immediately to a radiologist to review so that women who need a follow-up biopsy can have one taken the same day. If the average mammogram is 50 Mb, four mammogram images are taken per breast, and the bandwidth of the available internet is 3 Mb per second, how long would it take to transmit all of the images for one patient? If the internet is unstable and cuts out briefly on average every two minutes, would the data be successfully uploaded before the internet cuts out? How does this affect the ability to perform telehealth mammography?

Answer: If the average mammogram is 50 Mb and four images are taken per breast, then the total size of the data package is:

$$50 \text{ Mb} \times 4 \text{ images} \times 2 \text{ breasts} = 400 \text{ Mb}.$$

The size of the data package divided by the bandwidth is the time needed to perform the upload:

$$\frac{400 \text{ Mb}}{3 \frac{\text{Mb}}{\text{s}}} = 133 \text{ s} = 2.2 \text{ minutes}.$$

If the internet cuts out on average every two minutes, it would be challenging to complete the data upload between cutouts. If the upload has to be restarted each time the internet cuts out, it could be very challenging to send the entire data packet to the radiologist to review.

As already discussed, teleconsultations provide medical advice through video conferencing, phone calls, nursing call centers, text messaging, email, and other electronic technologies. Teleconsultations provide patients with information that will assess a particular healthcare problem, manage the problem through advice, or provide a referral to the patient for the appropriate service. Teleconsultations can be provided by nurses and/or physicians for a broad range of medical needs, including mental health evaluations, home-care follow-up appointments, and respiratory illness (Lewis et al., 2012).

Teleconsultations are being used by the US military to reduce costs associated with noncombat-related injuries, by distinguishing the appropriate treating facility prior to the solider leaving their post (Lewis et al., 2012).

Another example of telemedicine is the human diagnosis project, called Human Dx. The Human Dx system combines the expertise of physicians with machine learning to create care that is more accurate, less expensive, and more accessible. This is being implemented at top national medical organizations, including the American Medical Association, the American Board of Medical Specialties, and the Association of American Medical Colleges. Additionally, many academic centers, such as Harvard and MIT, as well as financial supporters such as the Moore Foundation, have invested in the Human Dx project.

Applying telemedicine technology to the delivery of integrated cancer care helps patients from diverse geographic locations to access treatment from physicians and oncologists without traveling to or waiting for an appointment. As much as 70 percent of US counties do not have an oncologist, limiting access for people who live within them. Better management of side effects, improved quality of life, and increased treatment access are just a few of the benefits teleoncology patients experience. There are benefits to the physicians as well, who may now be able to better focus on their patients, lowering costs, improving time to disease detection, and in doing so, make overall cancer care more personalized. Other related areas of development include telecytology and telepathology. In one model, robotic microscopes are used without an on-site cytotechnologist. In the second model, on-site cytotechnologists and pathologists can stream high-definition video microscopy at a high volume to a centrally located cancer facility. This underscores an important point. Telemedicine combined with point-of-care technologies that can replace the actual physician can further enhance access to high-quality healthcare (Sirintrapun and Lopez, 2018).

Deeper Look: Is Telehealth a Solution or a Problem?

Telehealth led to a massive shift in healthcare delivery at the height of the COVID-19 pandemic. Spending on telemedicine services during the first peak of the coronavirus pandemic in the US underscored its demand. In addition to federal spending through Medicare, nearly $4 billion was billed nationally for telehealth visits during March and April, compared to less than $60 million for the same two months of 2019, according to FAIR Health, a nonprofit group that analyzes private health insurance claims. Figure 10.5 shows the overall telehealth trends. Claims rose from less than 1 percent of all claims before the pandemic to a peak of

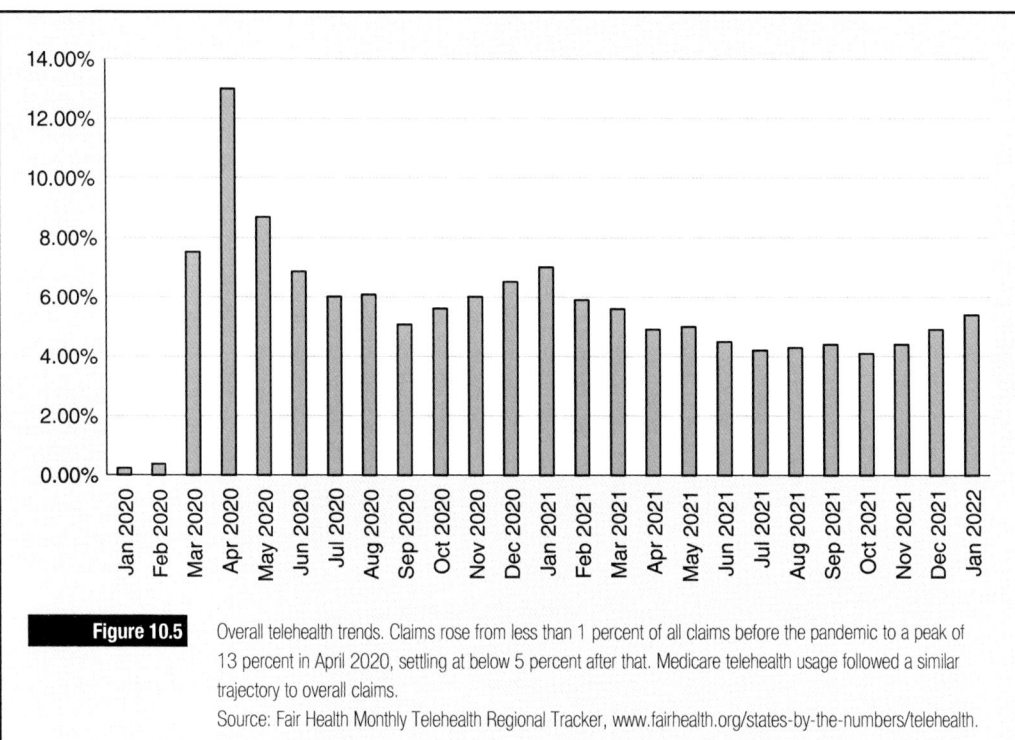

Figure 10.5 Overall telehealth trends. Claims rose from less than 1 percent of all claims before the pandemic to a peak of 13 percent in April 2020, settling at below 5 percent after that. Medicare telehealth usage followed a similar trajectory to overall claims.
Source: Fair Health Monthly Telehealth Regional Tracker, www.fairhealth.org/states-by-the-numbers/telehealth.

13 percent in April 2020, settling at below 5 percent after that. Medicare telehealth usage followed a similar trajectory to overall claims.

Telehealth can lead to a significant return on investment. One study estimated that the reduced time commitment for these visits, and reduced time off work, could lead to savings of $89 billion per year. Further, an expansion of telehealth could lead to a shift away from fee-for-service payment value-based care. There are several challenges, however, that will make it hard to scale telehealth. Higher utilization may not improve, or may worsen, health outcomes and inevitably lead to higher costs. In the US, physicians and hospitals have substantial influence on the volume, intensity, and price of care – more so than patients do in most cases. If telehealth visits are paid at the same rate as in-office visits, it would also drive up overall healthcare costs and defeat any potential benefit telehealth might have to reduce costs in select circumstances, and be highly problematic for the goal of appropriately aligning incentives. Yet another problem is misrepresenting the virtual services being provided – for example, billing for services that were not provided or using a reimbursement code that charges more for the visit. Therefore, for telehealth to be an effective return on health investment, these issues must be pre-emptively addressed.

Telehealth, while important, can inadvertently increase health inequities, particularly to those without internet access. According to the Pew Research Center, 28 percent of rural residents lack home broadband access, compared to 21 percent of suburban residents. Even those with broadband access may struggle to afford data plans. A 2021 study estimated that 18.1 million unconnected households have access to the internet but cannot afford low-cost broadband plans. These disparities also cut across racial lines. Eight in 10 white adults reported having a broadband connection, compared to fewer than 7 in 10 Black and Hispanic adults. Digital literacy is yet another problem. Older patients may be less comfortable with video technologies, and may be more inclined to use audio-only telephone calls instead. Resolving these digital inequities is essential to making telehealth more accessible to our most vulnerable populations.

There are a number of challenges associated with the growth of telemedicine. For example, misdiagnosis can occur in both face-to-face and virtual interactions, though it will likely be higher in the case of the latter. Hence, the risk of misdiagnosis owing to a potential decrease in quality of handling could lead to more malpractice lawsuits. Even if a telemedicine encounter is more efficient than a face-to face visit, the relative ease with which virtual visits can be accessed could lead to increased numbers of visits and, therefore, overuse of healthcare services. Virtual care can also challenge traditional conceptions of teamwork and collaboration that are required, particularly in oncology, given the different types of specialists that need to coordinate with each other to ensure effective patient care. As with any change, ushering in a new era of telemedicine will challenge the current healthcare systems in ways that can improve patient care yet have unintended consequences that could lead to ethical, legal, and regulatory concerns.

Addressing Healthcare Disparities in Low- and Middle-Income Countries

In developed countries, telemedicine is used to augment conventional healthcare, while in developing countries it has the potential to profoundly impact healthcare when budgets are overextended and physicians, particularly specialists, are scarce. Moreover, while telemedicine programs in developed countries have resources to easily deploy an emergency strategy, such as sending out a helicopter to transport a patient to the nearest hospital, this is simply impractical in less affluent countries. Telemedicine in developing countries could be leveraged to provide the population with basic healthcare services and to close the distance between rural areas and specialized hospitals that are located in big cities. Telemedicine does not typically involve a direct interaction between the provider and patient in low-resource settings. Rather, the main mode of communication is between specialists and nurses, midwives, or community health workers (CHWs).

Prior to the pandemic, the ratio of healthcare workers to population in LMICs was well below the minimum recommended by the WHO. A Global Burden of Disease Study in 2017 estimated that only half of all

Healthcare in the Twenty-First Century

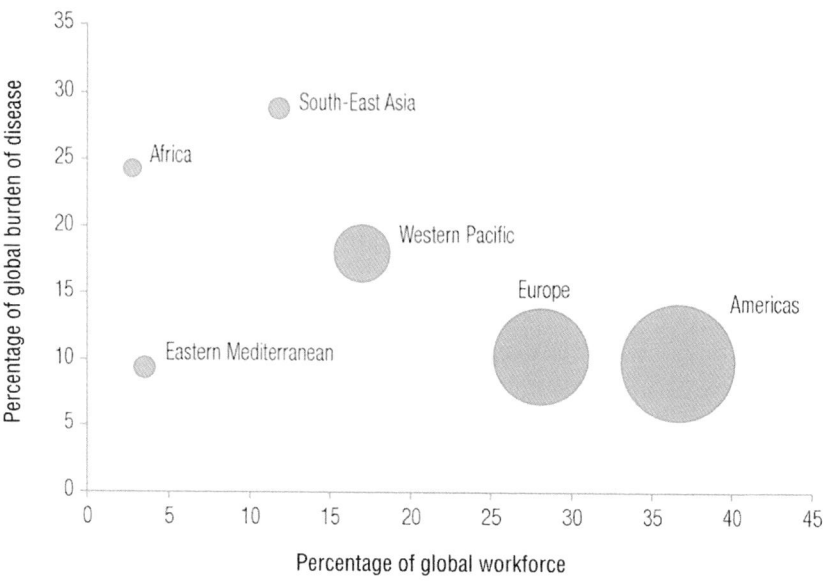

Figure 10.6 Distribution of health workers by level of health expenditure and burden of disease, by WHO region. The global health workforce is unevenly and inequitably distributed. The WHO region of the Americas, with 10 percent of the global burden of disease, has 37 percent of the world's health workforce, whereas the African region, with a 24 percent disease burden, has only 3 percent.
Source: World Health Organization, "Working together for health: The World Health Report 2006."

countries have the requisite health workforce required to deliver quality healthcare services, with many LMICs having the least. Figure 10.6 shows the percentage of the global workforce distributed by country. The global health workforce is unevenly and inequitably distributed. The WHO region of the Americas, with 10 percent of the global burden of disease, has 37 percent of the world's health workforce, whereas the African region, with a 24 percent disease burden, has only 3 percent. The further loss of healthcare workers to COVID-19 and the disruption of transportation because of lockdowns exacerbated this problem. Digital technology innovators leveraged their existing platforms to adapt to the new challenges that arose during the pandemic.

Given the disproportionately low number of health providers in LMICs, information and communication technologies (ICTs) are essential to filling this gap. The Millennium Development Goals (MDGs) established by the UN in 2000 initiated this step. Eight MDGs were established, with universally agreed objectives for tackling global inequities such as poverty, disease, hunger, lack of education, and gender equality by 2015. One of the MDGs, MDG 8, emphasized the inclusion of the "available benefits of new technologies, especially information and information and communications technologies (ICTs)."

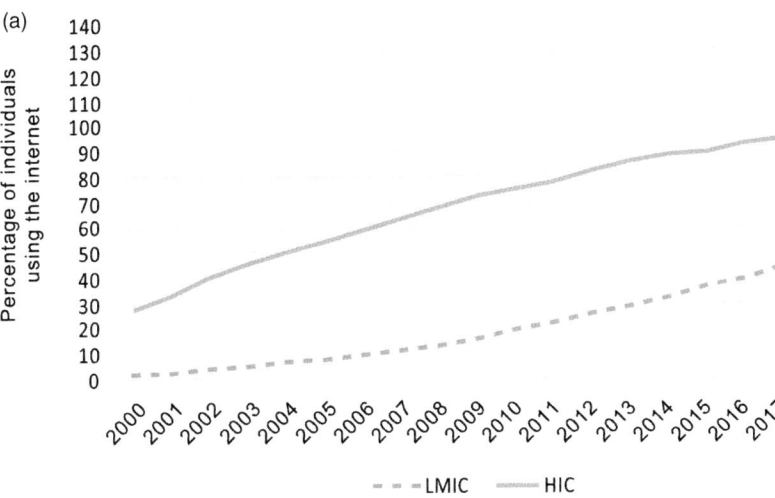
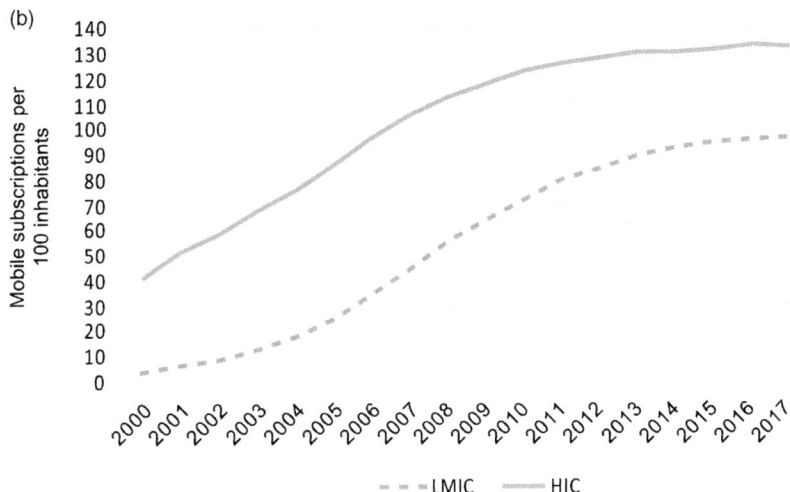

Figure 10.7

Internet users and mobile phone subscriptions in HICs and LMICs between 2000 and 2017. (a) The percentage of households with access to fixed internet; (b) the number of mobile/cellular subscriptions per 100 individuals (World Bank, 2018). Source: Kumm et al. (2022).

The three indicators for MDG 8 were fixed telephone lines, cellular phone subscriptions, and internet users per 100 inhabitants. Since 2000 there has indeed been a dramatic rise in the use of mobile ICT worldwide, and developing countries have had the greatest increase. Internet penetration has grown from just over 6 percent of the world's population in 2000 to 43 percent in 2015, translating to 3.2 billion people. The number of cell phone subscriptions has grown almost 10-fold in the last 15 years: from 738 million in 2000 to over 7 billion in 2015. Figure 10.7 shows internet users and mobile phone subscriptions in HICs and LMICs between 2000 and 2017. Figure 10.7(a) shows the percentage of households with access to fixed internet; Figure 10.7(b) shows the number of mobile/cellular subscriptions per 100 individuals (World Bank, 2018).

> **Example: Mobile Phone Use in LMICs**
>
> Question: The availability of telehealth depends in part on access to mobile phones and internet. During what period between 2000 and 2017 was the growth of mobile phone use the fastest in LMICs? What about internet use? Why may one have preceded the other?
>
> Answer: Growth of mobile phone use was the fastest from around 2005 to 2012, whereas growth of internet use was the fastest from 2013 to 2017. Because one of the major sources of access to the internet is mobile phone use, it makes sense that there was an uptick in internet access following increased access to mobile phones.

The exponential increase in mobile phone penetration has the potential to reach more people in resource-limited settings than the traditional forms of healthcare provision. The reduction in maternal mortality is an excellent example in which mHealth has played – and continues to play – an integral role. Specifically, it is important in reducing the **"three stages of delay"** – delay in the decision to seek care (e.g., poor understanding of complications and risk factors in pregnancy and when to seek medical help), delay in reaching care (e.g., lack of transportation), and the delay in getting adequate healthcare (e.g., lack of access to skilled health providers). By connecting rural health workers with urban specialists, and patients to the healthcare system, ICT can reduce overall mortality rates across a range of health services.

One approach to alleviate the burden placed on health workers was to engage consumers directly. What was distinct about the creation of these digital public goods was that much of this was driven by local innovators who were at the level of the problem. These organizations knew the local environment for which they were creating solutions, and the solutions were in many cases built on digital technologies that they were already using to support healthcare. This accelerated the pace of development and the uptake of digital services was greater than that compared to the pre-pandemic period.

Praekelt.org, a South African nonprofit organization, had 12 years of experience developing apps to target aspects of various health crises, and was poised to rapidly adapt its technology to the COVID-19 pandemic. One of their previous digital platforms, MomConnect, a mobile health initiative launched in 2014 in partnership with the South African Department of Health, helped women gain access to vital information and care needed to help ensure a safe and healthy pregnancy and labor. MomConnect was one of the first programs to pilot WhatsApp's enterprise solution in December 2017, adapting to meet the needs of the women it supported. In its first two years, MomConnect grew into the largest program of its kind, serving approximately 65 percent of women in South Africa.

Based on the success of MomConnect, the organization, in collaboration with the South African Department of Health, launched a COVID-19 service called HealthConnect for COVID-19, a set of services to support patients and health workers. Now over 20 million people globally engage with their health systems via HealthConnect for COVID-19, making it one of the world's largest digital health services. HealthConnect's symptom screening feature also provides a useful feedback loop, building an early-warning heatmap for governments on emerging COVID-19 hotspots. The infrastructure used to support these features is applicable across many other public health scenarios, including offering digital vaccine passports and immunization reminders. Utilizing this expertise, Praekelt.org and the WHO worked together to develop WHO HealthAlert, a dedicated messaging service in 11 languages, which had 12.6 million users in the first two months and has the potential to reach two billion people across the world.

Another way in which digital technologies have played an important role in the pandemic is delivery of care through CHWs. Living Goods helps governments strengthen and professionalize their community health systems. Specifically, they recruit, train, equip, and manage government-recognized networks of local CHWs who go door to door within their neighborhoods, providing health education, diagnoses, medicines, and health products that improve and save lives. These CHWs focus on high-impact areas where they make the biggest difference at a low cost, including pregnancy and newborn care, malaria, pneumonia, diarrhea, nutrition, immunization, and family planning.

To respond to the COVID-19 coronavirus pandemic, Living Goods equipped its CHW workforce with a diagnostic mobile application, the SmartHealth^{TM} app, which Living Goods co-developed with technology partner Medic Mobile. It allows CHWs to register, track, and follow-up with patients, ensuring data-driven performance management, as well as real-time data collection. Clients can also receive messages on their mobile phones with care reminders. In addition, CHWs used telemedicine via their cell phones to ensure that families continued to receive essential primary care during this time – making technology, internet connectivity, and the work of CHWs more important than ever.

A third way in which digital technologies can play an important role in healthcare is to manage medical supply inventory. mTrac is a real-time location-tracking app with several uses, including sharing your location with family and friends, tracking vehicles, etc. mTrac is part of a growing digital health revolution across much of the developing world, leap-frogging traditional infrastructural challenges to help impoverished communities receive healthcare. mTrac was used by health facility workers to submit routine, weekly health surveillance data by SMS using their own mobile phones.

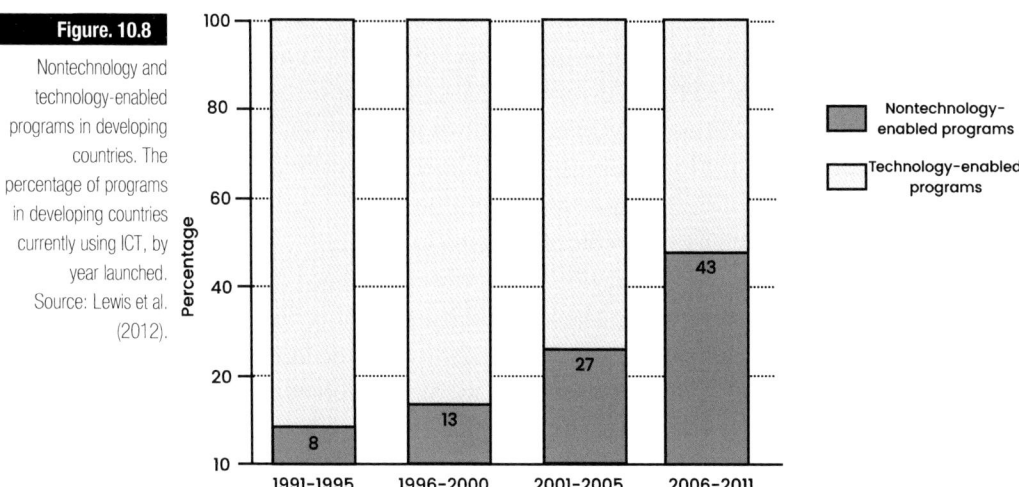

Figure. 10.8 Nontechnology and technology-enabled programs in developing countries. The percentage of programs in developing countries currently using ICT, by year launched. Source: Lewis et al. (2012).

mTrac indicators included notifiable diseases, stock levels for eight tracer medicines, and maternal and neonatal deaths, to name a few examples. When a preset threshold of cases is reached, an SMS alert is sent to every member of the district health management team for immediate response.

Developing countries are experiencing an unprecedented increase in the number of users of cell phone and internet technologies, as well as a decline in the price of devices and services. Figure 10.8 shows nontechnology and technology-enabled programs in developing countries by year launched (Lewis et al., 2012). Many health program implementers and policymakers are exploring the extent to which telemedicine can help address the challenges faced by resource-constrained health markets in terms of the availability, quality, and financing of healthcare. This increasing interest is evidenced by the growing number of events, websites, and literature focused on eHealth, including the Saving Lives at Birth Grand Challenge, the recent *Health Affairs* issue on eHealth in the developing world, the mHealth summits in Washington, DC, and Cape Town, South Africa, and the survey recently conducted by the WHO on the use of mHealth by its member states.

Deeper Look: The HOPE Program for Cervical Cancer Screening – Saving Women's Lives Through an Entrepreneurial Framework

For decades, CHWs – lay workers trained to provide basic health services to their neighbors – have served as a trusted source of primary healthcare in communities around the world. Despite the life-saving work they perform, CHWs have long been subject to global debate about their compensation. A perception exists among donors and Ministry of Health officials in many countries that CHW salaries are not "sustainable." As such, a global workforce of unpaid health workers has not been uncommon over the last 40 years. However, there is an opportunity to foster CHWs to be entrepreneurs. This is the case with the HOPE Peru Project.

HOPE is a social enterprise aiming to provide early screening for cervical cancer by reaching women in their homes, workplaces, and communities. Based at the Universidad Peruana Cayetano Heredia and led by former health minister Dr. Patty Garcia, HOPE partners with CHWs to deliver molecular human papilloma virus (HPV) self-testing kits and health promotion on reproductive health. HPV is the virus that causes cervical cancer.

In the social component, women from the communities (known as HOPE Ladies) are trained to promote cervical cancer screening through HPV self-sampling and to guide other women through the screening pathway in their communities. Figure 10.9 shows a HOPE lady receiving a HPV self-testing kit at her workplace in the market in Pachacutec, Peru. The HOPE model uses microfinancing coupled with tiered pricing for the private sector for sustainability. HOPE Ladies sell the self-testing kits for 10 PEN – about $3 – and keep a small profit of 5 PEN. HOPE Ladies report financial empowerment and autonomy with even this modest additional income. They invest the money in education for their children, better nutrition for their families, and better healthcare for themselves and other family members. Some HOPE Ladies say they have been able to spend the additional income on household expenditures or recreation. Evidence from around the world shows investments in education and women's agency lead to more inclusive economies, and the HOPE model is one such example of how CHWs can do good for society, and at the same time good for their families.

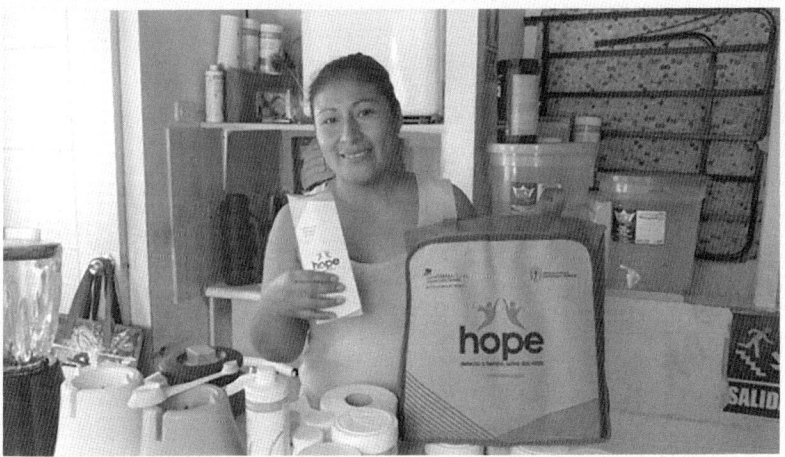

Figure 10.9 A HOPE Lady receives an HPV self-testing kit at her workplace in the market in Pachacutec, Peru. The HOPE model uses microfinancing coupled with tiered pricing for the private sector for sustainability. HOPE Ladies sell the self-testing kits for 10 PEN – about $3 – and keep a small profit of 5 PEN.
Source: Project HOPE, Peru; Calla Health.

Looking Ahead

It is apt to close this book by reflecting on the evolution of healthcare over the last 150 years. This book opened with the evolution of healthcare over the twentieth century and how the growing sophistication of medical technologies and specialists widened the gap in equitable healthcare.

The practice of medicine in the mid nineteenth century looked very little like modern hospitals – most physicians made house calls.

The digital revolution is poised to address this important gap, and perhaps in ways that don't require the significant investment it would take to build sufficient capacity of the primary care physician workforce.

In the past 100 years our healthcare system has become exponentially larger, more specialized, and more technological with far greater capacity to treat and manage disease. It has also become more complex, fragmented, and depersonalized. Physicians are trained to practice in sanitized, corporate environments and are expected to prioritize cost efficiencies, thereby limiting the amount of time they spend with each patient, which can be as little as 10 minutes. A major influencer of this evolution is advances in medical innovation.

Paradoxically, technology, which many have decried as a contributing factor to the speed and complexity of our clinical practice, is now serving us in a variety of remote monitoring situations. It is clear that an increasing number of clinical providers are extending their services to patients directly into the comfort of their homes. By leveraging our collective expertise and the power of modern technology, telemedicine can revive a once common feature of modern medicine – the house call – to deliver much of the care that many patients need, virtually.

SUMMARY

The number of primary care physicians, the gatekeepers of healthcare, has decreased at a disproportionate rate in the US. At the same time, the number of specialists has grown, largely due to the improved compensation that is commensurate with a physician who is an expert with respect to one organ system or disease. Of American physicians practicing in 1928, the vast majority were general practitioners. By 1942, the percentage of general practitioners had decreased by 50 percent. This decline continued, and in 1980, while there were 403,000 physicians in America, only 15 percent were primary care providers. This problem is exacerbated in LMICs, where physicians leave in droves to benefit from the resources in HICs. In both situations there is a scarcity of providers who can reach the largest swath of the population.

Digital health or eHealth is divided into a number of areas, in particular telehealth, telemedicine, telecare; mHealth – which corresponds to the use of mobile devices – cuts across all of these areas. Telehealth refers to a broader scope of remote healthcare services than telemedicine. While telemedicine refers specifically to remote clinical services, telehealth can refer to remote nonclinical services, such as provider training, administrative meetings, and continuing medical education. Telecare is the term for offering remote care to elderly and physically less able people, providing the reassurance needed to allow them to live independently. While telemedicine can enable more efficient and broader healthcare delivery in the US, reducing healthcare expenditures and improving patient satisfaction, telemedicine is essential to populations in LMICs. Physicians are woefully lacking in these areas and telemedicine can extend the impact of cell phone technology, which has transformed the way communication and transactions occur in developing countries.

The book began with a discussion of societal, medical, and engineering forces that led to the modern healthcare system. Breast cancer was described as a case study to provide context. This was followed by the potential for portable and affordable technologies to change the health delivery paradigm by bringing care to the people as a way of reducing deaths from cervical cancer. This narrative set the stage for Chapters 4–6, which were dedicated to a variety of innovative technologies that could be synergistic and used across the cancer care continuum. This was followed by a chapter on statistical testing and clinical trial design, which are critical elements in assuring regulatory bodies such as the FDA that these solutions offer benefit with minimal risk. The next two chapters address another critical point – the need for experts who can interpret data, even if the technology can be accessed at the point of care. A variety of data analytics methods from simple linear and logistic regression models to more complex neural networks can be leveraged, depending on the question posed. Telemedicine can be the conduit through which data and knowledge are exchanged, allowing decisions to be made.

PROBLEMS

The Growing Shortage of Healthcare Experts in Clinical Deserts

1. Why is there a primary care shortage in the US?
2. What are the three ways in which AI can extend the reach of telehealth?
3. What are five ways in which the performance of a healthcare system is measured? How does the US rank among the HICs?
4. What are professional shortage areas?
5. An elderly woman falls in her home and presses an alarm that alerts the hospital to send an ambulance. How can AI help?

6. The data in Figure 10.10 shows profit margins by healthcare sector by industry.
    a. Which industry will benefit most from preventive telemedicine and why?
    b. Which one will benefit the least from telemedicine and why?

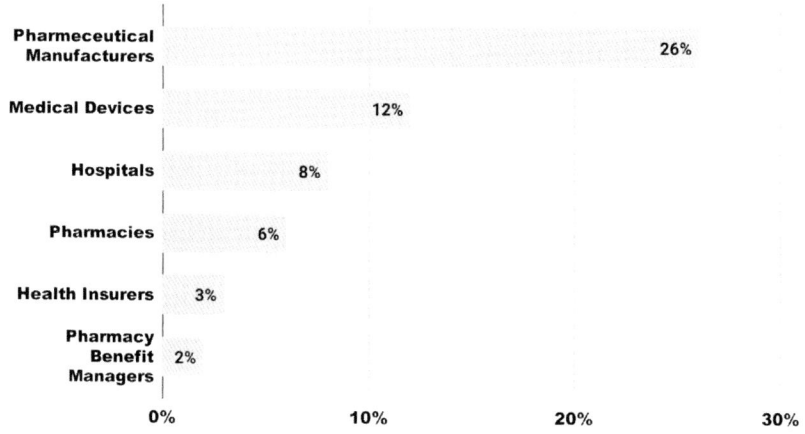

Figure 10.10 Profit margins in the healthcare sector by industry.

- Pharmeceutical Manufacturers: 26%
- Medical Devices: 12%
- Hospitals: 8%
- Pharmacies: 6%
- Health Insurers: 3%
- Pharmacy Benefit Managers: 2%

Addressing the Shortage of a Skilled Healthcare Workforce Through eHealth

7. Provide one example each of telemedicine, telehealth, and telecare in cancer prevention. Explain why these are representative examples.
8. A nurse in a community health setting uses a cell phone to image the oral cavity of a smoker for signs of oral cancer and sends the image to a remote physician for definitive diagnosis. What type of eHealth does this represent?
9. The US Centers for Disease Control and Prevention (CDC) estimates that eliminating three risk factors – poor diet, inactivity, and smoking – would prevent 80 percent of heart disease and stroke, 80 percent of type 2 diabetes, and 40 percent of cancers.
    a. Provide an example of how eHealth can improve prevention of each of these chronic diseases.
    b. Provide an example of how telemedicine can improve prevention of each of these chronic disease?
    c. Provide an example of how telecare can improve prevention of each of these chronic diseases
10. The effectiveness of telemonitoring on regulating blood sugar in diabetic patients is evaluated between two groups with 25 patients in each group – one without telemonitoring and one with telemonitoring. The nurse hypothesizes a higher percentage of the patients in the telemonitoring group will be at normal blood sugar levels.
    a. What is the null hypothesis?

b. What is the alternative hypothesis?
c. What statistical test would she use to test her hypothesis?

11. What is the time it will take for an X-ray image to be transferred from a mobile clinic to a health center in a rural setting with a DSL line (bandwidth is 3 Mb/s) vs. an urban setting where they use a Google Fiber (1,000 MB/s)? The typical size of an X-ray image is 20 Mb. How much faster (ratio of fast to slow download) is the Google Fiber compared to a DSL service?

12. A physician asks her patients to send her a message through a secure website if they have any severe side effects from a medication she has prescribed. Several of her elderly patients who had side effects do not send her a message, and she learns of this when her nurse follows up with each patient by phone. What assumption did the physician make and what ethical implication will it have?

13. Misdiagnosis is a serious but common medical error made during telemedicine. Give at least one example of how a patient, physician, and technology can cause a medical error in telemedicine.

14. A nurse performs a cervical cancer screening exam. She sends the image to the physician digitally and the physician renders a decision that the patient does not have cancer, when in fact she does. The patient is dismissed and later she dies of the disease. There are several reasons why this error could have occurred – degradation of the image during digital transmission, wrong annotation of the image by the community health provider, mistakenly assigning it to another patient, or an error made by the physician. The lawyers try to determine what type of malpractice occurred as defined by the 4Ds. Which of the following 4Ds (listed below) apply to each source of medical error?
    a. Degradation of image during digital transmission.
    b. Wrong annotation of the image by the community health provider.
    c. Physician mistakenly assigns the image to another patient.

Duty: the healthcare provider's duty of care – Physicians are required to uphold a certain standard of care for their patients.

Dereliction: dereliction of duty from the healthcare provider – Whenever doctors fail to maintain the agreed-upon relationship with a patient or overstep their boundaries, this is known as dereliction.

Direct causation: the negligence directly caused injury – Direct causation is the process of determining whether a physician's actions were the direct result of harm to the patient.

Damage: the damages you sustained – This includes physical harm, emotional harm, and wage loss.

Addressing Healthcare Disparities in Low- and Middle-Income Countries

15. What are three ways in which community health providers play an important role in telemedicine?
16. What was the purpose of establishing MDG 8 as part of the Millennium Development Goals?

17. How can telehealth reduce the three stages of delay?
18. What evidence is there that there has been an improvement in the use of internet and communication technologies in LMICs?
19. What three countries have the same disease burden but different percentages of the global workforce?
20. What two countries have different burdens of disease but the same percentage of the global workforce?

REFERENCES

Kaboli, P. J., Augustine, M. R., Rose, D. E., et al. 2021. Call center remote triage by nurse practitioners was associated with fewer subsequent face-to-face healthcare visits. *Journal of General Internal Medicine*, 36, 2315–2322. https://doi.org/10.1007/s11606-020-06536-0.

Kumm, A.J., Viljoen, M., & de Vries, P.J. 2022. The digital divide in technologies for autism: feasibility considerations for low- and middle-income countries. *Journal of Autism and Developmental Disorders*, 52, 2300–2313. https://doi.org/10.1007/s10803-021-05084-8.

Lewis, T., Synowiec, C., Lagomarsino, G., & Schweitzer, J. 2012. E-health in low-and middle-income countries: findings from the Center for Health Market Innovations. *Bulletin of the World Health Organization*, 90, 332–340.

Sirintrapun, S. J., & Lopez, A. M. 2018. Telemedicine in cancer care. *American Society of Clinical Oncology Educational Book*, 38, 540–545.

Van Dyk, L. 2014. A review of telehealth service implementation frameworks. *International Journal of Environmental Research and Public Health*, 11(2):1279–1298. https://doi.org/10.3390/ijerph110201279.

World Bank. 2018, Mobile cellular subscriptions (per 100 people) [Online]. Available: https://data.worldbank.org/indicator/IT.CEL.SETS.P2 (accessed April 16, 2024).

Index

ablation
    ablative zone, 198–200, 202, 204, 215–216
    chemical ablation, 195, 205
        ethanol ablation, 205
        photodynamic therapy, 186, 205–206, 214, 216
    thermal ablation, 195–196
abscopal effect, 210–211
activation function, 312–316, 320, 322, 338, 340
adjunct therapies, 63
adjuvant therapy, 63
Allison, James, 67
antibody test, 121
antigen presenting cells, 186
artificial intelligence, 349
artificial neural networks, 266, 309
ASSURED criteria, 131, 203–204
autoimmune deficiency syndrome, 122, 127
average pooling, 326, 341

backward propagation, 311–312
barriers to vaccination, 92
basic reproduction number, 190
Bayes' theorem, 278–279
Bayesian classifiers, 273–274, 303
bias error, 330, 332
biomarker, 120, 122, 128–130, 132–134, 137–138, 140–141, 145, 147, 247, 304
Bland–Altmann plot, 241
blinding, 252–253
block randomization, 252–253
boundary surface, 134, 171, 183
bounded rationality, 269–270
box plots, 220–221
brain tumors, 140
breast cancer, 31, 37, 329, 365
    BRCA1, 51
    BRCA2, 51
    ductal carcinoma in situ (DCIS), 33–34
    invasive ductal carcinoma, 33–34
    lumpectomy, 38, 71, 283–284
    mastectomy, 37–38, 51
    receptor subtypes
        estrogen receptor, 50, 63, 271
        human epidermal growth factor receptor, 50, 271
        triple negative breast cancer, 50, 61
    sentinel nodes, 45

cancer stage, 33–34
capacitor, 175–178, 183
carcinoma in situ (CIS), 70, 76–77, 202
cellular death
    apoptosis, 192–194, 201, 205–206
    autophagy, 192–194
    necrosis, 48, 193
cellular receptor, 4
Cervarix, 91, 98
cervical cancer, 1, 68, 74–84, 86, 89–92, 94–100, 102–104, 108, 110–115, 119, 122, 133, 140, 146–147, 167–168, 180, 185, 191, 202, 204, 213, 259, 265, 279, 296, 305–306, 342, 362–363, 365, 367
    cervical intraepithelial neoplasia, 78
    CIN I, 79
    CIN II, 79
    CIN III, 79
chimeric antigen receptor T-cell therapy, 67
circulating tumor cells, 142–144, 146–147, 341
circulating tumor DNA, 53, 120, 142–144, 146
clinical trials, xiii, 196, 213, 219–220, 223, 240, 250, 254–255, 257
cluster randomized trial, 251
clustering, 285–286, 303
cold knife conization, 202–203
colon cancer, 139–140, 147, 150
colposcopes, 81–84, 87, 90, 111, 165–170, 180–181, 183, 257, 265, 338, 342
    Callascope, 168, 181
    Pocket colposcope, 165–166, 168–170
    portable colposcopes, 165
common rule, 80–81
confidence interval, 242, 245, 260
conjugated antibody, 124
continuous, 220

control group, 220, 251–252, 254–255
convolutional neural networks, 266, 302, 311, 321–322
    convolution, 323–324
    convolutional layer, 322
cost function, 283, 317
covariance matrix, 292, 294, 307
Crane, Margaret, 118, 120, 130
cross validation, 298, 307
    k-fold, 298
    leave-one-out, 299
cryotherapy, 48, 104, 202, 204–205
Curie, Marie, 47
Curie, Pierre, 47

data analytics, xiii, 1, 257, 265–267, 271, 288–289, 301–302, 309, 349, 365
    descriptive analytics, 267–268, 302
    diagnostic analytics, 267–268, 302
    predictive analytics, 267–268, 302
    prescriptive analytics, 267–268, 302, 304
decision trees, 273–274, 283, 285, 303
deep learning, 309
DeepVariant, 310
degrees of freedom, 227, 230–231, 233, 239
dependent variable, 275
determinant, 293
diagnosis, 32–33, 86, 355
    diagnostic tests, 32
        colposcopy, 86, 103
        diagnostic biopsy, 33, 35, 70, 148
    molecular diagnostics, 48
disability adjusted life years (DALY), 104–106, 108–110, 112, 115
Dr. Harald zur Hausen, 90–91
dropout method, 332

early stopping, 332
ectocervix, 76–77, 104, 111
effective reproduction number, 190
eHealth, 344
eigenvalues, 292–295, 307
eigenvectors, 292–295, 307
electromagnetic radiation, 39–41, 44, 47–48, 69–70
    electromagnetic waves
        amplitude, 40, 171–172
        frequency, 40–41, 43, 96, 150–151, 171–172, 177
        penetration depth, 41, 44, 70, 111, 172, 181, 204, 214
        period, 8, 31, 40, 94, 113, 171–172, 253, 262, 301, 360
        wavelength, 40–43, 69–70, 152, 159, 171–172, 205
    gamma rays, 39
    ionizing radiation, 44–48, 62, 179
        free radicals, 46
        reactive oxygen species (ROS), 46, 205–206, 214
    microwaves, 40, 196–200, 203–204, 214
    radio waves, 40
    X-rays, 13–15, 39–40, 43–44, 46, 300
electron carrier, 42
electroporation, 195
ELISA
    competitive ELISA, 123
    direct ELISA, 122
    indirect ELISA, 122
    sandwich ELISA, 123
empirical medicine, 2, 4–5, 26, 83
endemic, 190
endocervix, 76–77
endoscopes, 161
    capsule endoscope, 163–164, 182
    fiber optic bundle, 162
    flexible endoscope, 139, 162–163
    high-resolution microendoscope, 169–170
    rigid endoscope, 162
energy generation
    capacity factor, 10
    coal, 8–10
    natural gas, 9–10, 28
    nuclear energy, 9
    petroleum, 9, 10
    renewable, 2, 9–11, 13
enzyme-linked immunosorbent assays. *See* ELISA
epithelium, 76–79, 112
ethyl cellulose, 212
Euler's number, 41, 106
evidence-based medicine, 2, 4, 26, 90, 96
experimental group, 220

false negatives, 35–36, 54–55, 98, 133, 148, 247–248, 282
false positives, 35, 69, 131, 247–248, 263, 296
feature extraction, 290
feature selection, 289
fecal immunochemical test, 140
fecal occult blood test, 140
flattening, 328
fluorescence in situ hybridization. *See* FISH
focal length, 152–156, 182
forward propagation, 311–312
Francis Collins, 55
fully connected layer, 322

G2 checkpoint, 77–78
Gardasil, 91, 98
Genetic Information Nondiscrimination Act, 52
genome-wide association studies (GWAS), 7
Ghebreyesus, Tedros Adhanom, 102
Global Alliance for Vaccines and Immunization, 93
gradient descent algorithm, 317
grand mean, 227, 232, 234
granulomatous inflammation, 208
gross domestic product, 24, 192, 213

Hans Hinselmann, 82–84, 111
health disparities, x, xii, 2, 6, 27–28, 76, 99–101, 114, 345
health equality, 100
health equity, 100–102, 114, 346
health inequity, 100–101
health insurance, xii, 15, 17, 23
    bundled payments, 20
    capitation, 19
    chargemaster, 22
    fee-for-service, 17–19, 23, 349, 356
    Medicaid, 17–18, 23
    Medicare, 17–18, 23–25, 346, 355–356
    Patient Protection and Affordable Care Act, 17
    pay for performance, 20
    shared savings, 20
    value-based care, 18, 349
HealthConnect, 361
Heaviside step function, 315
hematopoietic stem cell, 65–67
hepatitis B, 91, 122, 185, 214–215
herd immunity, 186, 190, 215
heritable cancers, 48
heuristics, 269–270
hidden layers, 311
histograms, 220–221
holdout set. *See* test set
Human Development Index
    high-income countries (HICs), 1, 31, 81, 348
    low-and middle-income countries (LMICs), xii, 1, 31, 119, 348, 357
    low-income countries (LICs), 1
    middle-income countries (MICs), 1
human immunodeficiency virus (HIV), 80, 122–123, 125–127, 131, 145, 147, 297, 353
human papilloma virus (HPV), 75, 77–80, 90–96, 98–99, 102–104, 110–114, 119, 122, 140, 146–147, 180, 185, 187–189, 191–192, 214–215, 363

hyperplane, 279–281, 303, 305
hypotheses, 220, 227–229, 250, 258
    alternative hypothesis, 228–229, 231, 233, 236, 238, 248, 258, 367
    null hypothesis, 227–233, 236, 238–239, 246, 248–249, 258, 260, 262, 366
hypothesis testing, 219–220
hysterectomy, 202

identity matrix, 293
imaging technologies
    CT, 14, 27, 39, 44, 46, 69, 71, 143, 150, 151, 178–179, 182, 216
    gamma probe, 45–46
    magnetic resonance imaging (MRI), 11, 14, 22, 27, 39–40, 44, 46, 56–58, 69, 71, 143, 150, 182, 341
    optical imaging, 40, 43
        absorption, 41–42, 44, 53, 124, 134, 152, 157–158, 181
        fluorescence, 40, 42, 53, 124, 126, 133–136, 151–152, 159–161, 181–182, 206
        scattering, 41–42, 44, 134, 152, 158, 182
        transmission, 41–42, 123, 159–160, 172–173, 183, 367
    positron emission tomography (PET), 14, 39–40, 44–46, 56–58, 69, 71, 143, 150
        FDG-PET, 45, 57–58
        fluorodeoxyglucose (FDG), 44
        radioactive tracer, 44
        radioisotope, 44
    ultrasound, 14, 44, 151, 170, 173, 178–181, 183
        doppler ultrasound, 42–43
    X-ray, 14–15, 43–44, 69, 367
imbalanced datasets, 296
immune checkpoints, 67
immune system, 15, 32, 53, 63, 65–67, 69, 71, 121–123, 145, 186–187, 190, 193–194, 201, 205, 208, 210–211, 214–215
    adaptive immunity, 65–67, 186
    antibodies, 15, 32, 53, 58, 63, 65, 67, 69, 71, 120–126, 129–133, 144–145, 147, 161, 186–187, 190, 193, 201, 205, 208, 210–211, 215
    IgA, 121
    IgG, 121–122, 125, 147
    IgM, 121–122, 125, 147

immune system (cont.)
  antigens, 53, 58, 66, 122, 129, 131, 145, 186–187, 194, 211, 290
    tumor associated antigens, 194
  innate immunity, 65–67
immune system cells
  B cells, 65, 67, 121, 145–146, 187–188, 210, 215
  dendritic cells, 65–67, 186–187, 210–211
  macrophages, 65–67, 194–195
  memory B cells, 67
  memory T cells, 67
  T cells, 65–67, 186–188, 210–211
    cytotoxic T lymphocytes, 187–188, 215
    helper T cells, 187
impedance, 172
independent variable, 275
input layer, 311
institutional review board, 80–81
internal combustion engine, 8
interventional radiologist, 197
intuitive medicine, 2–4, 26
irreducible errors, 330

kernel, 324–327, 341–342
k-means clustering algorithms, 286

Lasso regression, 334
lateral flow assays, 118, 129–133, 140, 142, 144–145, 147
level of significance, 228, 230, 249–250, 261, 263
light emitting diodes (LEDs), 160, 165, 181, 206
linear discriminant analysis, 290
liquid biopsy, 142, 146
liver cancer, 91, 185, 192, 198, 215–216
local cancer therapies
  ablation, 39–40, 48, 68–70, 104–105, 114, 145, 185–186, 192, 195–205, 207–216
    high-intensity focused ultrasound, 48
    microwave, 48
    radiofrequency, 48, 196–200, 204, 214
  radiation therapy, 4, 15, 62
  surgery, 13, 15, 18–19, 21–22, 28, 32–33, 35, 37–38, 60, 63, 70, 86, 114, 140, 142, 162, 180, 185, 192, 199, 213–214, 230, 233, 236, 238
logistic function, 315
logistic regression, 267, 273–275, 277–278, 303, 305, 316, 365

loop electro excision procedure (LEEP), 81–82, 86, 104, 202–203
loss function, 311, 316–317, 320, 330, 333
lung cancer, 3–6, 23, 74, 139, 242, 263

machine learning, xiii, 265–268, 272–273, 289, 295, 297, 301–304, 307, 309–311, 322, 328–331, 337, 344, 355
Marion Sims, James, 82–83, 85, 111
maximum likelihood estimation, 317, 320
maximum pooling, 326–327
mean squared error, 275–276, 305, 317, 320
metastases, 140, 142–143, 194, 199, 207, 210–212, 214
micro-electro-mechanical system, 175–177, 182
microfluidics, 120–129, 135–136, 148
microscope
  brightfield microscope, 157, 159, 182
  cell phone microscopes, 160
  condenser, 156–157
  darkfield microscope, 157–158
  epi-illumination, 159
  eye piece, 154–157
  fluorescence microscopy, 159
  foldscope, 160–161
  light microscope, 70, 156–157
  objective lens, 156–157, 165
  oblique illumination, 159
molecular tests, viii, 48–49, 128
  DNA testing, 49, 94
    FISH, 50, 53–55, 70, 285
    gene expression, 50, 53, 341
    NGS, 55–56
    PCR, 49–51, 53, 55, 69, 110, 120–122, 130, 144–147
      annealing, 49–50
      denaturation, 49–50, 208
      extension, 49–50, 133, 334
    RT-PCR, 50, 130–131
  mass spectrometry, 56
  molecular imaging, 32, 56–58, 70
  omics, 32, 48, 55, 58, 69–70, 127–128, 141–142, 265
    genomics, 55
    metabolomics, 55–56
    microbiomics, 55
    proteomics, 55–56
  protein testing
    ELISA, 53, 55, 120–127, 129, 131–133, 144–146

Index

IHC, 53–55, 70, 141–142, 161, 285
   protein expression, 49, 53, 70, 142
MomConnect, 360
Mullis, Kary, 49
multiple comparison bias, 225
multiple linear regression, 275

negative reinforcement learning, 273
neoadjuvant therapy, 63
nominal, 220, 260
normal distribution, 222–223, 230, 242, 257
nucleic acid amplification tests, 122

object detection networks, 323
optical axis, 152–154, 157, 182
optical biosensors, 146
ordinal, 220, 260
ordinary least squares regression, 273–274
os, 76
output layer, 311
overfitting, 330

p53, 77–78
Papanicolaou, George, 82, 83
paper assays, 120, 129, 136, 144, 146
pathologist, 86
Pennes model, 199
percutaneous ethanol injection, 207
P-hacking, 239–240
photosensitizer, 205, 207
   protoporphyrin, 205, 207
physician to resident ratio, 347
piezoelectric effect, 151, 170–171, 175–176
   direct effect, 171
   reverse effect, 171
placebo, 219, 250, 252, 254–255, 262
plasmonic technologies, 129, 134
   Raman scattering, 134
   surface plasmon resonance, 134–136
   surface-enhanced Raman scattering, 134
pneumonia, 31, 178–179, 361
point of care technologies, 26, 42
polymerase chain reaction. *See* PCR
pooling layers, 322
population mean, 221–223, 307
population standard deviation, 222
portable ultrasound system, 175
positive reinforcement learning, 273
power calculation, 220, 248–249, 258
precision medicine, 2, 5–6, 15, 27, 96, 265
predicate device, 256, 263

primary antibody, 124
principal component analysis (PCA), 273, 290, 294
prognosis, 33–34, 39, 51, 60, 64, 161
Project ECHO, 353
prospective studies, 250, 258
prostate cancer, 140

randomized controlled trials, 251, 258
ray tracing, 152–153, 155–156, 182
real images, 153
reducible errors, 330
regularization, 334
reinforcement learning, 267, 270, 272–274
residual error, 275
retrospective studies, 250, 258
ridge regression, 334

sample mean, 222–223, 227, 233, 242, 246, 259, 292, 307
sample standard deviation, 222, 242, 245
screening, xi, xiii, 31–33, 35, 38–39, 46, 68–70, 74–76, 78, 80–82, 84, 89–90, 92, 94–96, 98–99, 102–104, 110–114, 119–120, 135, 138–140, 145–148, 150, 167, 180, 185, 203, 213, 259, 265, 310, 361–363, 367
   screening tests, 32–33, 81–82, 90, 94, 98, 114, 150
      mammography, 33–34, 39, 44, 148, 354
      Pap smear, 75, 81–87, 90, 94–96, 98–99, 103, 111–114, 161
      visual inspection with acetic acid, 103–104, 265
secondary detection antibody, 124
silhouette scores, 286–287, 306
Simon, Herbert, 269
speculum, 81–83, 85, 87, 104, 111, 151, 165, 167–168, 181
spike proteins, 187, 195
standard error, 222, 226, 230, 259
statistical analysis, 220
statistical error
   type I error, 228, 248–249
   type II error, 248
statistical power, 248, 250, 288
statistical significance, 202–203, 220, 223–224, 226–227, 229, 235, 241, 250, 253, 260, 267, 290
statistical tests, 220–225, 227, 246
   Bland–Altmann test, 225
   correlation tests, 225
   multi-comparison test, 225